# Veterinary Laboratory Medicine

*Guest Editor*

MARY M. CHRISTOPHER, DVM, PhD

# CLINICS IN LABORATORY MEDICINE

www.labmed.theclinics.com

*Consulting Editor*
ALAN WELLS, MD, DMSc

March 2011 • Volume 31 • Number 1

SAUNDERS an imprint of ELSEVIER, Inc.

**W.B. SAUNDERS COMPANY**
*A Division of Elsevier Inc.*

1600 John F. Kennedy Boulevard • Suite 1800 • Philadelphia, Pennsylvania 19103-2899

http://www.theclinics.com

**CLINICS IN LABORATORY MEDICINE Volume 31, Number 1**
**March 2011 ISSN 0272-2712, ISBN-13: 978-1-4557-0464-4**

Editor: Katie Hartner
Developmental Editor: Donald Mumford

*Reprints.* For copies of 100 or more, of articles in this publication, please contact the Commercial Reprints Department, Elsevier Inc., 360 Park Avenue South, New York, New York 10010-1710. Tel. (212) 633-3813, Fax: (212) 462-1935, E-mail: reprints@elsevier.com.

*Clinics in Laboratory Medicine* (ISSN 0272-2712) is published quarterly by Elsevier Inc., 360 Park Avenue South, New York, NY 10010-1710. Months of issue are March, June, September, and December. Business and Editorial offices: 1600 John F. Kennedy Blvd., Suite 1800, Philadelphia, PA 19103-2899. Periodicals postage paid at NewYork, NY and additional mailing offices. Subscription prices are $225.00 per year (US individuals), $364.00 per year(US institutions), $120.00(US students), $273.00 per year (Canadian individuals), $460.00 per year (foreign institutions), $165.00 (foreign students). Foreign air speed delivery is included in all Clinics subscription prices. All prices are subject to change without notice. POSTMASTER: Send address changes to *Clinics in Laboratory Medicine*, Elsevier Health Sciences Division, Subscription Customer Service, 3251 Riverport Lane, Maryland Heights, MO 63043. **Customer Service: 1-800-654-2452 (US). From outside of the US and Canada, call 1-314-447-8871. Fax: 1-314-447-8029. E-mail: journalscustomerservice-usa@elsevier.com (for print support) or journalsonlinesupport-usa@elsevier.com (for online support).**

*Clinics in Laboratory Medicine* is covered in *EMBASE/Exerpta Medica, MEDLINE/PubMed (Index Medicus), Cinahl, Current Contents/Clinical Medicine, BIOSIS and ISI/BIOMED.*

Printed and bound by CPI Group (UK) Ltd, Croydon, CR0 4YY

Transferred to Digital Print 2011

# Contributors

## CONSULTING EDITOR

**ALAN WELLS, MD, DMSc**
Department of Pathology, University of Pittsburgh, Pittsburgh, Pennsylvania

## GUEST EDITOR

**MARY M. CHRISTOPHER, DVM, PhD**
Diplomate, American College of Veterinary Pathologists; Diplomate, European Societies of Veterinary Clinical Pathology; Professor of Clinical Pathology, Microbiology, and Immunology, School of Veterinary Medicine, University of California–Davis, Davis, California

## AUTHORS

**A. RICK ALLEMAN, DMV, PhD**
Professor of Clinical Pathology, Department of Physiological Sciences, University of Florida College of Veterinary Medicine, Gainesville, Florida

**CLAIRE B. ANDREASEN, DVM, PhD**
Diplomate, American College of Veterinary Pathologists; Associate Dean for Academic and Student Affairs; Professor and Director of Pathology Laboratory Services, Department of Veterinary Pathology, College of Veterinary Medicine, Iowa State University, Ames, Iowa

**HOLLY S. BENDER, DVM, PhD**
Diplomate, American College of Veterinary Pathologists; Professor, Department of Veterinary Pathology, College of Veterinary Medicine, Iowa State University, Ames, Iowa

**DOROTHEE BIENZLE, DVM, PhD**
Diplomate, American College of Veterinary Pathologists; Department of Pathobiology, University of Guelph, Guelph, Ontario, Canada

**DORI L. BORJESSON, DVM, PhD**
Diplomate, American College of Veterinary Pathologists; Associate Professor, Department of Pathology, Microbiology and Immunology, School of Veterinary Medicine, University of California, Davis, California

**MARJORY B. BROOKS, DVM**
Diplomate, American College of Veterinary Internal Medicine; Senior Research Associate; Director of Comparative Coagulation, Department of Population Medicine and Diagnostic Sciences, College of Veterinary Medicine, Cornell University, Ithaca, New York

**JAMES L. CATALFAMO, PhD**
Senior Research Associate, Department of Population Medicine and Diagnostic Sciences, College of Veterinary Medicine, Cornell University, Ithaca, New York

**CAROLYN CRAY, PhD**
Professor of Clinical Pathology and Microbiology and Immunology, Division of Comparative Pathology, Department of Pathology, University of Miami Miller School of Medicine, Miami, Florida

**JARED A. DANIELSON, PhD**
Assistant Professor; Director of Curricular and Student Assessment, Department of Veterinary Pathology, College of Veterinary Medicine, Iowa State University, Ames, Iowa

**AMY E. DECLUE, DVM, MS**
Diplomate American College of Veterinary Internal Medicine; Assistant Professor of Veterinary Internal Medicine, Department of Veterinary Medicine and Surgery, College of Veterinary Medicine, University of Missouri, Columbia, Missouri

**STINE JACOBSEN, DVM, PhD**
Associate Professor of Large Animal Surgery, Department of Large Animal Sciences, Faculty of LIFE Sciences, University of Copenhagen, Taastrup, Denmark

**MADS KJELGAARD-HANSEN, DVM, PhD**
Associate Professor of Veterinary Clinical Pathology, Department of Small Animal Clinical Sciences, Faculty of LIFE Sciences, University of Copenhagen, Frederiksberg C, Denmark

**JOHN F. PERONI, DVM, MS**
Diplomate, American College of Veterinary Pathologists; Associate Professor of Large Animal Surgery, Department of Large Animal Medicine, College of Veterinary Medicine, University of Georgia, Athens, Georgia

**BIRGIT PUSCHNER, DVM, PhD**
Diplomate, American Board of Veterinary Toxicology; Professor of Veterinary Toxicology, Department of Molecular Biosciences, School of Veterinary Medicine, University of California, Davis, California

**SHASHI K. RAMAIAH, DVM, PhD**
Diplomate, American College of Veterinary Pathologists; Diplomate, American Board of Toxicology; Biomarker Lab Head, Pfizer-Biotherapeutics Research Division, Drug Safety Research and Development, Cambridge, Massachusetts

**RENATE REIMSCHUESSEL, VMD, PhD**
Research Biologist, Center for Veterinary Medicine, Office of Research, Food and Drug Administration, Laurel, Maryland

**KATHERINE A. SAYLER, MEd**
Senior Biological Scientist, Department of Physiological Sciences, University of Florida College of Veterinary Medicine, Gainesville, Florida

**LESLIE C. SHARKEY, DVM, PhD**
Associate Professor, Veterinary Clinical Sciences Department, University of Minnesota College of Veterinary Medicine, St Paul, Minnesota

**NICOLE I. STACY, DrMedVet**
Adjunct Clinical Assistant Professor, Department of Large Animal Clinical Sciences, Aquatic Animal Health, University of Florida College of Veterinary Medicine, Gainesville, Florida

**TRACY STOKOL, BVSc, PhD**
Diplomate, American College of Veterinary Pathologists; Associate Professor, Department of Population Medicine and Diagnostic Sciences, College of Veterinary Medicine, Cornell University, Ithaca, New York

**WILLIAM VERNAU, DVM, DVSc, PhD**
Diplomate, American College of Veterinary Pathologists; Department of Pathology, Microbiology and Immunology, School of Veterinary Medicine, University of California, Davis, California

**MAXEY L. WELLMAN, DVM, MS, PhD**
Professor, Department of Veterinary Biosciences, The Ohio State University, Columbus, Ohio

**CHARLES E. WIEDMEYER, DVM, PhD**
Diplomate, American College of Veterinary Pathologists; Assistant Professor of Veterinary Clinical Pathology, Department of Veterinary Pathobiology, College of Veterinary Medicine, University of Missouri, Columbia, Missouri

**PAMELA A. WILKINS, DVM, MS, PhD**
Diplomate, American College of Veterinary Internal Medicine-Large Animal; Diplomate, American College of Veterinary Emergency and Critical Care; Professor of Equine Internal Medicine and Emergency/Critical Care, Section Head and Chief of Service, Equine Medicine and Surgery, Department of Veterinary Clinical Medicine, College of Veterinary Medicine, University of Illinois at Champaign-Urbana, Urbana, Illinois

# Contents

> Diagnostic cytology is a core veterinary pathology service involving specimens from domestic animals, laboratory animals, and exotic species. Evidence-based application of cytopathology involves management of preanalytical factors, and thorough evaluation of the diagnostic accuracy of the technique in each species and for all specimen types. Unique to veterinary medicine is the reliance on cytology as the basis for crucial medical decisions such as humane euthanasia, especially when the patient is critically ill or when financial considerations limit diagnostic and therapeutic options. This article reviews the cytologic criteria for the diagnosis of selected neoplastic and infectious diseases.

> Lymphoma in dogs is a heterogeneous cancer with highly variable prognosis. Many types of canine lymphoma have similar counterparts in the World Health Organization classification of human lymphoid tumors. The most common variant of canine lymphoma is diffuse large B-cell lymphoma, which, if treated with multiagent chemotherapy, has a survival time of approximately 12 months. T-cell lymphomas are more heterogeneous and high- and low-grade variants are common, which necessitates classification beyond B- versus T-cell lineage.

> Glucose levels in dogs and cats with diabetes mellitus can be monitored using a variety of techniques. Selecting the best monitoring technique requires involvement of the pet owner, communication between the owner and veterinarian, and practicality of the method. Some of the techniques typically used in dogs and cats are identical to those used in human diabetic patients. The use of modern technology designed specifically for people is being used increasingly for the management of diabetes in dogs and cats and offers a new mechanism for monitoring glucose in diabetic animals.

> The use of major acute-phase proteins (APPs) for assessment of health and disease in companion animals has increased within the last decade

because of increased knowledge in the field and increased access to appropriate assay systems for detection of relevant APPs, which are highly species specific. Despite evidence being restricted almost solely to proven excellent overlap performance of these markers in detecting inflammatory activity, clinically relevant studies at higher evidence levels do exist. The available body of literature shows a clear, but seemingly untapped, potential for more extended routine clinical use of major APP testing in companion animal medicine.

Pet bird ownership and the veterinary diagnostic market for avian and exotic species testing have grown markedly during the past 20 years. Birds present with both unique infectious diseases and other diseases that are known to the human medical community, including aspergillosis, mycobacteriosis, chlamydophilosis, and bornavirus infection, some of which have clear zoonotic implications. Although diagnostic testing for these avian infectious diseases has grown considerably and includes the newer technology of polymerase chain reaction as well as traditional serologic testing, guidelines for the use and interpretation of these tests and standardization of tests among veterinary laboratories remains an unmet challenge.

The hematologic evaluation of reptiles is an indispensable diagnostic tool in exotic veterinary practice. The diversity of reptile species, their characteristic physiologic features, and effects of intrinsic and extrinsic factors present unique challenges for accurate interpretation of the hemogram. Combining the clinical presentation with hematologic findings provides valuable information in the diagnosis and monitoring of disease and helps guide the clinician toward therapy and further diagnostic testing. This article outlines the normal and pathologic morphology of blood cells of reptile species. The specific comparative aspects of reptiles are emphasized, and structural and functional abnormalities in the reptilian hemogram are described.

This article focuses on the emerging field of equine regenerative medicine with an emphasis on the use of mesenchymal stem cells (MSCs) for orthopedic diseases. We detail laboratory procedures and protocols for tissue handling and MSC isolation, characterization, expansion, and cryopreservation from bone marrow, fat, and placental tissues. We provide an overview of current clinical uses for equine MSCs and how MSCs function to heal tissues. Current laboratory practices in equine regenerative medicine mirror those in the human field. However, the translational use of autologous and allogeneic MSCs for patient therapy far exceeds what is currently permitted in human medicine.

Rapid evaluation and intervention is a requirement and a characteristic of patient management in neonatal intensive care units, and this applies for equine neonates also. Appropriate interventions are based on solid knowledge of age, maturity, and species-specific differences in reference ranges. Point-of-care (POC) testing devices speedup decision making regarding treatments and interventions. However, there are potential limitations of these devices when applied to age groups and species beyond those they were specifically developed for. This article discusses the age-specific differences in the reference ranges and the potential limitations of POC devices currently used, which may affect delivery of care.

This article provides an overview of animal model systems to include their strengths and limitations in the study of hemostasis. Specific examples of spontaneous and engineered animal models are described in the context of cell-based hemostasis. The article concludes with a review of the comparative aspects of 3 laboratory assays of cell-based hemostasis: thromboelastography, thrombin generation, and flow cytometric assessment of platelet activation.

Currently, no serum biomarkers, including the biochemical gold standard alanine aminotransferase, can differentiate drug-induced from non–drug-related liver injury, can differentiate liver injury mediated by a specific drug or mechanism, or can accurately predict the progression and outcome of hepatic injury. Efforts have been made by veterinary clinical pathologists, toxicologists, and other scientists to address the gaps in hepatic biomarkers faced during drug development; although there have been no breakthroughs, several novel biomarker candidates have been identified. Efforts to address the gaps in translatable hepatic biomarkers and the challenges and hurdles faced during this process are highlighted in this review.

The current detection system for animal diseases requires coordination between veterinarians; veterinary medical laboratories; and state, federal, and international agencies, as well as associated private sector industries. Veterinary clinical pathologists in clinical and governmental laboratories often have responsibilities and expertise in one or more laboratory disciplines involved in diagnosing zoonotic and/or emerging diseases and diseases exotic to the United States that are important to animal and human health and the nation's food supply. The knowledge and roles of all veterinary laboratory professionals are vital to detect, monitor, and confirm diseases and conditions that affect animal and human health and the nation's animal food supply.

Birgit Puschner and Renate Reimschuessel

Several major pet-food and human-food safety incidents occurred worldwide between 2003 and 2008, causing illnesses and deaths in children, cats, dogs, and pigs. During the 2007 outbreak of renal failure in dogs and cats in the United States, veterinary diagnostic laboratories helped identify melamine and melamine analogues as contaminants in implicated food. In 2008, thousands of infants developed renal failure from exposure to melamine alone. Management of these outbreaks depends on the collaboration of veterinary and human laboratories and clinics, government agencies, academic institutions, and food industries, along with prompt communication and sharing of data.

Holly S. Bender and Jared A. Danielson

The Diagnostic Pathfinder was designed to help students learn diagnostic problem solving by supporting them in explaining relationships among history and physical examination findings, data abnormalities, and the underlying mechanisms of disease. The Pathfinder has been used to teach diagnostic problem solving to veterinary students since 2001 and is currently in use at 10 colleges of veterinary medicine. This article describes how the Pathfinder works and summarizes results from studies exploring the effect of Pathfinder use on learning and satisfaction. Pathfinder characteristics are described in terms of their influence on cognitive load, and strategies are provided for effective implementation.

## THE CLINICS ARE NOW AVAILABLE ONLINE!

Access your subscription at:
**www.theclinics.com**

# Preface

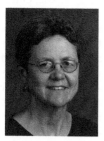

Mary M. Christopher, DVM, PhD
*Guest Editor*

It is my great pleasure to introduce Veterinary Laboratory Medicine, which, like its counterpart in the medical profession, is a discipline that bridges basic science and clinical practice. This theme issue brings the best of the field to the audience of *Clinics in Laboratory Medicine,* demonstrating the diversity, strengths, and challenges of laboratory medicine in animals and highlighting its many important links with human health. The authors are veterinary clinical pathologists[a] as well as clinicians, toxicologists, and other scientists who are actively engaged in diagnostic pathology, translational and clinical research, clinical medicine, education, and basic research involving animal models. Their expertise is impressive and wide-ranging and conveys a commitment to improving the quality of animal health through research and practice in clinical pathology. I hope you will gain new perspectives on the ways in which veterinary and medical laboratories and testing overlap but also diverge, stimulating new ideas about your own work and facilitating cooperative research in the future.

The articles in this issue highlight several key areas in which veterinary laboratory medicine is making major contributions to the understanding, diagnosis, and treatment of animal (and human) health and disease.

---

[a] Veterinary clinical pathology is a board-certified specialty within the American College of Veterinary Pathologists (www.acvp.org). Three-year residency programs exist at most of the 33 schools of veterinary medicine in the United States and Canada and include training in hematopathology, coagulation, immunopathology, clinical chemistry, endocrinology, cytopathology, surgical pathology, molecular diagnostics, general pathology, and laboratory management and quality assurance. Veterinary clinical pathologists work in academia, diagnostic and research laboratories, and the pharmaceutical and biotech industries, where they contribute to the advancement of laboratory medicine in domestic, zoo and wildlife, and laboratory animals. Organizations such as the American (www.asvcp.org) and European (www.esvcp.org) Societies of Veterinary Clinical Pathology bring together veterinary clinical pathologists with other clinical and laboratory professionals to advance the discipline through scientific conferences, consensus papers, training and educational materials, and publication of *Veterinary Clinical Pathology,* an international journal.

Clin Lab Med 31 (2011) xiii–xvi
doi:10.1016/j.cll.2011.01.001
0272-2712/11/$ – see front matter © 2011 Elsevier Inc. All rights reserved.

## COMPANION ANIMAL HEALTH AND NOVEL THERAPEUTIC MODALITIES

Laboratory medicine for companion animals, including dogs, cats, horses, birds, and reptiles, has experienced enormous growth and technological advancement over the past two decades, paralleling laboratory medicine in people, but with important species differences, unique neoplasms and disease manifestations, added challenges in test validation, and outcomes that often depend on the cost-benefit of diagnosis and treatment. Sharkey and Wellman explain the routine use cytopathology in evaluating cancer and infectious diseases in animals and its important role in providing rapid and accurate decision support for clinicians and animal owners. Lymphoma, one of the most frequently diagnosed cancers in dogs, has stimulated extensive research and the development of advanced diagnostic modalities for classification and phenotyping, as elucidated by Bienzle and Vernau. Wiedmeyer and DeClue have met an important challenge by adapting the use of continuous glucose monitoring devices for diabetic dogs and cats, thereby avoiding the complications of stress from hospitalization and repeated handling and restraint (those of you who have had to take your cat to the veterinarian can appreciate this). Kjelgaard-Hansen and Jacobsen have been at the forefront of expanding the use of acute-phase proteins for monitoring and establishing prognosis in animals with immune-mediated, infectious, and surgical diseases. Cray focuses on the current status of diagnostic testing for important infectious and zoonotic diseases of pet birds, and Stacy and coworkers have taken advantage of a large and diverse reptile caseload in their teaching hospital to add extensively to our knowledge of reptile hematology for evaluating diseases in turtles, alligators, lizards—and yes, dragons.

One of the most exciting new areas of veterinary laboratory specialization has been the development of regenerative medicine laboratories for stem cell-based therapy. Borjesson and Peroni describe the extensive translational use of mesenchymal stem cells for equine orthopedic injuries and the laboratory procedures and protocols required to support this. Specialized intensive care laboratories have emerged to meet point-of-care testing needs for critically ill neonatal foals (see the article by Pamela A. Wilkins elsewhere in this issue for further exploration of this topic), in which the variables of species and age add to the challenges inherent in "stall-side" analysis. Specialized veterinary laboratories devoted, for example, to coagulation testing in animals (see the article by Brooks and colleagues elsewhere in this issue for exploration of this topic) provide essential diagnostic and consultation services to veterinarians and animal owners, as well as develop and validate new tests and support clinical and translational research.

## COMPARATIVE MEDICINE AND ANIMAL MODELS

Veterinary clinical pathology plays a critical role in the identification and laboratory investigation of animal models of human disease, in drug discovery, and in the selection, development, and interpretation of diagnostic tests for laboratory animals used in preclinical drug safety assessment, especially rodents, nonhuman primates, and dogs. Ramaiah cogently describes the need for new translatable hepatic biomarkers that differentiate drug-induced from other types of liver injury and effectively predict outcome in laboratory animals and ultimately in humans. Brooks and coworkers comprehensively detail the many spontaneous and engineered animal models of hemostatic disorders—including platelet and coagulation factor defects in species ranging from mice to pigs to whales—and the laboratory assays developed to assess them. As described above, spontaneous diseases in companion animals, such as canine lymphoma and equine orthopedic diseases, also provide unique and important models and opportunities for evaluating new diagnostic and treatment modalities that contribute to our understanding and treatment of disease in humans.

## GLOBAL ANIMAL, ENVIRONMENTAL, AND PUBLIC HEALTH

Veterinary diagnostic laboratories are at the forefront of preventing the introduction of foreign animal diseases, helping ensure the health of farm animals and the safety of food products, and identifying zoonotic diseases and toxicoses that threaten human and animal health, including wildlife. Andreasen provides a useful overview of the state diagnostic laboratory system, the coordination required between government laboratories and agencies, and the knowledge needed to detect, monitor, and confirm emerging infectious agents in production animals. Zoonotic diseases also can be transmitted to people by pets (see the articles by Sharkey and Wellman, and Carolyn Cray elsewhere in this issue for further exploration of this topic), increasing the onus on veterinary pathologists for making accurate diagnoses. Puschner and Reimschuessel detail the dramatic recent example of pet food contamination with melamine and melamine analogues, and the veterinary laboratory and toxicologic investigations that helped resolve this global crisis. Theirs is a riveting story that begins with an increased incidence of acute renal failure in dogs and cats in the United States and ends with nephropathy in children in China, removing any doubt you may have had about the intrinsic and complex relationships between human and animal health and food safety.

## LABORATORY QUALITY ASSURANCE AND STANDARDS

Quality assurance and the ability to create and maintain laboratory and test-specific standards are huge challenges for veterinary laboratories, where species-specific reagents and tests may not be available, proficiency testing is not always feasible, and regulatory guidelines may be lacking. As Andreasen points out, an accreditation system is mandated for state veterinary laboratories; however, quality assurance programs in other veterinary laboratories are voluntary (albeit often rigorous and of high quality) and fragmented, and medical laboratories that analyze animal samples may fail to appreciate species differences or reporting requirements. In birds and reptiles, the huge diversity of species confounds the development of test performance parameters, reference intervals, and disease-defining criteria (see the articles by Stacy and colleagues, and Carolyn Cray elsewhere in this issue for further exploration of this topic). Sharkey and Wellman emphasize the need for an evidence-based approach to cytology, and as noted by Wilkins, improved assessment of point-of-care devices is needed for specific animal applications. Kjelgaard-Hansen and Jacobson provide a valuable analysis of the steps involved in validating the analytical and clinical performance of assay systems, and point to the achievements gained with acute phase protein tests for animals, where a high level of evidence in clinically relevant studies appears to warrant their routine inclusion in clinical chemistry panels.

## EDUCATION IN CLINICAL PATHOLOGY

Clinical pathology courses in veterinary curricula often provide the first opportunity for students to develop diagnostic reasoning skills, in conjunction with didactic knowledge about laboratory tests and basic laboratory skills. Bender and Danielson have taken excellent teaching and educational pedagogy to a higher level by developing a novel software program with a demonstrated ability to facilitate learning by veterinary students as they tackle the interpretation of laboratory data. The Pathfinder has been applied in veterinary schools nationally and internationally and has strong potential for use as a flexible and extensible learning tool in diverse disciplines.

I hope the articles in this issue stimulate your interest, contribute to your understanding of veterinary laboratory medicine, and encourage you to identify and build on areas of common interest with veterinarians engaged in laboratory medicine research, diagnostic practice, and education. The connections between animal and human health are inextricable and growing; this issue of *Clinics in Laboratory Medicine* is intended to strengthen those connections, to the benefit of both animals and people.

Mary M. Christopher, DVM, PhD
Department of Pathology,
Microbiology, and Immunology
School of Veterinary Medicine
University of California–Davis
One Shields Avenue
Davis, CA 95616, USA

E-mail address:
mmchristopher@ucdavis.edu

# Diagnostic Cytology in Veterinary Medicine: A Comparative and Evidence-Based Approach

Leslie C. Sharkey, DVM, PhD[a],*, Maxey L. Wellman, DVM, MS, PhD[b]

KEYWORDS

• Cytology • Neoplasia • Infectious disease • Evidence-based
• Veterinary

Cytology is a core diagnostic pathology service that involves specimens from domestic animals, laboratory animals, and exotic species spanning the phylogenetic spectrum from invertebrates to marine mammals. Veterinarians in general practice perform in-clinic cytologic examination of routine lesions such as exudative ears or subcutaneous masses, which comprise approximately 50% of the samples collected.[1] More complicated lesions usually are evaluated by board-certified veterinary clinical pathologists in veterinary diagnostic laboratories and academic teaching hospitals, which contributes to increased confidence of the clinician in the diagnosis.[1] As the level of sophistication of veterinary medicine has advanced, driven by veterinary medical research, ecological and public health concerns, exponential growth of veterinary specialists (eg, in oncology, neurology, dermatology), and the human-animal bond, client expectations for veterinary pathology services also have increased, resulting in the expansion of veterinary diagnostic laboratories. In response, training programs in veterinary clinical pathology also have expanded, with increasing emphasis on diagnostic proficiency and quality assurance.[2]

Species and breed differences in the prevalence and biology of neoplastic, inflammatory, and degenerative diseases in animals present unique and fascinating

Disclosure: Both authors are paid consultants of IDEXX Laboratories.
[a] Veterinary Clinical Sciences Department, University of Minnesota College of Veterinary Medicine, 1352 Boyd Avenue, St Paul, MN 55108, USA
[b] Department of Veterinary Biosciences, The Ohio State University, 1925 Coffey Road, Columbus, OH 43210, USA
* Corresponding author.
E-mail address: Shark009@umn.edu

Clin Lab Med 31 (2011) 1–19
doi:10.1016/j.cll.2010.10.005
0272-2712/11/$ – see front matter © 2011 Elsevier Inc. All rights reserved.

labmed.theclinics.com

challenges for veterinary cytopathologists. In this review, the authors share some of these diagnostic challenges by focusing on selected neoplasms and infectious diseases that are unique to animals and/or that provide important examples of comparative disease relevant to humans. The authors hope to emphasize both the important contributions of medical pathology to veterinary pathology and the important role and knowledge base of veterinary clinical pathologists in making cytologic diagnoses in animals. Where possible, the evidence available for the diagnosis and classification of these disorders is presented, and areas are identified where additional research is needed.

## EVIDENCE-BASED APPROACH TO VETERINARY CYTOLOGY

In veterinary medicine, as in human medicine, fine-needle aspiration cytology is widely accepted as an initial diagnostic option for animals with mass lesions, internal organs with ultrasonographic abnormalities, and other samples, such as effusions. However, the clinical utility of fine-needle aspirates depends on obtaining a high-quality specimen with adequate cellularity that will be interpreted by an experienced cytopathologist,[3] and ultimately on evidence-based medicine (EBM) that supports the diagnostic accuracy and clinical relevance of cytology for specific lesions.[4] Increased demand for EBM in veterinary cytology—based on clearly defined studies and comparison with a reference method—has resulted in part because of rapid advances in veterinary medical science, newer diagnostic modalities, increased health care costs for animals, and easier access of clients to electronic media.[4] Progress in veterinary EBM has been impeded by limited funding for controlled studies; the small numbers of animals usually evaluated; few multi-institutional studies; the variable impact of species, breed, and geographic location; and obtaining client consent to enroll their animals in a clinical trial or to collect tissues from their pets for biospecimen repositories or for research purposes.

Guidelines for evidence-based medical cytology, a relatively new branch of EBM, often include the need for information about sampling and specimen adequacy, because these may have a significant impact on interpretation of results.[4] For example, the sensitivity of sputum cytology increases when samples are obtained over several consecutive days,[5,6] and inadequate sampling and improper specimen handling are major causes of false-negative results in cytologic evaluation of the cervix.[7] Similarly, in dogs, sample cellularity has been shown to be an important determinant of sensitivity and specificity of fine-needle aspirates of bone lesions and mammary masses in the diagnosis of osteosarcoma and mammary tumors, respectively.[8,9] Criteria to determine the adequacy of fine-needle aspirates include the numbers of intact cells, cell clusters, and cells within a group; cell types; and blood or bacterial contamination.[4,8,9]

Results of cytologic evaluation often are compared with those of histologic evaluation of biopsy specimens to determine sensitivity and specificity, using histopathology as the reference method.[4,8,9] However, assessment of cytologic and histopathologic specimens by cytopathologists may have a lower interobserver agreement than is desirable.[4] Development of specific cytologic criteria of malignancy for particular cell types, which are well developed in medical cytopathology but have been described only for a few animal organs,[10–13] may improve diagnostic accuracy, as can the use of ancillary tests such as immunocytochemistry, immunohistochemistry, and flow cytometry. Various expert computer systems based on Bayesian belief networks, artificial neural networks, and logistic regression analysis have been developed for a more objective approach to analysis of cytologic and histopathologic specimens, such as discrimination between benign and malignant lesions. In veterinary medicine, computerized assessment of mean nuclear morphometry in fine-needle aspirates has been used to differentiate between benign and malignant mammary gland tumors and to predict local recurrence of basal cell carcinomas in dogs.[14-16]

A pathology report that clearly and consistently communicates the cytopathologist's interpretation is an important component of evidence-based cytology. Optimum content and format can be in the form of an open-ended report or checklist.[4] Defined terminology and use of consistent vocabulary to express the probability or likelihood of cytologic diagnosis may improve communication and the quality of data in cytology reporting.[17] It is important for the clinician to understand the cytopathologist's degree of certainty in the diagnosis of the lesion. Numerical reporting schemes have been established in human medicine for some lesions,[18] but have not been widely applied in veterinary medicine.

Determination of positive predictive values and other indicators of diagnostic accuracy, including correlation with histology and clinical outcome, can improve quality assurance of cytopathology. In veterinary medicine, correlation between cytologic and histologic diagnoses depends on the tissue and type of lesion. Correlation is 70% to 90% for skin masses in dogs and cats,[13] but only 38% to 60% for splenic lesions.[19] In dogs with neoplastic bone lesions, the correlation between cytologic and histopathologic diagnoses was 92%, but there was only a 27% correlation for dogs with nonneoplastic lesions.[8] In dogs with benign mammary gland tumors the correlation between cytologic and histologic diagnoses was 93%, whereas the correlation for dogs with malignant tumors was only 81%.[9] Critical evaluation of correlation studies between cytology and histopathology can be enhanced by using standards for reporting studies of diagnostic accuracy. Several medical journals have adopted the Standard for Reporting of Diagnostic Accuracy (STARD), including *Veterinary Clinical Pathology*,[20] wherein many studies and cases are reported that involve cytology in animals. Such criteria facilitate complete reporting of methodology and data, optimize comparison of conclusions with data from similar studies, and ultimately contribute to the advancement of evidence-based cytology in veterinary medicine.[8]

## DIAGNOSTIC APPLICATION OF CYTOLOGY IN VETERINARY MEDICINE

The advantages of using cytology as a diagnostic modality in animals are similar to those in humans but often take on an even greater importance in veterinary medicine. Noninvasive collection methods lower the risk of complications, and rapid availability of results facilitates triage and timely clinical decisions. Superficial lesions can be sampled with minimal physical or chemical restraint, compared with biopsy, which requires local or general anesthesia. Most tissues can be sampled by fine-needle aspiration, and the increased availability of ultrasonography in the veterinary private practice setting has contributed to increased sampling of internal organs and lesions for cytologic evaluation. The relatively low cost of routine cytology compared with histopathology, advanced imaging, and other ancillary testing also is a particular benefit in veterinary medicine, where financial limitations can be a significant consideration when formulating a diagnostic plan. Unique to veterinary medicine is the fact that cytologic diagnoses can form the basis for advising owners about euthanasia as a humane option for their pets. In some cases, cytology may be the major or even the sole basis for such crucial medical decisions, especially if the patient is critically ill or suffering, or if there are financial considerations that limit additional diagnostic or therapeutic options. These situations emphasize the importance of high standards for training and certification of veterinary clinical pathologists, quality assurance guidelines, and a comprehensive understanding of the diagnostic sensitivity and specificity of cytology, which may vary with the type of lesion or pathologic process.[21]

Cytology often is very useful in differentiating between neoplastic and infectious processes, and in some cases provides an etiologic diagnosis that is helpful in instituting a specific chemotherapeutic plan. Most samples for cytologic evaluation in veterinary medicine are collected by fine-needle aspiration, although impression smears of biopsy specimens or scrapings of ulcerated or superficial lesions also are evaluated. Rather than the predominant use of Papanicolaou stain as in medical pathology, veterinary laboratories and practices typically air-dry samples and use Romanowsky-type stains for routine evaluation. Papanicolaou staining requires a multistep procedure and has limitations for evaluating inflammatory reactions, whereas Romanowsky-type stains like Wright Giemsa stain are rapid, easy to use, and result in adequate staining of inflammatory and neoplastic cells.[22] The differentiation between inflammatory and neoplastic lesions often is a critical step in client communications and determination of additional diagnostic testing.

Numerous additional diagnostic techniques are used to increase the diagnostic utility of cytologic specimens from animals. Cytochemical stains such as nonspecific esterase and alkaline phosphatase have been used to support diagnoses of histiocytic sarcoma and osteosarcoma, respectively.[23,24] Immunocytochemical staining and flow cytometric analysis are used routinely to determine cell lineage in tumors of hematopoietic, epithelial, melanocytic, or mesenchymal origin, and to distinguish between lymphoma involving B or T lymphocytes, which may have therapeutic and prognostic relevance in dogs.[25–36] DNA-based testing such as polymerase chain reaction (PCR) for antigen receptor rearrangement often is done using fine-needle aspirate specimens to differentiate lymphoid hyperplasia from lymphoid neoplasia, and to determine whether lymphoid neoplasms are of B- or T-cell origin[35,36] (see the article by Bienzle and Vernau elsewhere in this issue for further exploration of this topic). Although identifying genetic abnormalities in neoplastic cells from most veterinary species is in its infancy, this information likely will become important in the future diagnosis and prevention of disease in animals, especially because breeding options allow the potential of modifying genetic predisposition for some diseases.[37]

## CYTOLOGIC DIAGNOSIS OF SELECTED NEOPLASMS IN ANIMALS

When establishing a cytologic diagnosis of neoplasia in animals, numerous species differences in occurrence, prevalence, manifestation, and biologic behavior of the neoplasms must be considered. Demographic factors such as age, sex and reproductive status, geography, physical traits such as coat (skin) color, and genetic factors reflected in breeds or strains within species, add an additional challenge to interpretation. This section describes the cytologic and comparative features of transmissible tumors, histiocytic neoplasms, melanocytic tumors, and squamous cell carcinoma affecting different species of animals. These neoplasms are unique to animals or affect animals in unique ways that contrast with the comparable disease in humans. All of these neoplasms are diagnosed routinely by veterinary cytopathologists.

### Transmissible Tumors

Only two known naturally occurring malignancies can be transmitted by direct engraftment of neoplastic cells between tumor-bearing individuals, and both affect animals: canine transmissible venereal tumor (TVT) and Tasmanian Devil facial disease (TDFD). Canine TVT is commonly observed on the face and external genitalia of dogs in populations where there are large numbers of sexually intact, free-roaming animals.

Cytologic diagnosis is based on identification of a population of round cells with abundant lightly basophilic and highly vacuolated cytoplasm, single round nuclei with coarse chromatin, and one or two prominent nucleoli (**Fig. 1**). Lesions may spontaneously regress, although chemotherapy is successful for persistent lesions and metastasis has been observed in untreated or immunocompromised dogs. The cell type involved in TVT remains an unsolved mystery. Genetic analysis suggests the tumor arose from a single point of origin somewhere between 7800 and 78,000 years ago, likely from wolves.[38] Neoplastic cells have fewer chromosomes (2n = 57–59) compared with normal canine cells (2n = 76). This chromosomal abnormality is uniform in TVTs affecting dogs across the globe,[39] the result of gene fusion and rearrangement as well as unique genetic mutations in the tumor. Tumor cells express vimentin and CD45, and are positive for lysozyme and $\alpha$1-antitrypsin, suggesting macrophage lineage. During the growth phase of the tumor, major histocompatibility complex (MHC) class I and II are not highly expressed; however, regression in immunocompetent dogs appears to be associated with increased MHC expression, possibly triggered by cytokines from infiltrating lymphocytes. Likewise, the tumor's ability to suppress natural killer cells and B cells and to prevent dendritic cell maturation diminishes over time as the tumor succumbs to both cell-mediated and humoral immune responses in the host, with persistent immunity after tumor regression.

The second transmissible neoplasm, TDFD, is predicted to lead to the imminent extinction in the wild of its host species, the Tasmanian Devil, a marsupial carnivore native to the island of Tasmania. In contrast to the long period of coevolution between TVT and dogs, TDFD was first observed in the mid-1990s. Cytologically, the tumor cells are large, pleomorphic, and round to spindloid, with large, central, single nuclei.[38]

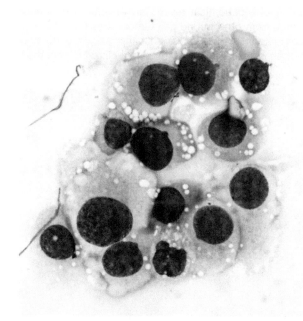

**Fig. 1.** Transmissible venereal tumor from the prepuce of a dog. Note the round-cell morphology, clear cytoplasmic vacuoles, and moderate anisokaryosis. The cell of origin of this sexually transmitted neoplasm unique to dogs remains uncertain (Wright Giemsa stain ×100 oil immersion).

The cell of origin has recently been reported to be a Schwann cell.[40] The cells are biologically aggressive in this rapidly progressive and fatal disease, which may be transmitted by bite wounds. In contrast to TVT, in which more severe disease is observed in immunocompromised individuals, Tasmanian Devils that succumb to TDFD are generally immunocompetent. The precise reasons for the difference in biologic behavior of the two tumors have not been completely elucidated; however, MHC complexes have low levels of sequence divergence in Tasmanian Devils, which may allow allograft transmission.

### Canine Histiocytic Tumors

Canine cutaneous histiocytoma is a frequently diagnosed round cell tumor that is unique to dogs. Histiocytomas are single, hairless domed lesions that often occur in young dogs, with a predilection for the head, ear pinnae, limbs, and trunk, but lesions may occur anywhere on the body and occasionally are multiple. The diagnosis frequently is based on the classic clinical presentation and gross appearance, in combination with characteristic cytologic findings of numerous individual round cells with moderately abundant basophilic cytoplasm that sometimes contains a few small clear vacuoles (**Fig. 2**). Each cell contains a single round, oval, or indented nucleus with finely stippled chromatin and occasional small nucleoli. Anisocytosis and aniso-karyosis are mild to moderate. The relatively immature appearance of the cells can lead cytopathologists unfamiliar with this tumor to be concerned about malignancy, especially because there often is histopathologic evidence of epidermal invasion, leading to potential confusion with epidermotropic cutaneous lymphoma. Immunohis-tochemical staining indicates an epidermal Langerhans cell origin, as the cells are positive for CD1a, MHC class II, CD11c/CD18, and often cadherin, and negative for CD4 and Thy-1. Immunohistochemical results are helpful in differentiating canine cutaneous histiocytoma from other round cell tumors. Canine cutaneous histiocyto-mas frequently undergo spontaneous remission within a few months of onset, similar to TVT. Regression often is associated with transient enlargement of the lesion due to

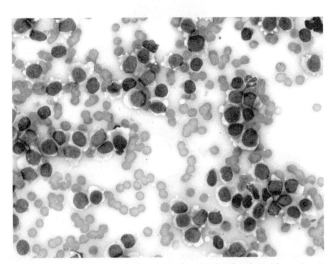

**Fig. 2.** Canine cutaneous histiocytoma from the forelimb of a dog. These benign neoplasms usually regress spontaneously, and sometimes are associated with a lymphocytic infiltrate (Wright Giemsa stain, ×50 oil immersion objective).

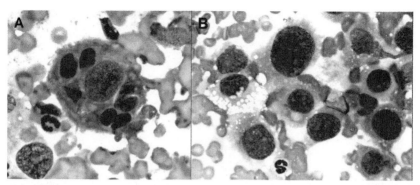

**Fig. 3.** Histiocytic sarcoma in a dog. (*A*) Cytophagic cell in the spleen and (*B*) cellular pleomorphism in the bone marrow (Wright Giemsa stain, ×100 oil immersion objective).

massive recruitment of CD8$^+$ $\alpha\beta$ T lymphocytes,[41] such that cytologic specimens can contain large numbers of lymphocytes that in some cases outnumber tumor cells. Down-regulation of E-cadherin expression also has been documented during regression.[42]

Canine cutaneous histiocytoma is one of a group of proliferative histiocytic diseases that are most common in dogs, infrequently described in cats, and rare or absent in other animal species. Recent reviews describe the full spectrum of these disorders in animals.[41,43] In contrast to histiocytomas, which are relatively benign lesions, histiocytic sarcoma complex (HS) is a rapidly progressive and fatal disease with a significant breed predilection for Bernese Mountain Dogs, although Rottweilers, flat-coated retrievers, and Golden retrievers are also predisposed. Primary lesions occur in the spleen, lymph node, lung, bone marrow, skin and subcutis, and in the periarticular tissues of the limbs, all sites that are sampled routinely by fine-needle aspiration for making a cytologic diagnosis.[41] Regardless of the site of origin, the cytologic features include large pleomorphic mononuclear cells with scant to abundant basophilic cytoplasm, variable cytophagia, large immature nuclei, multinucleation, and bizarre mitotic figures (**Fig. 3**). A hemophagocytic variant of HS exhibits a more diffuse distribution within affected organs and is often associated with regenerative anemia and thrombocytopenia, which may lead to a temporary misdiagnosis of Evan's syndrome.[41] Distinguishing among HS, other round cell tumors, mesenchymal malignancies, and non-neoplastic hemophagocytic syndrome in cytologic specimens is augmented by immunophenotyping: HS cells express CD1, CD11c/CD18, and MHCII, with substitution of CD11d for CD11c in the hemophagocytic form. HS cells are CD3-negative, distinguishing them from the large-cell form of T-cell lymphoma, and also typically are negative for mast cell markers (CD18 variable, CD45$^+$, CD45A$^+$, tryptase$^+$, c-kit$^+$).[41]

## Melanocytic Tumors in Horses and Dogs

Melanomas are routinely diagnosed and staged in animals using cytologic methods. Melanocytic tumors are common in dogs, horses, and some breeds of pigs, less common in cats and cattle, and rare in sheep and goats.[44] Melanocytic lesions are divided into benign melanocytomas and malignant melanomas. Cutaneous melanocytomas are common in horses older than 5 years with gray or dilute coat color; the number of tumors increases with age.[45] In addition, benign single to confluent lesions of the deep dermis, concentrated in the perineum, ventral tail, and external genitalia, can progress over time to multiple malignant tumors in both the skin and internal

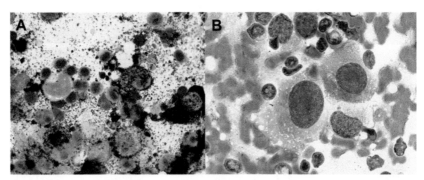

**Fig. 4.** Metastatic melanoma in fine-needle aspirate specimens of canine lymph nodes. (*A*) Highly pigmented melanoma cells and abundant background pigment granules are admixed with small lymphocytes (Wright Giemsa stain, ×50 objective). (*B*) An amelanotic melanoma with marked cellular pleomorphism and no apparent melanin pigment. Cell origin was verified by immunohistochemical staining for S-100 and Melan A (Wright Giemsa stain, ×100 oil immersion objective).

organs. In contrast, horses with nondilute coat color can have benign or malignant melanomas that are randomly distributed. Recently, a rare equine melanocytic tumor resembling human intradermal common melanocytic nevi, cellular blue nevi, and combined cellular blue nevus has been described.[45]

Certain breeds of dogs have higher (eg, Vizsla, Schnauzer, Chesapeake Bay retriever) or lower (eg, Siberian husky, Old English Sheepdog, Bichon Frise) statistical risk of developing melanocytic tumors. In all dogs, benign lesions tend to occur in the skin and are often black, whereas malignant lesions tend to occur in the oral cavity and nail bed and have variable pigmentation. Prognosis depends on both the anatomic location of the lesion and the degree of differentiation.[46] Cytologically, well-differentiated melanomas consist of numerous round to polyhedral cells with abundant melanin pigment and small condensed and uniform nuclei. The less differentiated and more malignant forms are highly variable cytologically. Malignant melanocytes generally have marked cellular pleomorphism and can resemble round cells, epithelial cells, or spindle cells. Pigmentation ranges from heavy to a barely perceptible light-gray dusting in isolated cells. Nuclei are often large, with marked anisokaryosis, variable nuclear to cytoplasmic ratios, and large prominent nucleoli (**Fig. 4**). As in humans, balloon cell variants of melanoma are rare but have been described in dogs and cats. These variants are difficult to distinguish cytologically from other cell types with abundant clear cytoplasm, such as sebaceous cell carcinoma and liposarcoma, and special stains or ultrastructural studies may be needed for definitive diagnosis.[47]

### Squamous Cell Carcinoma in Animals

Squamous cell carcinomas (SCC) have wide species distribution and are relatively common tumors in horses, cattle, cats, and dogs. Exposure to solar radiation is a risk factor in all species, but especially in cattle breeds such as Hereford and Simmental, which lack pigmentation in the poorly haired circumocular region. Some breeds of dogs appear to have higher genetic risk for SCC, and white or piebald dogs with extensive exposure to the sun are also predisposed.[44] SCC occurs in the nail bed of dogs and in the oral cavity of many species, and is the most common tumor of llamas and horses, where it originates in the squamous epithelium-lined portion of the stomach.[48,49] SCC often is diagnosed cytologically, although well-differentiated

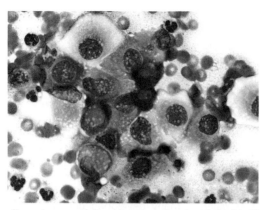

**Fig. 5.** Squamous cell carcinoma of the pharynx of a dog (Wright Giemsa stain, ×50 oil immersion objective). Cohesive clusters of polygonal to angular cells are visible, some of which appear to be keratinizing.

tumors may be difficult to distinguish from marked reactive epithelial hyperplasia or dysplasia, especially when only superficial impression smears are collected and when there is abundant concurrent inflammation. In the latter cases, histopathology is required for a definitive diagnosis. Cytologic features of SCC include variably cohesive polyhedral cells in which some or all cells have glassy clear to aqua cytoplasm indicating keratinization; perinuclear vacuolization is noted in some cases (**Fig. 5**). Nuclei are round and central, and asynchronous nuclear and cytoplasmic maturation and a range of immature to well-differentiated squamous epithelial cells often is observed. Keratinized debris and secondary suppurative inflammation is relatively common, and there may be secondary bacterial infection or overgrowth of commensal organisms.

## CYTOLOGIC DIAGNOSIS OF SELECTED INFECTIOUS DISEASES IN ANIMAL SPECIES

Similar to neoplasms, there are numerous species differences in prevalence, manifestation, and biologic behavior of infectious diseases, and in some cases important breed differences have been recognized. Etiologic agents that can be recognized in cytologic specimens include bacteria, fungi, protozoa, rickettsia, and mycoplasma; viral inclusions; and endo- and ectoparasites. Accurate recognition of infectious agents is important in diagnosing disease outbreaks in kennels, breeding or research facilities, herds, and zoos. Diagnosis of zoonotic infections is important in food safety and security, and in preventing spread of disease to human beings. Although culture, serology, DNA-based testing, and other sensitive or specific assays can be used to confirm the diagnosis of most of these infectious diseases, cytology often is the first diagnostic step and thus can be important in making an initial differential or etiologic diagnosis. This section describes the cytologic appearance of mycobacteria, the yeast form of cryptococcosis, the tachyzooites of toxoplasmosis, and the morulae of erhlichiosis, all of which infect animals and people, with either similar or unique syndromes associated with infection.

### Mycobacteria

Mycobacteria include several groups and individual species of organisms that vary markedly in host affinity and pathogenicity. In cytologic specimens, these organisms appear as negatively stained intra- and extracellular rods with Romanowsky stains, but are red to magenta when stained with acid-fast stains (**Fig. 6**). Acid-fast staining of cytologic specimens from infected tissues can be helpful in making a rapid presumptive diagnosis of mycobacteriosis. Mycoplasma infections in animals cause bronchopneumonia, pulmonary nodules, and hilar lymphadenopathy, although granulomas in other tissues and disseminated disease also can occur. Several mycobacteria have zoonotic potential, and recognition of infection is important for prognosis, treatment, and prevention (see the article by Carolyn Cray elsewhere in this issue for further exploration of this topic).

*Mycobacterium tuberculosis* is a highly pathogenic organism for which human beings are the only reservoir host.[50] Infections in dogs and cats are examples of anthroponoses because the source, replication, and primary means of transmission occur in humans; spread of this organism from dogs or cats back to people has not been reported. Although the prevalence of human and animal infections with *M tuberculosis* has been decreasing in many developed countries, prevalence has been increasing in underdeveloped countries, and in some countries wildlife has become endemically infected from close contact with human habitats, serving as reservoirs for further human infection.[50] The majority of reported canine cases of tuberculosis are caused by *M tuberculosis*, likely acquired from inhalation of microorganisms in households shared with tubercular people. The cytology of lesions involving the lungs, tracheobronchial lymph nodes, and pleura is characterized by a mixed population of inflammatory cells that includes vacuolated histiocytic cells containing acid-fast bacilli. The characteristic multinucleated Langerhans cells seen in tubercular lesions in people are seen less commonly in dogs.[51]

Infection in people and domestic animals with *Mycobacterium bovis* is rare, due to successful eradication programs in ruminants; however, wildlife hosts have become a reservoir of infection in some areas. Tuberculosis from *M bovis* is endemic in white-tailed deer in the northeastern portion of the lower peninsula in Michigan, and domestic cats have been infected with this organism by ingestion of tissues from infected deer.[52] Calcospherites and granular caseous debris have been described in a dog with *M bovis* infection, similar to what has been described in people with *M tuberculosis* infection, but have not been described in other types of mycobacterial infection in dogs and cats.[53]

Other mycobacterial species often are referred to as atypical mycobacteria. Most of these organisms are ubiquitous and potentially pathogenic. *Mycobacterium avium*

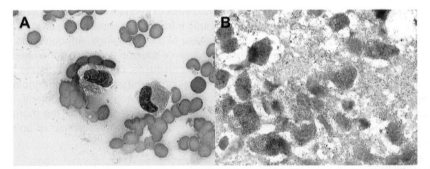

**Fig. 6.** Fine-needle aspirate of a subcutaneous mass from a cat with mycobacteriosis (*Mycobacterium* sp). (*A*) Intracellular nonstaining rods can be seen within macrophages (Wright Giemsa stain, ×100 oil immersion objective). (*B*) Numerous acid-fast intra- and extracellular organisms appear as magenta rods (Ziehl-Neelsen stain, ×50 oil immersion objective).

infections are common in wild, domestic, and captive birds, but are rare in mammals. Siamese and Abyssinian cats, Basset Hounds, and Miniature Schnauzers may be predisposed to infection with an opportunistic group of mycobacteria called *M avium-Mycobacterium intracellulare*.[53–55] In humans, these mycobacteria usually infect only immunocompromised individuals. There is no other evidence of spread of these particular mycobacteria from people to animals or animals to people.[50] Cutaneous lesions characterized by neutrophils, macrophages, lymphocytes, and plasma cells caused by rapidly growing mycobacteria species such as *Mycobacterium fortuitum*, *Mycobacterium chelonei*, and *Mycobacterium smegmatis* have been described in dogs and cats,[22] and infection with *M fortuitum* transmitted by bites from domestic animals has been reported in people.[56] *M avium* subsp *paratuberculosis* causes a chronic inflammatory intestinal disease in cattle called Johne's disease, and has been implicated as a cause of Crohn disease in people.[57]

Mycobacteria that infect animals but not people include *Mycobacterium lepramaemurium*, which causes murine leprosy, and an unnamed mycobacterium that causes canine leproid granuloma.[58] Feline leprosy syndrome can be caused by several species of mycobacteria, including *M lepramaemurium* in cats that become infected after being bitten by an infected rodent.[50] Lymphadenitis and peritonitis caused by *Mycobacterium xenopi* infection have been reported in a cat,[59] and systemic mycobacteriosis due to *Mycobacterium marinum* complex has been reported in *Xenopus* frogs.[60] Rapid identification of mycobacteria using cytology is integral to minimizing zoonotic risk and further spread of disease. In addition to acid-fast stains, other stains such as auramine O/acridine orange fluorescent staining have been used to detect mycobacteria. However, none of these stains is as sensitive as immunohistochemical or PCR analysis in detecting infection.[61]

## Local and Systemic Fungal Infections

The characteristic morphology of some fungal organisms allows them to be recognized in cytologic specimens, although more sensitive and specific assays often are performed for a definitive diagnosis. Some fungal organisms such as *Cryptococcus* are sapronotic, whereby people and animals acquire infections directly from the environment. Diagnosis of the infection in animals can therefore be important in recognizing contaminated environments and preventing similar exposure and infection in people. Other fungal infections such as sporotrichosis and dermatophytosis can be acquired from the environment, or from a scratch or close contact with an infected animal.

Cryptococcosis occurs in cats, dogs, ferrets, horses, goats, sheep, cattle, dolphins, birds, koalas, and other marsupials. Most infections occur in dogs and cats, and cats are more commonly affected than dogs. Infection in dogs and cats most commonly is due to *Cryptococcus neoformans* and *Cryptococcus gattii*, which are likely primary pathogens.[62] *Cryptococcus* has worldwide distribution and cryptococcosis is an important fungal disease of immunocompromised human patients, who usually develop meningoencephalitis. Dogs and cats with cryptococcosis most often present with clinical signs of nasal cavity infection, although progression to the central nervous system is not uncommon and gastrointestinal tract infection has been described.[63] Koalas may have respiratory tract infections or have asymptomatic colonization of the nasal passages and skin with *C gattii*. Subclinical infection and nasal colonization with *C gattii* in dogs and cats has been described in evaluation of the recent outbreak of cryptococcosis in people and animals on Vancouver Island in British Columbia, Canada.[64] Various tree species may be environmental sources for these organisms in Australia[65,66] and Canada.[67]

*Cryptococcus* is a dimorphic fungus that exists in the yeast phase in tissues. The wide capsule is a critical virulence factor but also is important in recognition of the organism in cytologic specimens.[68] The yeast is round and 4 to 40 μm in diameter, depending on the width of the capsule, which appears clear with routine Romanowsky stains. Narrow-based budding of the organism may be apparent and is important for differentiating *Cryptococcus* from *Blastomyces* sp in cytologic specimens (**Fig. 7**).[69] New methylene blue and India ink may be used to enhance visibility of the capsule,[22] which may be distorted with routine Romanowsky stains. Poorly encapsulated *Cryptococcus* strains are more difficult to recognize in cytologic specimens, and may resemble *Sporothrix schenckii* or *Histoplasma capsulatum*. Infection may be associated with granulomatous or pyogranulomatous inflammation, although there may be minimal inflammation in some animals. Eosinophilic pleocytosis has been described with meningoencephalitis caused by *C neoformans* infection.[70] A negative cytologic examination does not exclude a diagnosis of cryptococcosis. A sensitive and specific latex agglutination test to detect the capsular antigen in serum is commercially available, and has been used to monitor response to treatment.[70]

Sporotrichosis occurs most commonly in dogs and cats, and can be transmitted to immunocompromised human hosts. Infection is caused by *S schenckii*, a dimorphic fungus that occurs as a yeast form in tissues and a telomorph form in soil and on bushes and trees.[71] Infection of both animals and people most often is caused by skin wounds infected with contaminated soil or plant material, resulting in cutaneous lesions that can progress to lymphadenitis or occasionally systemic infection. Cats with sporotrichosis often have multiple draining lesions that typically contain numerous organisms; these facilitate cytologic diagnosis but can be an important source of zoonotic infection for people, even in the absence of a skin-penetrating lesion.[71] Transmission from dogs to people is less likely because dogs have fewer lesions with fewer organisms. Cytologic preparations of lesions caused by *S schenckii* are characterized by a mixed cell population of neutrophils, macrophages, lymphocytes, and eosinophils, and may contain numerous (cats) or rare (dogs) intra- and extracellular and intracellular yeasts. The organisms can occur extracellularly or within neutrophils and macrophages.[71,72] With Romanowsky stains, the yeast organisms are round, oval, or cigar-shaped, 3 to 5 μm wide and 5 to 9 μm long (**Fig. 8**).[69] The

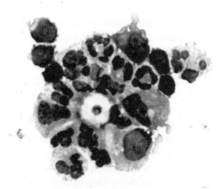

**Fig. 7.** Cerebrospinal fluid from a cat. A single *Cryptococcus neoformans* organism with a wide, nonstaining capsule is surrounded by neutrophils, large mononuclear cells, and lymphocytes (Wright Giemsa stain, ×100 objective).

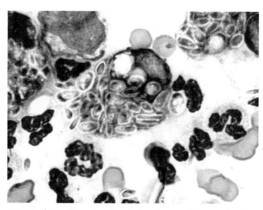

**Fig. 8.** Impression smears from an ulcerated lesion on the nose of a domestic shorthair kitten. Numerous cigar-shaped *Sporothrix schenckii* organisms can be seen within macrophages. Several neutrophils also are present, consistent with pyogranulomatous inflammation (Wright Giemsa stain, ×100 objective).

organism may be surrounded by a clear halo that resembles a capsule. Differential diagnoses include *H capsulatum* and poorly encapsulated *C neoformans*. Definitive diagnosis is by culture of the exudate from a draining tract or macerated tissue from a lesion.[71,72]

### Protozoal and Rickettsial Diseases

Toxoplasmosis can affect all warm-blooded animals, including people. Rats, cattle, horses, and Old World monkeys are relatively resistant to infection, whereas Australian marsupials and New World monkeys are susceptible to severe and often fatal infection. Toxoplasmosis is caused by an obligate intracellular coccidian parasite called *Toxoplasma gondii*. Infectious oocysts are excreted in feces of domestic cats and other Felidae, which are definitive hosts.[73] Tissue cysts containing the infectious stages (tachyzoites and bradyzoites) occur in other animals, including people, which are intermediate hosts.[73] Transmission most commonly is congenital, or occurs by ingestion of cysts in infected tissues (eg, meat), or ingestion of oocysts in contaminated food, water, or feces from recently infected cats.[73] Tachyzoites can be detected using routine staining of fine-needle aspirates of various infected tissues and body fluids, and rarely have been identified in circulating neutrophils and monocytes.[74] Infection may be associated with a mixed inflammatory response that includes neutrophils and macrophages.[75] Tachyzoites are oval, spindloid, or crescent-shaped structures, 2 to 4 μm long, with light-blue cytoplasm and reddish-purple nuclei that may be eccentric (**Fig. 9**).[73,75,76] The organisms occur extracellularly or intracellularly within macrophages or epithelial cells.[75] Tachyzoites are similar in morphology to *Neospora caninum* and *Sarcocystis neurona* organisms.[74,77] Synchronous fluorescent illumination or immunocytochemical staining of cytologic samples may be helpful in facilitating detection of tachyzoites.[78] Serologic tests are available, but the results may be difficult to interpret. PCR assays for DNA in infected tissues is available for definitive diagnosis.[73,74]

Ehrlichia organisms are obligate intracellular gram-negative bacteria transmitted by ticks that feed on infected mammalian wildlife, which may serve as reservoirs for disease.[79] There are several different Ehrlichial organisms with variable geographic distributions, vectors, wildlife reservoirs, and infected cell types that can cause

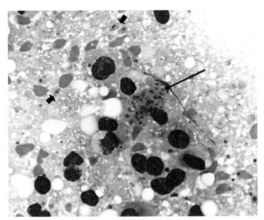

**Fig. 9.** Impression smear of lung parenchyma from a cat with *Toxoplasma gondii* infection. Several crescent-shaped tachyzoites can be seen inside a macrophage (*long arrow*) and several extracellular tachyzoites are also present (*short arrows*) (Wright Giemsa stain, ×100 objective).

disease in animals and people. *Ehrlichia chaffeensis* can infect multiple species[79,80] and is considered an emerging infection in people.[81] *Ehrlichia canis* and *Ehrlichia ewengii* can infect dogs and people. The small coccoid bacteria occur intracellularly, in clusters called morulae, which sometimes can be detected in peripheral blood leukocytes or cells in aspirates of infected tissues. In dogs with *E canis*, infection morulae are detected in lymphocytes and monocytes in peripheral blood and lymph node aspirates from the majority of dogs evaluated.[82] In dogs with *E ewengii* infection, morulae have been identified in neutrophils, peripheral blood, and synovial fluid.[80] With routine stains, morulae are tightly to loosely packed round, purple, mulberry-like granular structures, one to several micrometers in diameter, within a vacuole (**Fig. 10**).[79–82] Although the cytology of the morulae is characteristic and offers a rapid

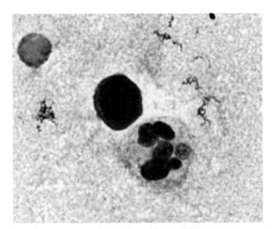

**Fig. 10.** Synovial fluid from a mixed-breed puppy with *Ehrlichia ewingii* infection. The neutrophil contains an intracellular morula (Wright Giemsa stain, ×100 objective).

diagnosis, few morulae may be present. Definitive diagnosis by serology or PCR is important because infections are responsive to appropriate antirickettsial agents.

## SUMMARY

In this article the authors provide a historical perspective on the development of veterinary cytology and brief context in comparison with human cytopathology. Veterinary cytopathologists must consider several unique entities such as directly transmissible tumors, as well as extensive species and breed differences in prevalence and diagnostic factors, for a variety of neoplastic and infectious diseases common to animals and humans. Similar to human cytopathology, advances in molecular diagnostics contribute to increasing the utility of cytology as a sole diagnostic modality. As both human and veterinary cytopathology evolve, clinicians continue to strive for a rigorous evidence-based approach to best serve their patients.

## REFERENCES

1. Christopher MM, Hotz CS, Shelly SM, et al. Use of cytology as a diagnostic method in veterinary practice and assessment of communication between veterinary practitioners and veterinary clinical pathologists. J Am Vet Med Assoc 2008; 232:747–54.
2. Christopher MM, Schultze AE, Bird KE. Postgraduate training programs in veterinary clinical pathology in the United States and Canada (1998–2002). Vet Clin Pathol 2003;32(3):121.
3. Nasuti JF, Gupta PK, Baloch ZW. Diagnostic value and cost-effectiveness of on-site evaluation of fine needle aspiration specimens: review of 5,688 cases. Diagn Cytopathol 2002;27:1–4.
4. Dey P. Time for evidence-based cytology. Cytojournal 2007;4:1–9.
5. Johnston WW. Fine needle aspiration biopsy versus sputum and bronchial material in the diagnosis of lung cancer: a comparative study of 168 patients. Acta Cytol 1998;32:641–8.
6. Johnston WW. Ten years of respiratory cytopathology of Duke University Medical Center III. The cytopathologic diagnosis of lung cancer during the years 1970–1974 noting the significance of specimen number and type. Acta Cytol 1981;25:103–7.
7. McGoogan E, Colgan TJ, Ramzy I, et al. Cell preparation methods and criteria for sample adequacy. IAC Task force summary. IAC TASK FPRCE NO 21. Acta Cytol 1998;42:25–32.
8. Berzina I, Sharkey LC, Matise, et al. Correlation between cytologic and histopathologic diagnoses on bone lesions in dogs: a study of the diagnostic accuracy of bone cytology. Vet Clin Pathol 2008;37:332–8.
9. Simon D, Schoenrock D, Nolte I, et al. Cytology examination of fine-needle aspirates from mammary gland tumors in the dog: diagnostic accuracy with comparison to histopathology and association with postoperative outcome. Vet Clin Pathol 2009;38:521–8.
10. Stockhaus C, Van Den Ingh T, Rothuizen J, et al. A multistep approach in the cytologic evaluation of liver biopsy samples of dogs with hepatic diseases. Vet Pathol 2004;41:461–70.
11. Masserdotti C, Bonfanti U, De Lorenzi D, et al. Cytologic features of testicular tumours in dog. J Vet Med A Physiol Pathol Clin Med 2005;52:339–46.
12. De Lorenzi D, Mandara MT, Tranquillo M, et al. Squash-prep cytology in the diagnosis of canine and feline nervous system lesions: a study of 42 cases. Vet Clin Pathol 2006;35:208–14.

13. Ghisleni G, Roccabianca R, Ceruti R, et al. Correlation between fine-needle aspiration cytology and histopathology in the evaluation of cutaneous and subcutaneous masses from dogs and cats. Vet Clin Pathol 2006;35:24–30.

14. Simeonov R, Simeonov G. Computerized morphometry of mean nuclear diameter and nuclear roundness in canine mammary gland tumors on cytologic smears. Vet Clin Pathol 2006;35:88–90.

15. Simeonov R, Simeonov G. Fractal dimension of canine mammary gland epithelial tumors on cytologic smear. Vet Clin Pathol 2006;35:446–8.

16. Simeonov R, Simeonov G. Comparative morphometric analysis of recurrent and nonrecurrent canine basal cell carcinomas: a preliminary report. Vet Clin Pathol 2009;39:96–8.

17. Christopher MM, Hotz CS. Cytologic diagnosis: expression of probability by clinical pathologists. Vet Clin Pathol 2004;33:84–93.

18. Kocjan G, Chandra A, Cross P, et al. BSCC Code of Practice—fine needle aspiration cytology. Cytopathology 2009;20:283–96.

19. Ballenger EA, Forrest LJ, Dickinson RM, et al. Correlation of ultrasonographic appearance of lesions and cytologic and histologic diagnoses in splenic aspirates from dogs and cats: 32 cases (2002–2005). J Am Vet Med Assoc 2007; 230:690–6.

20. Bossuyt PM, Reitsman JB, Bruns DE, et al. Towards complete and accurate reporting of studies of diagnostic accuracy: the STARD initiative. Vet Clin Pathol 2007;36:8–12.

21. Sharkey LC, Dial SM, Matz ME. Maximizing the diagnostic value of cytology in small animal practice. Vet Clin North Am Small Anim Pract 2007;37:351–72.

22. Raskin RE. Skin and subcutaneous tissue. In: Raskin RE, Meyer DJ, editors. Canine and feline cytology. 2nd edition. St Louis (MO): Saunders Elsevier; 2010. p. 36.

23. Wellman ML, Krakowka S, Jacobs RM, et al. A macrophage-monocyte cell line from a dog with malignant histiocytosis. In Vitro Cell Dev Biol 1988;24:223–9.

24. Barger A, Graca R, Bailey K, et al. Use of alkaline phosphatase staining to differentiate canine osteosarcoma from other vimentin-positive tumors. Vet Pathol 2005;42:161–5.

25. Comazzi S, Gelain ME, Spagnolo V, et al. Flow cytometric patterns in blood from dogs with non-neoplastic and neoplastic hematologic diseases using double labeling for CD18 and CD45. Vet Clin Pathol 2006;35:47–54.

26. Höinghaus R, Mischke R, Hewicker-Trautwein M. Use of immunocytochemical techniques in canine melanoma. J Vet Med A Physiol Pathol Clin Med 2002;49: 198–202.

27. Höinghaus R, Hewicker-Trautwein M, Mischke R. Immunocytochemical differentiation of neoplastic and hyperplastic canine epithelial lesions in cytologic imprint preparations. Vet J 2007;173:79–90.

28. Höinghaus R, Hewicker-Trautwein M, Mischke R. Immunocytochemical differentiation of canine mesenchymal tumors in cytologic imprint preparations. Vet Clin Pathol 2008;37:104–11.

29. McManus PM. Classification of myeloid neoplasms: a comparative review. Vet Clin Pathol 2005;34:189–212.

30. Ponce F, Magnol JP, Marchal T, et al. High-grade canine T-cell lymphoma/leukemia with plasmacytoid morphology: a clinical pathological study of nine cases. J Vet Diagn Invest 2003;15:330–7.

31. Suter SE, Vernau W, Fry MM, et al. CD34+, CD41+ acute megakaryoblastic leukemia in a dog. Vet Clin Pathol 2007;36:288–92.

32. Tasca S, Carli1 E, Caldin M, et al. Hematologic abnormalities and flow cytometric immunophenotyping results in dogs with hematopoietic neoplasia: 210 cases (2002–2006). Vet Clin Pathol 2009;38:2–12.
33. Thilakaratne DN, Mayer MN, MacDonald VS, et al. Clonality and phenotyping of canine lymphomas before chemotherapy and during remission using polymerase chain reaction (PCR) on lymph node cytologic smears and peripheral blood. Can Vet J 2010;51:79–84.
34. Vernau W, Moore PF. An immunophenotypic study of canine leukemias and preliminary assessment of clonality by polymerase chain reaction. Vet Immunol Immunopathol 1999;69:145–64.
35. Avery A. Molecular diagnostics of hematologic malignancies. Top Companion Anim Med 2009;24:144–50.
36. Lana SE, Jackson TL, Burnett RC, et al. Utility of polymerase chain reaction for analysis of antigen receptor rearrangement in staging and predicting prognosis in dogs with lymphoma. J Vet Intern Med 2006;20:329–34.
37. Breen M, Modiano JF. Evolutionarily conserved cytogenetic changes in hematological malignancies of dogs and humans–man and his best friend share more than companionship. Chromosome Res 2008;16:145–54.
38. Murchison EP. Clonally transmissible cancers in dogs and Tasmanian devils. Oncogene 2009;27:S19–30.
39. Rebbeck CA, Thomas R, Breen M, et al. Origins and evolution of a transmissible cancer. Evolution 2009;63:2340–9.
40. Murchison EP, Tovar C, Hsu A, et al. The Tasmanian Devil transcriptome reveals Schwann cell origins of a clonally transmissible cancer. Science 2010;327:84–7.
41. Moore PF. Histiocytic proliferative diseases. In: Weiss DJ, Waldrop KJ, editors. Schalm's veterinary hematology. 6th edition. Ames (IA): Wiley Blackwell Publishers; 2010. p. 540–9.
42. Baines SJ, McInnes EF, McConnell I. E-cadherin expression in canine cutaneous histiocytomas. Vet Rec 2008;162:509–13.
43. Fulmer AK, Mauldin GE. Canine histiocytic neoplasia: an overview. Can Vet J 2007;48:1041–50.
44. Goldschmidt MH, Hendrick MJ. Tumors of the skin and soft tissues. In: Meuten DJ, editor. Tumors in domestic animals. 4th edition. Ames (IA): Blackwell Publishing; 2002. p. 45–118.
45. Schöniger S, Summers BA. Equine skin tumours in 20 horses resembling three variants of human melanocytic naevi. Vet Dermatol 2009;20:165–73.
46. Esplin DG. Survival of dogs following surgical excision of histologically well differentiated melanocytic neoplasms of the mucous membranes of the lips and oral cavity. Vet Pathol 2008;45(6):889–96.
47. Wilkerson MJ, Dolce K, DeBey BM, et al. Metastatic balloon cell melanoma in a dog. Vet Clin Pathol 2003;32:31–6.
48. Sartin EA, Waldridge BM, Carter DW, et al. Gastric squamous cell carcinoma in three llamas. J Vet Diagn Invest 1997;9:103–6.
49. Taylor SD, Haldorson GJ, Vaughan B, et al. Gastric neoplasia in horses. J Vet Intern Med 2009;5:1097–102.
50. Greene CE, Gunn-Moore DA. Infections caused by slow-growing mycobacteria. In: Greene CE, editor. Infectious diseases of the dog and cat. 2nd edition. St Louis (MO): Saunders Elsevier; 2006. p. 462–77.
51. Turinelli V, Ledieu D, Guilbaud L, et al. Mycobacterium tuberculosis infection in a dog from Africa. Vet Clin Pathol 2004;33:177–81.

52. Kaneene JB, Bruning-Fann CS, Dunn J, et al. Epidemiology investigation of *Mycobacterium bovis* in a population of cats. Am J Vet Res 2002;63:1507–11.
53. Bauer NB, O'Neill E, Sheahan BJ, et al. Calcospherite-like bodies and caseous necrosis in tracheal mucus from a dog with tuberculosis. Vet Clin Pathol 2004; 33:168–72.
54. Bauer N, Burkhardt S, Kirsch A, et al. Lymphadenopathy and diarrhea in a miniature Schnauzer. Vet Clin Pathol 2002;31:61–4.
55. Blauvelt M, Weiss D, McVey A, et al. Space-occupying lesion within the calvarium of a cat. Vet Clin Pathol 2001;31:19–21.
56. Ngan N, Morris A, de Chalain T. *Mycobacterium fortuitum* infection caused by a cat bite. N Z Med J 2005;118(1211):U1354.
57. Hermon-Taylor J. *Mycobacterium avium* subspecies paratuberculosis, Crohn's disease and the doomsday scenario. Gut Pathog 2009;1:1–15.
58. Foley JE, Borjesson D, Gross TL, et al. Clinical microscopic, and molecular aspects of canine leproid granuloma in the United State. Vet Pathol 2002; 39:234–9.
59. MacWilliams PS, Whitley N, Moore F. Lymphadenitis and peritonitis caused by *Mycobacterium xenopi* in a cat. Vet Clin Pathol 1998;27:50–3.
60. Tarigo J, Linder K, Neel J, et al. Reluctant to dive: coelomic effusion in a frog. Vet Clin Pathol 2006;35:341–4.
61. Huntley JFJ, Whitlock H, Bannantine JP, et al. Comparison of diagnostic methods for *Mycobacterium avium* subsp. *paratuberculosis* in North American Bison. Vet Pathol 2005;42:42051.
62. Taboada J, Grooters AM. Cryptococcosis. In: Ettinger SJ, Feldman EC, editors. Veterinary internal medicine. 7th edition. St Louis (MO): Saunders Elsevier Publishing; 2010. p. 988–92.
63. Graves TK, Barger AM, Adams B, et al. Diagnosis of systemic cryptococcosis by fecal cytology in a dog. Vet Clin Pathol 2005;34:409–12.
64. Duncan C, Stephen C, Lester S, et al. Sub-clinical infection and asymptomatic carriage of *Cryptococcus gattii* in dogs and cats during an outbreak of cryptococcosis. Med Mycol 2005;43:511–6.
65. Krockenberger MB, Canfield PJ, Malik R. *Cryptococcus neoformans* in the koala (*Phascolarctos cinereus*): colonization by *C n. var. gattii* and investigation of environmental sources. Med Mycol 2002;40:263–72.
66. Krockenberger MB, Canfield PJ, Malik R. *Cryptococcus neoformans* var. *gattii* in the koala (*Phascolarctos cinereus*): a review of 43 cases of cryptococcosis. Med Mycol 2003;41:225–34.
67. Galanis E, MacDougall L, Kidd S, et al. Epidemiology of *Cryptococcus gattii*, British Columbia, Canada, 1999–2007. Emerg Infect Dis 2010;16(2):251–7.
68. Malik R, Krockenberger M, O-Brien CR, et al. Cryptococcosis. In: Greene CE, editor. Infectious diseases of the dog and cat. 2nd edition. St Louis (MO): Saunders Elsevier; 2006. p. 584–98.
69. Radin MJ, Wellman ML. Interpretation of canine and feline cytology. Wilmington (DE): The Gloyd Group for Ralston Purina Company; 2001. p. 20.
70. Walker DB, Pierce KR, Boone L. What is your diagnosis? A 4 year old male dachshund. Vet Clin Pathol 1997;26:71 94–5.
71. Rossner EJ, Dunstan RW. Sporotrichosis. In: Greene CE, editor. Infectious diseases of the dog and cat. 2nd edition. St Louis (MO): Saunders Elsevier; 2006. p. 608–12.
72. Bernstein JA, Cook HE, Gill AF, et al. Cytologic diagnosis of generalized cutaneous sporotrichosis in a hunting hound. Vet Clin Pathol 2007;36:94–6.

73. Dubey JP, Lappin MR. Toxoplasmosis and neosporosis. In: Greene CE, editor. Infectious diseases of the dog and cat. 2nd edition. St Louis (MO): Saunders Elsevier; 2006. p. 584–98.
74. Adkesson MJ, Gorman ME, Hsiao V, et al. *Toxoplasma gondii* inclusions in peripheral blood leukocytes of a red-necked wallaby (*Macropus rufogriseus*. Vet Clin Pathol 2007;36:97–100.
75. Poitout F, Weiss JD, Dubey JP. Lun aspirate from a cat with respiratory distress. Vet Clin Pathol 1998;27:10–1, 22.
76. Little L, Shokek A, Dubey JP, et al. *Toxoplasma gondii*-like organisms in skin aspirates from a cat with disseminated protozoal infection. Vet Clin Pathol 2005;34: 156–60.
77. Cowell RL, Tyler RD, Meinkoth JH, et al. Selected infectious agents. In: Cowell RL, Tyler RD, Meinkoth JH, et al, editors. Diagnostic cytology of the dog and cat. 3rd edition. St Louis (MO): Mosby Elsevier; 2008. p. 47–67.
78. Zaharopoulos P. Demonstration of parasites in toxoplasma lymphadenitis by fine-needle aspiration cytology: report of two cases. Diagn Cytopathol 2000;22:11–5.
79. Green CE. Ehrlichiosis, neorickettsiosis, anaplasmosis, and *Wolbachia* infection. In: Greene CE, editor. Infectious diseases of the dog and cat. 2nd edition. St Louis (MO): Saunders Elsevier; 2006. p. 203–32.
80. Gieg J, Rikihisa Y, Wellman M. Diagnosis of *Ehrlichia ewingii* infection by PCR in a puppy from Ohio. Vet Clin Pathol 2009;38:406–10.
81. Paddock CD, Childs JE. *Ehrlichia chaffeensis*: a prototypical emerging pathogen. Clin Microbiol Rev 2003;16:37–64.
82. Myolonakis ME, Koutinas AF, Billinis C, et al. Evaluation of cytology in the diagnosis of acute canine monocyte ehrlichiosis (*E. canis*): a comparison between five methods. Vet Microbiol 2003;91:197–204.

# The Diagnostic Assessment of Canine Lymphoma: Implications for Treatment

Dorothee Bienzle, DVM, PhD[a],*,
William Vernau, DVM, DVSc, PhD[b]

**KEYWORDS**

- Clonal antigen receptor polymerase chain reaction
- Flow cytometry • Immunohistochemistry • Lymphosarcoma
- Veterinary • WHO classification

Lymphoma in dogs is a heterogeneous cancer with highly variable prognosis. Many types of canine lymphoma have similar counterparts in the WHO classification of human lymphoid tumors. The most common variant of canine lymphoma is diffuse large B cell lymphoma, which, if treated with multi-agent chemotherapy, has a survival time of approximately 12 months. T cell lymphomas are more heterogeneous and high and low grade variants are common, which necessitates classification beyond B- versus T-cell lineage.

## EPIDEMIOLOGY, ETIOLOGY, CLINICAL FEATURES, AND GENETICS

The incidence of lymphoma in dogs appears to be relatively high, though large-scale recent epidemiologic data are lacking. In a Norwegian population study of cancer in animals, lymphoma was the most common malignancy in all dogs younger than 2 years, and second only to mast cell tumors in male and neutered female dogs younger than 6 years.[1] In comparable regions of Norway, among all cancers the overall incidence of lymphoma was 3.4% in dogs and 3.1% in people.[1] Data from

This work was supported by grants from the Pet Trust Foundation at the University of Guelph and the Canada Research Chairs Program.
The authors declare no financial interest or conflict of interest.
[a] Department of Pathobiology, University of Guelph, Guelph, Ontario N1G 2W1, Canada
[b] Department of Pathology, Microbiology and Immunology, School of Veterinary Medicine, University of California, Davis, CA 95616, USA
* Corresponding author.
E-mail address: dbienzle@uoguelph.ca

Clin Lab Med 31 (2011) 21–39
doi:10.1016/j.cll.2010.10.001
0272-2712/11/$ – see front matter © 2011 Elsevier Inc. All rights reserved.

pedigree dogs in the United Kingdom suggested a lower incidence of lymphoma at 0.8%,[2] but the analysis included predominantly very young (and insured) dogs. Previous surveys from North America[3] and the Netherlands[4] indicated incidence rates of 24 and 33 per 100,000 dogs, respectively. Hence, though precise and current figures on the epidemiology of canine lymphoma are incomplete, lymphoma is sufficiently common to be regularly encountered by general veterinary practitioners, and to comprise a large proportion of the caseload in specialized veterinary oncology practices.

Dogs are diagnosed with lymphoma most commonly between 6 and 9 years of age, with some variation according to breed and type of lymphoma.[1,2,5,6] Considering that humans live 6 to 8 times longer than dogs, the age of highest lymphoma incidence in dogs would correspond to 42 to 63 years of age in people. Breeds reported to have lymphoma at a younger age include Golden Retrievers, Bullmastiffs, and Bulldogs, but these are large dog breeds that have a naturally shorter lifespan.[2,7] Cutaneous epitheliotropic lymphoma is more commonly diagnosed in older dogs (mean 9–11 years), whereas thymic lymphoma is more commonly diagnosed in younger dogs (mean 5.8 years).[8–10]

Certain dog breeds have a higher incidence of lymphoma than others. Dogs have been selectively bred for more than 100 years to achieve breed-specific appearance and behavior, which has resulted in dramatic phenotypic variation as illustrated by the more than 80-fold difference in weight between Irish Wolfhounds and Chihuahuas. Concomitantly, breeding efforts have reduced genetic heterogeneity within breeds and have increased the incidence of breed-associated genetic conditions, including cancer susceptibility.[11] Breeds recognized in multiple surveys to have a significantly increased incidence of lymphoma are Boxers, Bulldogs, Bullmastiffs, Golden Retrievers, Bernese Mountain Dogs, Flat-coated Retrievers, and Rottweilers.[1,2,5] Conversely, breeds with a lower relative risk of lymphoma are Bichon Frise dogs, poodles, German shorthaired pointers, West Highland white terriers, and German Shepherds.[1,2,5] While such data may apply regionally, breed-specific epidemiologic data should be interpreted cautiously, due to global variation in breed popularity and definition. The genetic basis for breed-specific susceptibility to lymphoma is unknown.

Lymphoma in dogs is considered to be a sporadic cancer. Etiologic agents analogous to Epstein-Barr herpesvirus or T-lymphotropic retrovirus in humans have not been convincingly demonstrated in dogs, nor has immunodeficiency been identified as a contributing factor. In France, correlation of the geographic location of waste incinerators, pollution, and radioactive waste storage with the frequency of diagnosing lymphoma in dogs and people suggested significant associations with each of these environmental factors.[6] An increased risk for lymphoma in dogs was also reported if owners applied 2,4-dichlorphenoxyacetic acid (2,4-D) herbicide to lawns,[12] and if dogs resided in industrial areas or with owners who applied lawn herbicides.[13] However, experimental studies did not replicate genotoxicity or carcinogenesis of 2,4-D; therefore, the potential of environmental toxin exposure to cause canine lymphoma remains unclear.[14]

The clinical features of lymphoma in dogs (and humans) vary by the type of lymphoma. In approximately 80% of dogs, lymphoma presents as a painless enlargement of multiple peripheral lymph nodes noticed by the owner or detected on physical examination by the veterinarian. This presentation is often associated with a history of vague illness or inappetence over days or a few weeks. This multicentric type of lymphoma is of B-cell origin in 60% to 70% of cases, and of T-cell origin in 30% to 40% of cases.[7,15] Other types of lymphoma in dogs involve primarily the skin, gastrointestinal system, central nervous system, liver/spleen, thymus, or other organs, and may present with clinical features reflecting dysfunction of the affected organ such as ulceration, vomition, seizure, or jaundice.[16] Characteristic laboratory abnormalities are uncommon in canine lymphoma, except for the presence of hypercalcemia in 20% to 40% of T-cell lymphomas, and detection of morphologically abnormal lymphocytes on routine blood smear review in 10% to 20% of both T- and B-cell lymphomas.[17,18]

A large survey of the incidence of B- versus T-cell lymphoma by dog breed indicated that ancestrally related groups of dog breeds may share susceptibility to a specific type of lymphoma.[5] For example, Spitz-type dogs such as the Siberian husky, Alaskan malamute, and Chinese Shar-Pei, as well as the Asian-origin lapdog breeds Shi Tzu and Lhaso Apso, have a higher incidence of T-cell lymphoma relative to mixed breed or all dogs.[5] Mastiff-type dogs such as Boxers have also been repeatedly identified to have a much higher incidence of T-cell lymphoma relative to the general canine population.[5,6,19] The basis for predilection of transforming events to occur in one type of lymphocyte versus another remains to be elucidated, but susceptibility to lineage-specific mutations appears to have been fixed in the canine genome prior to genetic selection of phenotypic traits characteristic for certain breeds.

A range of genetic changes has been identified in canine lymphoma. Cytogenetic evaluation has demonstrated that genomic gain is more common than genomic loss, that multiple chromosomal regions are involved in individual lymphomas, and that 32 of the 38 canine autosomes have genetic aberrations.[20] Gains on canine chromosomes 13 and 31, and loss on chromosome 14, are most common.[20] Canine chromosome 13 is evolutionarily related to regions on human chromosomes 8 and 4, which harbor the c-myc and c-KIT oncogenes, respectively. Breed-specific genetic changes such as deletions on chromosome 14 were more common in B-cell lymphoma of Golden retrievers relative to other dog breeds.[5] Subsequent analysis with higher resolution genetic techniques revealed that cells in Burkitt lymphoma, a less common type of lymphoma in the dog, contained a translocation of c-myc to a region containing the immunoglobulin heavy-chain enhancer, analogous to a common translocation in human Burkitt lymphoma.[11] Other cases of canine diffuse large B-cell lymphoma (DLBCL), the most common type of lymphoma in dogs, also had constitutive expression of Myc.[11]

Loss of chromosome 11 is a prevalent numeric abnormality in T-cell lymphoma.[20] Chromosome 11 harbors the p16 inhibitor of cyclin-dependent kinase (CDK)-4 and -6. Lack of p16 activity increases cell proliferation, which in turn results in hyperphosphorylation, and therefore hypofunction, of the retinoblastoma (Rb) suppressor protein. Loss of p16 is specific for lymphoblastic T-cell lymphoma, a more aggressive subtype of canine T-cell lymphoma, while Rb hyperphosphorylation is present in high-grade lymphoma of either B- or T-cell origin.[21] Recent investigation has focused on identifying microRNA (miRNA) signatures in various lymphomas relative to normal lymphoid tissue. Interrogation with a panel of 11 miRNA probes found up- and down-regulation of miR-17-5 p and miR-181a in canine B- and T-cell lymphoma, respectively, but no consistent difference in miRNA concentration was found between high- and low-grade lymphomas.[22] Both of the altered miRNAs regulate expression of the TCL1 oncogene, and thus are potential therapeutic targets. Progress clearly has been made in characterizing genetic abnormalities in canine lymphoma, and this remains an active area of investigation for comparative molecular biologists and geneticists. However, application of high-resolution and throughput methods to fine-map genetic changes, and to correlate these with morphologic type and response to therapy, remains to be done on a statistically meaningful number of cases.

## ROUTINE DIAGNOSTIC APPROACH

Ninety percent to 95% of canine lymphoma cases manifest with diffuse and homogeneous effacement of peripheral lymph nodes; hence, fine-needle biopsy (FNB) typically yields specimens suitable for cytopathologic interpretation. Fine-needle biopsy can be performed with manual or no restraint in most canine patients, whereas both incisional and excisional surgical biopsy of lymph nodes (or other tissues) require a general anesthetic. For these reasons, FNB is the most widely employed first-line diagnostic approach. However, FNB is unlikely to yield samples suitable for diagnosis from follicular and small cell lymphoma cases. Although the limitations of not assessing tissue architecture, and the unavailability of tissue blocks for further studies, are appreciated among veterinary specialists, economic and practical considerations generally outweigh these disadvantages. Furthermore, cytologic evaluation of canine lymphoma samples has high sensitivity and specificity,[23] and FNB samples are suitable for immunocytochemistry, flow cytometry, detection of clonal antigen receptor gene rearrangement, and genetic investigation, provided sufficient material is collected.[18,24–30]

## CLASSIFICATION OF CANINE LYMPHOMA

Using histopathology, canine lymphoma can be readily classified using schemes designed for human non-Hodgkin disease. Over time, the Rappaport, Kiel, and Working Formulation classification schemes have been applied to canine lymphomas.[4,18,31,32] Each of these schemes, using criteria similar to those for human tumors regarding architecture and morphology, has allowed for classification with few modifications (**Table 1**). Although the terminology applied to different categories varied among schemes, description of the most prevalent categories indicates that approximately 85% of canine lymphomas are high-grade tumors with diffuse or nearly diffuse architecture; approximately 10% are low-grade tumors with diffuse architecture composed of small cells; and the remainder comprises follicular or nodular tumors.[4,33] Further, the cytomorphology of most large-cell tumors consist of cells with large nuclei and single or multiple prominent large nucleoli.[4]

Application of antibodies that are reactive with formalin-fixed, paraffin-embedded tissue, and directed against CD79a, CD20, and CD3 epsilon, subsequently allowed preliminary classification of canine lymphoma into B- or T-cell origin.[4,34] Incorporation of this basic immunophenotype into morphologic classification schemes confirmed that most diffuse large-cell lymphomas are of B-cell origin, and also suggested that the cell origin of several cytomorphologic types of lymphoma could not be predicted without immunophenotyping.[17,35] In the early 1990s, the Revised European American Classification of Lymphoid Neoplasms (REAL) was established for human lymphoid neoplasms and incorporated morphology, immunophenotype, genetic features, clinical presentation, and disease course.[36] This classification was tested for broad applicability and clinical relevance, and thereafter developed into a consensus classification under the auspices of the World Health Organization (WHO), most recently updated in 2008.[36] Classification of canine lymphoid tumors according to morphology, immunophenotype, clinical presentation, and disease course into categories recognized within this WHO scheme was also readily accomplished, though limited immunophenotypic data and lack of genetic information for most categories was a major limitation.[32]

**Table 1**
**The most common types of canine lymphoma with morphologic and immunophenotypic similarity to human lymphoma, based on World Health Organization classification**

| Category of Lymphoma | Immunophenotypic Characteristics[a] | Anatomic and Histomorphologic Features |
|---|---|---|
| Diffuse large B-cell lymphoma (DLBCL), not otherwise specified (NOS) | $CD1^+$, $CD18^{low}$, $CD20^+$, $CD21^+$, $CD79a^+$, MHC II$^+$; $CD3^-$, $CD4^-$, $CD8^-$, $TCR^-$ | Generalized effacement of lymph nodes; round nuclei, high mitotic rate; single nucleolus = immunoblastic type; multiple nucleoli = centroblastic type |
| Marginal zone lymphoma (MZL) | $CD18^{intermed}$, $CD20^+$, $CD21^+$, $CD79a^+$, MHC II$^+$; $CD1^-$, $CD3^-$, $CD4^-$, $CD8^-$, $TCR^-$ | Nodal, splenic white pulp, or extranodal mucosal, origin; follicular pattern, small to intermediate cell size, low mitotic rate |
| Follicular lymphoma (FL) | $CD20^+$, $CD79a^+$; $CD3^-$ | Single or multiple nodal origin; follicular pattern, variable cell size, low mitotic rate |
| Mantle cell lymphoma (MCL) | $CD20^+$, $CD79a^+$; $CD3^-$ | Splenic white pulp origin; follicular pattern, small cell size, round to irregular nuclei, low mitotic rate |
| Peripheral T-cell lymphoma (PTCL), NOS | $CD3^+$, $CD4^+$ or $CD8^+$ or $CD4^+/CD8^+$ or $CD4^-/CD8^-$, $CD18^{high}$, $TCR\alpha\beta^+$ | Diffuse effacement of multiple lymph nodes, possible hypercalcemia; variable cell morphology and mitotic rate |
| Small T-cell lymphoma (T-zone lymphoma, TZL) | $CD3^+$; $CD20^-$, $CD79a^-$ | Nodal paracortical expansion with remnant follicles; small or intermediate cell size, round, cleaved, or indented nuclei |
| Primary cutaneous epitheliotropic lymphoma | $CD3^+$, $CD8^+$, $TCR\gamma\delta^+$ or $TCR\alpha\beta^+$; $CD4^-$, $CD45RA^-$ | Diffuse or aggregate, mucocutaneous site predilection, epitheliotropic; small to large cell size depending on disease stage |
| Hepatosplenic T-cell lymphoma | $CD3^+$, $CD8\alpha^+$, $CD11d^+$, $CD18^+$, $TCR\gamma\delta^+$; $CD79a^-$, $CD\beta^-$, $TCR\alpha\beta^-$ | Diffuse, splenic red pulp origin, extensive spread (liver, marrow), cytopenias; large cell size, cytoplasmic granules, high mitotic rate |

[a] Low, intermediate, high immunophenotypic characteristics refer to the relative frequency of the antigen as detected by flow cytometry.

## B-CELL LYMPHOMAS
### Diffuse B-Cell Lymphomas

The most common mature B-cell neoplasm in dogs is DLBCL—not otherwise specified (NOS). DLBCL typically occurs in 5- to 9-year-old dogs, affects multiple or all lymph nodes, and is composed of large cells with round nuclei greater than 15 μm in diameter, a moderate amount of basophilic cytoplasm, a frequent perinuclear clear zone, and prominent single or multiple nucleoli (**Fig. 1**). This group may be morphologically subdivided into immunoblastic and centroblastic variants, distinguished by single large nucleoli in the former and multiple, frequently peripheral, nucleoli in the latter.[32] The mitotic rate of most DLBCL is high. Response to multiagent chemotherapy is variable within DLBCL, which most likely indicates heterogeneity of genetic abnormalities underlying morphologically similar lymphomas, akin to the germinal center B-cell (GCB) and activated B-cell (ABC) types of human DLBCL.[36] In addition to positivity for CD20 and CD79a, which are usually detected as intracellular antigens by immunocytochemistry or immunohistochemistry, immunophenotypic evaluation of DLBCL with a wider range of antibodies by flow cytometry indicates cell surface expression of CD1, CD21, CD45RA, CD90, and major histocompatibility complex II (MHC II) (**Fig. 2**). Monotypic immunoglobulin light chain expression has also been implemented to diagnose and characterize B-cell neoplasms in dogs, but because in most domestic animals λ light chain gene usage is far more frequent than κ light chain gene usage, benign as well as malignant B lymphocytes typically express only λ light chains.[37] Hence, monotypic λ light chain detection is not a useful criterion for the diagnosis of lymphoma in dogs.

Other diffuse B-cell lymphomas rarely identified in dogs are T-cell–rich large B-cell lymphoma,[38] mediastinal lymphoma,[39] plasmacytoid lymphoma,[35] cutaneous nonepidermotropic lymphoma,[40] and intravascular lymphoma.[41] However, for the latter 3 types of lymphoma, T-cell origin is more common than B-cell origin. Each of these types of lymphoma has a counterpart with similar histomorphology within the WHO classification of human lymphoid tumors; but their frequency, immunophenotype, and response to therapy have not been thoroughly characterized in dogs.

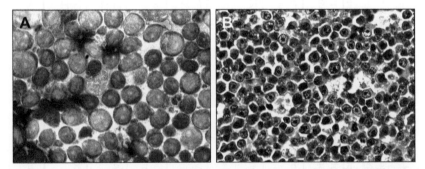

**Fig. 1.** Diffuse large B-cell lymphoma (DLBCL), not otherwise specified, immunoblastic type, in a 7-year-old Golden Retriever dog. (*A*) Cytologic preparation of a fine-needle biopsy of an enlarged lymph node (Wright stain, original magnification ×600). The cells are uniformly large and round with intensely blue cytoplasm, small perinuclear clear zones, and round nuclei with single central nucleoli. (*B*) Histologic section of same lymph node (hematoxylin and eosin stain, original magnification ×400). Lymphocyte nuclei are uniformly round with prominent central nucleoli.

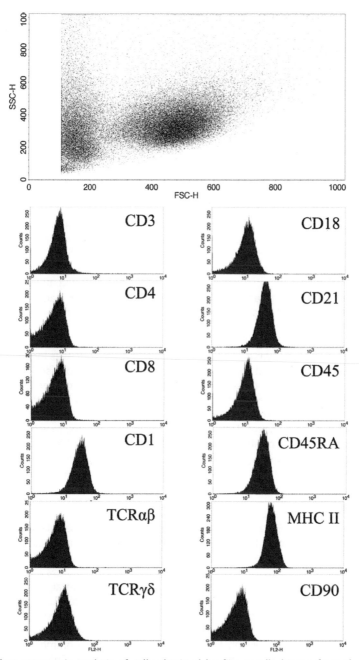

**Fig. 2.** Flow cytometric analysis of cells obtained by fine-needle biopsy from the dog in **Fig. 1**. The cells are large with high forward scatter (FSC-H) and express CD1, CD21, low levels of CD45RA, and MHC II antigens.

## Follicular B-Cell Lymphomas

Follicular or nodular lymphomas are diagnosed much less frequently than diffuse lymphomas, and comprise several distinct subtypes. Marginal zone lymphoma (MZL) is a nodular indolent type of lymphoma affecting older dogs (>9 years) with approximately 60 cases described in the literature.[15,31,39,42] This tumor occurs in lymphoid (lymph node, spleen, tonsil) and nonlymphoid organs such as the mucosa-associated lymphoid tissue (MALT) of the gastrointestinal system, eye, lung, or urinary tract.[43–45] Immunophenotyping of MZL cells clearly indicates B-cell origin (expression of CD20 and CD79a), but detailed immunologic or genetic analyses have not been reported. Involvement of a single or multiple lymph nodes is more common than involvement of the spleen[15,31]; however, splenic MZL, like other indolent lymphomas affecting the spleen, may not be detected clinically until the animal has advanced organomegaly. The cells of MZL are of small to intermediate in size with a low mitotic rate and single central nucleoli, and tumors have very gradual disease progression. MZL has been clearly identified in several surveys of canine lymphoma,[15,39,42] and single cases of extranodal lymphoma with histomorphologic features of MZL were reported in the urinary bladder and eye.[44,45]

Differing from the relatively high frequency in humans, follicular lymphoma (FL) is uncommon in dogs,[15,39] and involvement is typically restricted to one or a few nodes.[31] The histologic appearance of expanded follicles densely packed with homogeneous lymphocytes of small to large size, depending on the subtype, mirrors that of FL in humans.

Mantle cell lymphoma (MCL) is rarely diagnosed in dogs, with only 5 reported cases in dogs between 3 and 9 years of age.[31,39] In those cases, MCL was identified only in the spleen, where it occurred grossly as a solitary mass thought to arise from lymphoid tissue surrounding end arterioles.[31] Histologically, MCL consists of vaguely defined nodules that are located near small arterioles, and tumor cells are small to intermediate in size with densely staining nuclei, slightly irregular nuclear membranes, absent nucleoli, and a low mitotic rate. Translocations resulting in overexpression of cyclin D1 or hyperphosphorylation of Rb are characteristic of human MCL.[36] Similar overexpression has been identified in high- and low-grade canine lymphomas, suggesting that future investigation for specific association with MCL in dogs may be warranted.[7]

## Other B-Cell Neoplasms

Other canine tumors of B-cell origin with correlates in the WHO classification of human lymphoid tumors, but only briefly summarized here, are B-lymphoblastic leukemia, chronic lymphocytic leukemia, extraosseous plasmacytoma, and plasma cell myeloma.

Diagnosis of acute or chronic lymphocytic leukemia is usually straightforward based on routine hematology findings. Acute lymphoblastic leukemia (ALL) is a relatively uncommon neoplasm in dogs, and may be morphologically difficult to distinguish from some types of acute myeloid leukemia (AML). B-cell lineage as indicated by CD79a and/or CD21 expression has been identified more commonly than T-cell lineage[46–48]; genetic abnormalities in ALL are uncharacterized. Chronic lymphocytic leukemia (CLL), on the other hand, is not uncommonly reported in older dogs, and the morphology and immunophenotype have been well characterized.[48] Contrary to CLL in humans, 70% to 80% of canine CLL is of T-cell origin, and in most cases the neoplastic cells express CD8, $\alpha\beta$-T cell receptor (TCR) and CD11d, and frequently have cytoplasmic granules.[48] Anatomic origin of T-CLL is splenic red pulp, and the natural history of the neoplasm consists of very gradual disease progression. The remainder of canine CLL has a mature B-cell phenotype, frequently involves bone marrow, and may be accompanied by a monoclonal gammopathy.[49]

Solitary or multiple extraosseous plasma cell tumors are relatively common in dogs. Tumors have a predilection for limbs and head, and most behave in a benign manner curable by excision. Plasma cell tumors are readily diagnosed by cytopathology or histopathology, and nearly all are characterized by nuclear expression of multiple myeloma 1/interferon regulatory factor 4 (MUM/IRF-4), with cytoplasmic expression of CD79a and CD20 in approximately 60% and 20% of cases, respectively.[50] Multiple cases of myeloma involving bone and extraosseous tissues have been reported. The diagnosis of this neoplasm is not diagnostically challenging,[51] but as in people, myeloma in dogs is a heterogeneous disease with regard to immunoglobulin elaboration, biologic behavior, paraneoplastic effects, and response to therapy.

## T-CELL LYMPHOMAS

T-cell lymphomas in dogs comprise a wider range of less clearly defined entities than B-cell lymphomas. Although morphologic subtypes are recognized, etiologic agents, immunophenotype, and genetic changes are insufficiently characterized to allow consistent categorization. Hence, the grouping "peripheral T-cell lymphoma (PTCL)-NOS" includes a wide range of diverse entities (see **Table 1**).

In its most common presentation, canine T-cell lymphoma involves multiple lymph nodes ("nodal"), has a diffuse pattern, and is comprised of intermediate to large cells with irregularly shaped nuclei, finely dispersed chromatin, indistinct nucleoli, and a high mitotic rate.[17,18] This type of lymphoma is commonly termed "lymphoblastic" based on cytomorphologic criteria. Most tumors are characterized by expression of CD4 and $\alpha\beta$-TCR, and 40% to 60% of patients have hypercalcemia induced by tumor secretion of a parathyroid-like hormone.[18] Pleomorphic T-cell lymphomas are the next most common cytomorphologic category, and as in the lymphoblastic type, CD4 expression is more common than CD8 expression.[17] As the descriptive category implies, pleomorphic T-cell lymphomas are composed of a mixture of large and small lymphocytes, all of which express CD3. Coexpression of CD4 and CD8, or absence of either molecule despite CD3 expression, occurs in both lymphoblastic and pleomorphic types of T-cell lymphoma. Data linking T-cell immunophenotype with prognosis are lacking, but it has been suggested that pleomorphic lymphomas have a more aggressive course of disease than lymphoblastic lymphomas.[42]

A small-cell T-cell lymphoma, also termed "T-zone lymphoma" (TZL), is an uncommon indolent type of nodal lymphoma thought to arise from the paracortical region of the lymph node (**Fig. 3**).[31,32] Ten cases are described in the literature, and affected dogs ranged from 6 to 11 years old.[31] Architecturally, in TZL there is preservation but compression of follicles. The neoplastic cells have a low mitotic rate and may express CD8 or CD4 in conjunction with $\alpha\beta$-TCR (**Fig. 4**). The neoplasm is slowly progressive and may preferentially involve only one or a few lymph nodes.

Primary cutaneous T-cell lymphoma (PCTCL) is a well-recognized entity in dogs older than 9 years, with more than 50 reported cases. Variants of PCTCL described in dogs are mycosis fungoides, characterized by pronounced epitheliotropism; pagetoid reticulosis, with extensive epidermal involvement and patch-plaque stage lesions; and Sézary syndrome, with lymphadenopathy and circulating neoplastic cells.[8,9,52] Tumors are most often composed of lymphocytes expressing CD8 and $\gamma\delta$-TCR, a very different immunophenotype compared with the comparable tumor in humans. Tumors occur frequently at mucocutaneous junctions, and the neoplastic cells have tropism for hair follicles and apocrine sweat glands.[8]

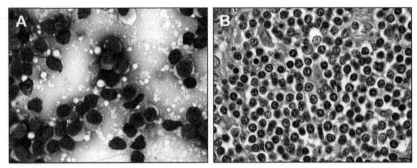

Fig. 3. Small-cell T-cell lymphoma in a 10-year-old mixed-breed dog. (*A*) Cytologic prepara-tion of a fine-needle biopsy of the mandibular lymph node (Wright stain, original magnifi-cation ×600). The cells are small to medium sized, have a moderate amount of clear cytoplasm, and dark, round to angular nuclei without apparent nucleoli. (*B*) Section of same lymph node (hematoxylin and eosin stain, original magnification ×400). Lymphocyte nuclei are small, round to indented, with nucleoli apparent in 20% to 30% of cells.

Cutaneous accumulation of small lymphocytes inducing minimal tissue disruption has been termed "cutaneous lymphocytosis." This type of indolent lymphoma has been described in 8 dogs ranging from 5 to 14 years old.[53] On histopathology, the tumor is located in the dermis and lacks epitheliotropism. Clinical tumor progression is very gradual over several months to years, but tumors may eventually progress to a more aggressive lymphoma.[53] Tumor cells more commonly express αβ-TCR than γδ-TCR, and either express CD8 or lack both CD4 and CD8 expression.

Hepatosplenic lymphoma is a distinct and aggressive rare T-cell lymphoma in dogs that is similar to its counterpart in people. Only 2 cases have been described in detail in dogs, but in both cases tumors extensively involved spleen, liver, and bone marrow with relative sparing of lymph nodes.[54,55] Neoplastic lymphocytes expressed γδ-TCR, CD8, and CD11d.[54] Diagnosis is typically established late in the course of disease, and response to therapy in the 2 cases reported has been poor.[54,55]

Other T-cell lymphomas described in dogs include tumors composed of granular lymphocytes that express cytoplasmic CD3 but lack CD4 and CD8, and are thought to be of natural killer cell phenotype; thymic lymphomas comprising CD4/8 double-positive lymphocytes; and gastrointestinal lymphomas.[17,35,42] In a recent survey of 30 dogs with gastrointestinal lymphoma, T-cell lineage was more common than B-cell lineage, and prognosis was poor for all lymphomas except those restricted to the colon or rectum.[43]

## ANCILLARY DIAGNOSTIC MODALITIES
### Flow Cytometry

Immunophenotypic characterization of neoplastic lymphocytes is a powerful tool in veterinary oncology, enabled by an expanding range of validated antibodies. Due to the prevailing diffuse architecture and homogeneous composition of most canine lymphomas, samples obtained by FNB of enlarged superficial lymph nodes, or of internal masses accessible through ultrasonic visualization, are readily analyzed by flow cytometry (see **Figs. 2** and **4**).[26,56] As in human medicine, it is paramount that the diagnosis of lymphoma be first established from microscopic assessment of tumor samples; flow cytometry should be retained for characterization and classification of the neoplasm. Nonspecific antibody binding, potential admixtures of inflammatory lymphocytes with nonneoplastic lymphocytes in FNB samples, sample hemodilution,

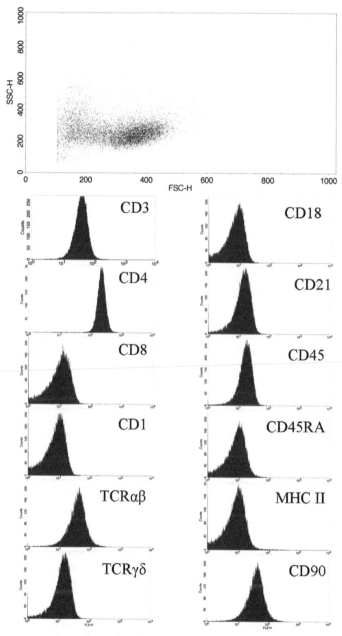

**Fig. 4.** Flow cytometric analysis of cells obtained by fine-needle biopsy from the dog in **Fig. 3**. The cells are small to intermediate in size with low side scatter (SSC-H) and forward scatter (FSC-H), and express CD3, CD4, αβ-TCR, and CD90.

and other factors render flow cytometry prone to artifact and error. Antibody panels applied at the first level of investigation and at a possible secondary level of investigation should be standardized, and immunophenotypic results must be interpreted in conjunction with clinical and morphologic findings. Nevertheless, more than 30 antibodies suitable for characterizing canine leukocytes are available, which allow for relatively refined classification of lymphoma and other hemic neoplasms.[57] Flow cytometry in veterinary oncology is currently available mainly in academic institutions, where integration of this technology into diagnostic laboratories is accompanied by implementation of essential quality control and quality assurance procedures.

### Detection of Clonal Antigen Receptors

Detection of clonal antigen receptor gene rearrangements, and hence a clonal population of lymphocytes, is a useful adjunct test when morphologic, architectural, and immunophenotypic features fail to reliably distinguish a reactive (polyclonal) from a neoplastic (monoclonal) lymphoid proliferation. This diagnostic dilemma can arise with most types of lymphoproliferative disease, but especially with indolent forms characterized by small, mature lymphocytes, where it can be particularly difficult to establish a definitive diagnosis. Diagnostic uncertainty is also common with endoscopic gastrointestinal biopsies and other "minimal" biopsies, and with incipient lymphomas. In human hematopathology, it is generally accepted that assessment and demonstration of clonality by molecular genetic analysis of antigen receptor gene rearrangement provides the most objective and accurate predictor of lymphoid neoplasia.[58–60] This methodology exploits the (physiologic) occurrence of molecular genetic rearrangements of the antigen receptor genes during T- and B-cell differentiation, and is contingent on knowledge of species-specific antigen receptor DNA sequence information.

Polymerase chain reaction (PCR)-based tests to assess clonality within lymphoid populations have been developed for the dog.[29,31,48,61] In one study assessing 77 canine lymphoid malignancies, the sensitivity of a PCR assay for clonality comprised of 3 different sets of primers directed to immunoglobulin heavy chain and $\gamma$-TCR sequences was 91%, a surprisingly high value considering that standardized clonality assays in people may require more than 50 primers to reach sensitivity exceeding 95%.[29,62,63] Assessment of nonmalignant tissues from 24 dogs yielded one clonal antigen PCR result, for a specificity of 96%.[29] More precise definition of sensitivity and specificity of PCR-based detection of clonal antigen receptors in dogs will require interrogation of samples using primers directed against additional components of the T- and B-cell receptor, assessment of samples from nonlymphoid tumors that may have rearrangement of lymphocyte receptors (such as myeloid leukemias), samples from dogs with infectious diseases that induce marked restricted lymphoid activation, and samples of neoplastic lymphocytes admixed with heterogeneous inflammatory lymphocytes. The use of primers designed to detect a specific clonal lymphocyte population (clonotypic primers), as has been described for people and now dogs, should result in higher analytical sensitivity of a particular type of lymphoma, and would be especially valuable for subsequent minimal residual disease detection.[62]

Although molecular clonality tests can be highly informative, they are not without limitations and pitfalls. False-negative results can occur for several reasons. First, recognition of all possible V, (D), and J rearrangements is unlikely with current primer sets.[62,64–66] Second, the occurrence of somatic hypermutations in rearranged immunoglobulin genes of B-cell malignancies can result in subsequent false negative results due to inadequate primer annealing.[63] The authors have observed this in canine lymphomas, where use of one set of primers yielded a clonal PCR product, but a second set of traditional primers directed to the framework 3 (FR3) region of the immunoglobulin gene did not yield a clonal product (W. Vernau, unpublished data, 2004–2010). A similar phenomenon has been shown in feline DLBCL.[64] In people, this problem has been approached by designing additional upstream consensus primers to Framework 1 (FR1) and FR2 regions, complemented by concurrent use of primers that amplify light chain rearrangements and rearrangements of the κ-deleting element (Kde).[63] Kde rearrangements are assumed to be free of somatic hypermutations and hence should represent more stable targets for PCR amplification.[63] FR1, FR2, and Kde primers have been developed for the dog (P.F. Moore, University of California-Davis, personal communication, 2010). FR1 primers amplify a region of more than 300 base pairs, which is suitable for application to DNA derived from FNB or frozen tissue, but which precludes their use on DNA derived from formalin fixed, paraffin-embedded material, where degradation frequently results in DNA fragments smaller than 300 base pairs in length.[67,68]

False-positive results may also occur, and if used to diagnose cancer may have disastrous consequences. False-positive results are primarily a problem when *TCRG* genes are used as PCR targets because of the more limited junctional diversity of *TCRG* rearrangements.[63] Because of this problem, analytical techniques of higher resolution than simple gel electrophoresis of amplicons have to be used. These methods include single-strand conformation polymorphism analysis, denaturing gradient gel electrophoresis, heteroduplex analysis, and gene scanning technologies.[69] Pseudoclonality is another cause of false-positive results that has been reported in humans, dogs, and cats.[31,63,64,70,71] In this case an apparent monoclonal amplicon is detected, but repeat amplification yields different size amplicons resulting from amplification of different rearrangements. The main causes of pseudoclonality are poor quality or limited template DNA, allowing for selective primer annealing in the initial rounds of PCR amplification. Hence, the optimal method for clonality assessment consists of duplicate or triplicate PCR amplifications analyzed in parallel with high-resolution techniques such as capillary electrophoresis (**Fig. 5**).[63]

PCR-based assays to detect antigen receptor gene rearrangement have been used to assign lymphoid lineage in dogs.[5] However, in people and dogs, clonal rearrangement of B- or T-cell antigen receptor genes does not consistently indicate B- or T-cell lineage, and comprehensive immunophenotyping is the preferred method for lineage assignment.[31,72–76]

In conclusion, given the limitations of PCR clonality assessment, and that clonality alone does not prove neoplasia, results of clonality assessment must always be interpreted together with clinical, morphologic and immunophenotypic findings.

## PROGNOSTIC INDICATORS AND TREATMENT

The prognosis for different types of canine B-cell lymphoma is relatively well established, and guidelines on how the response to therapy in lymphoma should be assessed were recently published.[77] Canine T-cell lymphoma is more variable, and the prognosis for the large group of nodal T-cell lymphomas is skewed negatively by the short survival times of the lymphoblastic subgroup.[78] Lymphoblastic T-cell lymphomas are more commonly associated with hypercalcemia and have a poorer response to multiagent chemotherapy than DLBCL. However, within the T-cell lymphoma group, as usually defined soley by expression of CD3, are also more indolent lymphomas that have slower disease progression, lack paraneoplastic hypercalcemia, and respond relatively well to chemotherapy. For these reasons, using available investigative modalities, it is particularly important to design prospective studies in dogs to correlate cytomorphology and immunophenotype of T-cell lymphomas with response to therapy.

Most canine lymphomas are responsive to intensive combination chemotherapy comprising vincristine, cyclophosphamide, doxorubicin, and prednisone, with or without L-asparaginase, with median remission and disease control times of

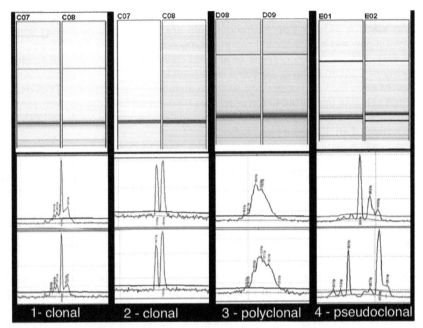

**Fig. 5.** Capillary electrophoresis (*top panel*) and BioCalculator (Qiagen, Valencia, CA, USA) software analysis plots (*bottom panel*) of antigen receptor gene arrangement PCR on DNA extracted from 4 different dogs (*1–4*). Major peaks reflect homogeneous amplicons, minor small peaks at the baseline reflect background DNA, and red markers are size indicators. Dog 1 is a 7-year-old mixed breed with peripheral T-cell lymphoma, not otherwise specified (PTCL-NOS), as confirmed using this assay. Dog 2 is a 1.5-year-old Dachshund with DLBCL, also confirmed with this assay. The PCR results from dogs 3 and 4 indicate a polyclonal (reactive) and pseudoclonal result, respectively.

approximately 13 and 9 months, respectively.[79] Established protocols involve alternating chemotherapy over 19 to 26 weeks; however, new protocols with shorter treatment periods are under investigation.[77] Dogs generally tolerate chemotherapy well, although side effects akin to those observed in human patients, such as nausea, vomiting, hair loss, bone marrow suppression, cardiotoxicity from doxorubicin, and sterile hemorrhagic cystitis from cyclophosphamide, may be observed. Virtually all dogs with DLBCL that achieve clinical remission will have recurrence of lymphoma and will eventually die of the disease.[80] Radiation therapy has been evaluated for treatment of lymphoma, and in combination with chemotherapy may yield longer survival times.[81] Bone marrow transplantation as therapy intended to cure lymphoma in dogs is available at select institutions.[79]

## SUMMARY

The diagnosis and treatment of canine lymphoma has been progressively refined over the past decades. Today the treatment of lymphoma in "our best friend" is commonplace and important, the dog genome has become refined as a blueprint to build molecular tools for investigation, and the value of cancers that are similar in dogs and humans is better appreciated. As a result, continued progress in defining the molecular basis of lymphoma and identifying better treatments can be expected.

## REFERENCES

1. Gamlem H, Nordstoga K, Glattre E. Canine neoplasia—introductory paper. APMIS Suppl 2008;125:5–18.
2. Edwards DS, Henley WE, Harding EF, et al. Breed incidence of lymphoma in a UK population of insured dogs. Vet Comp Oncol 2003;1:200–6.
3. Dorn CR, Taylor DO, Schneider R. The epidemiology of canine leukemia and lymphoma. Bibl Haematol 1970;36:403–15.
4. Teske E, Wisman P, Moore PF, et al. Histologic classification and immunophenotyping of canine non-Hodgkin's lymphomas: unexpected high frequency of T cell lymphomas with B cell morphology. Exp Hematol 1994;22:1179–87.
5. Modiano JF, Breen M, Burnett RC, et al. Distinct B-cell and T-cell lymphoproliferative disease prevalence among dog breeds indicates heritable risk. Cancer Res 2005;65:5654–61.
6. Pastor M, Chalvet-Monfray K, Marchal T, et al. Genetic and environmental risk indicators in canine non-Hodgkin's lymphomas: breed associations and geographic distribution of 608 cases diagnosed throughout France over 1 year. J Vet Intern Med 2009;23:301–10.
7. Modiano JF, Breen M, Valli VE, et al. Predictive value of p16 or Rb inactivation in a model of naturally occurring canine non-Hodgkin's lymphoma. Leukemia 2007; 21:184–7.
8. Moore PF, Affolter VK, Graham PS, et al. Canine epitheliotropic cutaneous T-cell lymphoma: an investigation of T-cell receptor immunophenotype, lesion topography and molecular clonality. Vet Dermatol 2009;20:569–76.
9. Fontaine J, Bovens C, Bettenay S, et al. Canine cutaneous epitheliotropic T-cell lymphoma: a review. Vet Comp Oncol 2009;7:1–14.
10. Day MJ. Review of thymic pathology in 30 cats and 36 dogs. J Small Anim Pract 1997;38:393–403.
11. Breen M, Modiano JF. Evolutionarily conserved cytogenetic changes in hematological malignancies of dogs and humans–man and his best friend share more than companionship. Chromosome Res 2008;16:145–54.
12. Hayes HM, Tarone RE, Cantor KP. On the association between canine malignant lymphoma and opportunity for exposure to 2,4-dichlorophenoxyacetic acid. Environ Res 1995;70:119–25.
13. Gavazza A, Presciuttini S, Barale R, et al. Association between canine malignant lymphoma, living in industrial areas, and use of chemicals by dog owners. J Vet Intern Med 2001;15:190–5.
14. Garabrant DH, Philbert MA. Review of 2,4-dichlorophenoxyacetic acid (2,4-D) epidemiology and toxicology. Crit Rev Toxicol 2002;32:233–57.
15. Ponce F, Marchal T, Magnol JP, et al. A morphological study of 608 cases of canine malignant lymphoma in France with a focus on comparative similarities between canine and human lymphoma morphology. Vet Pathol 2010;47:414–33.
16. Greenlee PG, Filippa DA, Quimby FW, et al. Lymphomas in dogs. A morphologic, immunologic, and clinical study. Cancer 1990;66:480–90.
17. Fournel-Fleury C, Ponce F, Felman P, et al. Canine T-cell lymphomas: a morphological, immunological, and clinical study of 46 new cases. Vet Pathol 2002;39:92–109.
18. Lurie DM, Milner RJ, Suter SE, et al. Immunophenotypic and cytomorphologic subclassification of T-cell lymphoma in the boxer breed. Vet Immunol Immunopathol 2008;125:102–10.
19. Lurie DM, Lucroy MD, Griffey SM, et al. T-cell-derived malignant lymphoma in the boxer breed. Vet Comp Oncol 2004;2:171–5.

20. Thomas R, Smith KC, Ostrander EA, et al. Chromosome aberrations in canine multicentric lymphomas detected with comparative genomic hybridisation and a panel of single locus probes. Br J Cancer 2003;89:1530–7.

21. Fosmire SP, Thomas R, Jubala CM, et al. Inactivation of the p16 cyclin-dependent kinase inhibitor in high-grade canine non-Hodgkin's T-cell lymphoma. Vet Pathol 2007;44:467–78.

22. Mortarino M, Gioia G, Gelain ME, et al. Identification of suitable endogenous controls and differentially expressed microRNAs in canine fresh-frozen and FFPE lymphoma samples. Leuk Res 2010;34:1070–7.

23. Teske E, van Heerde P. Diagnostic value and reproducibility of fine-needle aspiration cytology in canine malignant lymphoma. Vet Q 1996;18:112–5.

24. Caniatti M, Roccabianca P, Scanziani E, et al. Canine lymphoma: immunocytochemical analysis of fine-needle aspiration biopsy. Vet Pathol 1996;33:204–12.

25. Aulbach AD, Swenson CL, Kiupel M. Optimized processing of fine-needle lymph node biopsies for automated immunostaining. J Vet Diagn Invest 2010;22:383–8.

26. Gibson D, Aubert I, Woods JP, et al. Flow cytometric immunophenotype of canine lymph node aspirates. J Vet Intern Med 2004;18:710–7.

27. Sözmen M, Tasca S, Carli E, et al. Use of fine needle aspirates and flow cytometry for the diagnosis, classification, and immunophenotyping of canine lymphomas. J Vet Diagn Invest 2005;17:323–30.

28. Gentilini F, Turba ME, Calzolari C, et al. Real-time quantitative PCR using hairpin-shaped clone-specific primers for minimal residual disease assessment in an animal model of human non-Hodgkin lymphoma. Mol Cell Probes 2010;24: 6–14.

29. Burnett RC, Vernau W, Modiano JF, et al. Diagnosis of canine lymphoid neoplasia using clonal rearrangements of antigen receptor genes. Vet Pathol 2003;40: 32–41.

30. Starkey MP, Murphy S. Using lymph node fine needle aspirates for gene expression profiling of canine lymphoma. Vet Comp Oncol 2010;8:56–71.

31. Valli VE, Vernau W, de Lorimier LP, et al. Canine indolent nodular lymphoma. Vet Pathol 2006;43:241–56.

32. Valli VE, Myint MS, Barthel A, et al. Classification of canine malignant lymphoma according to the World Health Organization Criteria. Vet Pathol 2010. [Epub ahead of print].

33. Fournel-Fleury C, Magnol JP, Bricaire P, et al. Cytohistological and immunological classification of canine malignant lymphomas: comparison with human non-Hodgkin's lymphomas. J Comp Pathol 1997;117:35–59.

34. Jubala CM, Wojcieszyn JW, Valli VE, et al. CD20 expression in normal canine B cells and in canine non-Hodgkin lymphoma. Vet Pathol 2005;42:468–76.

35. Ponce F, Magnol JP, Marchal T, et al. High-grade canine T-cell lymphoma/ leukemia with plasmacytoid morphology: a clinical pathological study of nine cases. J Vet Diagn Invest 2003;15:330–7.

36. Jaffe ES, Harris NL, Stein H, et al. Classification of lymphoid neoplasms: the microscope as a tool for disease discovery. Blood 2008;112:4384–99.

37. Sitnikova T, Su C. Coevolution of immunoglobulin heavy- and light-chain variable-region gene families. Mol Biol Evol 1998;15:617–25.

38. Aquino SM, Hamor RE, Valli VE, et al. Progression of an orbital T-cell rich B-cell lymphoma to a B-cell lymphoma in a dog. Vet Pathol 2000;37:465–9.

39. Vezzali E, Parodi AL, Marcato PS, et al. Histopathologic classification of 171 cases of canine and feline non-Hodgkin lymphoma according to the WHO. Vet Comp Oncol 2010;8:38–49.

40. Day MJ. Immunophenotypic characterization of cutaneous lymphoid neoplasia in the dog and cat. J Comp Pathol 1995;112:79–96.
41. McDonough SP, Van Winkle TJ, Valentine BA, et al. Clinicopathological and immunophenotypical features of canine intravascular lymphoma (malignant angioendotheliomatosis). J Comp Pathol 2002;126:277–88.
42. Guija de Arespacochaga A, Schwendenwein I, Weissenböck H. Retrospective study of 82 cases of canine lymphoma in Austria based on the working formulation and immunophenotyping. J Comp Pathol 2007;136:186–92.
43. Frank JD, Reimer SB, Kass PH, et al. Clinical outcomes of 30 cases (1997–2004) of canine gastrointestinal lymphoma. J Am Anim Hosp Assoc 2007;43:313–21.
44. Vascellari M, Multari D, Mutinelli F. Unicentric extranodal lymphoma of the upper eyelid conjunctiva in a dog. Vet Ophthalmol 2005;8:67–70.
45. Kessler M, Kandel-Tschiederer B, Pfleghaar S, et al. Primary malignant lymphoma of the urinary bladder in a dog: longterm remission following treatment with radiation and chemotherapy. Schweiz Arch Tierheilkd 2008;150:565–9.
46. Tasca S, Carli E, Caldin M, et al. Hematologic abnormalities and flow cytometric immunophenotyping results in dogs with hematopoietic neoplasia: 210 cases (2002–2006). Vet Clin Pathol 2009;38:2–12.
47. Williams MJ, Avery AC, Lana SE, et al. Canine lymphoproliferative disease characterized by lymphocytosis: immunophenotypic markers of prognosis. J Vet Intern Med 2008;22:596–601.
48. Vernau W, Moore PF. An immunophenotypic study of canine leukemias and preliminary assessment of clonality by polymerase chain reaction. Vet Immunol Immunopathol 1999;69:145–64.
49. Workman HC, Vernau W. Chronic lymphocytic leukemia in dogs and cats: the veterinary perspective. Vet Clin North Am Small Anim Pract 2003;33:1379–99, viii.
50. Ramos-Vara JA, Miller MA, Valli VE. Immunohistochemical detection of multiple myeloma 1/interferon regulatory factor 4 (MUM1/IRF-4) in canine plasmacytoma: comparison with CD79a and CD20. Vet Pathol 2007;44:875–84.
51. Giraudel JM, Pagès JP, Guelfi JF. Monoclonal gammopathies in the dog: a retrospective study of 18 cases (1986–1999) and literature review. J Am Anim Hosp Assoc 2002;38:135–47.
52. Moore PF, Olivry T, Naydan D. Canine cutaneous epitheliotropic lymphoma (mycosis fungoides) is a proliferative disorder of CD8 + T cells. Am J Pathol 1994;144:421–9.
53. Affolter VK, Gross TL, Moore PF. Indolent cutaneous T-cell lymphoma presenting as cutaneous lymphocytosis in dogs. Vet Dermatol 2009;20:577–85.
54. Fry MM, Vernau W, Pesavento PA, et al. Hepatosplenic lymphoma in a dog. Vet Pathol 2003;40:556–62.
55. Cienava EA, Barnhart KF, Brown R, et al. Morphologic, immunohistochemical, and molecular characterization of hepatosplenic T-cell lymphoma in a dog. Vet Clin Pathol 2004;33:105–10.
56. Comazzi S, Gelain ME. Use of flow cytometric immunophenotyping to refine the cytological diagnosis of canine lymphoma. Vet J 2010. [Epub ahead of print].
57. Allison RW, Brunker JD, Breshears MA, et al. Dendritic cell leukemia in a Golden Retriever. Vet Clin Pathol 2008;37:190–7.
58. Weiss LM, Spagnolo DV. Assessment of clonality in lymphoid proliferations. Am J Pathol 1993;142:1679–82.
59. Griesser H, Tkachuk D, Reis MD, et al. Gene rearrangements and translocations in lymphoproliferative diseases. Blood 1989;73:1402–15.

60. Knowles DM. Immunophenotypic and antigen receptor gene rearrangement analysis in T cell neoplasia. Am J Pathol 1989;134:761–85.
61. Dreitz MJ, Ogilvie G, Sim GK. Rearranged T lymphocyte antigen receptor genes as markers of malignant T cells. Vet Immunol Immunopathol 1999;69:113–9.
62. Yamazaki J, Takahashi M, Setoguchi A, et al. Monitoring of minimal residual disease (MRD) after multidrug chemotherapy and its correlation to outcome in dogs with lymphoma: a proof-of-concept pilot study. J Vet Intern Med 2010;24: 897–903.
63. van Dongen JJ, Langerak AW, Brüggemann M, et al. Design and standardization of PCR primers and protocols for detection of clonal immunoglobulin and T-cell receptor gene recombinations in suspect lymphoproliferations: report of the BIOMED-2 Concerted Action BMH4-CT98-3936. Leukemia 2003;17:2257–317.
64. Werner JA, Woo JC, Vernau W, et al. Characterization of feline immunoglobulin heavy chain variable region genes for the molecular diagnosis of B-cell neoplasia. Vet Pathol 2005;42:596–607.
65. Greiner TC, Raffeld M, Lutz C, et al. Analysis of T cell receptor-gamma gene rearrangements by denaturing gradient gel electrophoresis of GC-clamped polymerase chain reaction products. Correlation with tumor-specific sequences. Am J Pathol 1995;146:46–55.
66. Davis TH, Yockey CE, Balk SP. Detection of clonal immunoglobulin gene rearrangements by polymerase chain reaction amplification and single-strand conformational polymorphism analysis. Am J Pathol 1993;142:1841–7.
67. Signoretti S, Murphy M, Cangi MG, et al. Detection of clonal T-cell receptor gamma gene rearrangements in paraffin-embedded tissue by polymerase chain reaction and nonradioactive single-strand conformational polymorphism analysis. Am J Pathol 1999;154:67–75.
68. Langerak AW, Szczepański T, van der Burg M, et al. Heteroduplex PCR analysis of rearranged T cell receptor genes for clonality assessment in suspect T cell proliferations. Leukemia 1997;11:2192–9.
69. Kneba M, Bolz I, Linke B, et al. Analysis of rearranged T-cell receptor beta-chain genes by polymerase chain reaction (PCR) DNA sequencing and automated high resolution PCR fragment analysis. Blood 1995;86:3930–7.
70. Elenitoba-Johnson KS, Bohling SD, Mitchell RS, et al. PCR analysis of the immunoglobulin heavy chain gene in polyclonal processes can yield pseudoclonal bands as an artifact of low B cell number. J Mol Diagn 2000;2:92–6.
71. Hoeve MA, Krol AD, Philippo K, et al. Limitations of clonality analysis of B cell proliferations using CDR3 polymerase chain reaction. Mol Pathol 2000;53: 194–200.
72. Szczepański T, Beishuizen A, Pongers-Willemse MJ, et al. Cross-lineage T cell receptor gene rearrangements occur in more than ninety percent of childhood precursor-B acute lymphoblastic leukemias: alternative PCR targets for detection of minimal residual disease. Leukemia 1999;13:196–205.
73. Pelicci PG, Knowles DM, Dalla Favera R. Lymphoid tumors displaying rearrangements of both immunoglobulin and T cell receptor genes. J Exp Med 1985;162: 1015–24.
74. Cheng GY, Minden MD, Toyonaga B, et al. T cell receptor and immunoglobulin gene rearrangements in acute myeloblastic leukemia. J Exp Med 1986;163: 414–24.
75. Kyoda K, Nakamura S, Matano S, et al. Prognostic significance of immunoglobulin heavy chain gene rearrangement in patients with acute myelogenous leukemia. Leukemia 1997;11:803–6.

76. Rovigatti U, Mirro J, Kitchingman G, et al. Heavy chain immunoglobulin gene rearrangement in acute nonlymphocytic leukemia. Blood 1984;63:1023–7.
77. Vail DM, Michels GM, Khanna C, et al. Veterinary Cooperative Oncology Group. Response evaluation criteria for peripheral nodal lymphoma in dogs (v1.0)—a Veterinary Cooperative Oncology Group (VCOG) consensus document. Vet Comp Oncol 2010;8:28–37.
78. Ettinger SN. Principles of treatment for canine lymphoma. Clin Tech Small Anim Pract 2003;18:92–7.
79. Chun R. Lymphoma: which chemotherapy protocol and why? Top Companion Anim Med 2009;24:157–62.
80. Marconato L. The staging and treatment of multicentric high-grade lymphoma in dogs: a review of recent developments and future prospects. Vet J 2010. [Epub ahead of print].
81. Lurie DM, Gordon IK, Théon AP, et al. Sequential low-dose rate half-body irradiation and chemotherapy for the treatment of canine multicentric lymphoma. J Vet Intern Med 2009;23:1064–70.

# Glucose Monitoring in Diabetic Dogs and Cats: Adapting New Technology for Home and Hospital Care

Charles E. Wiedmeyer, DVM, PhD[a],*, Amy E. DeClue, DVM, MS[b]

**KEYWORDS**

• Diabetes • Glucose • Monitoring • Dogs • Cats

Diabetes mellitus (DM) is one of the most common endocrinopathies in dogs and cats, and like in people, the incidence is rising substantially.[1] Although there are similarities in the clinical disease manifestation between dogs and cats, there are differences in pathogenesis and treatment. Using the classification scheme for human diabetes, the disease in dogs most resembles type 1 (insulin-dependent) DM, whereas cats may develop type 1 or type 2 (noninsulin-dependent) DM.[2–5] The suspected causes of DM in dogs include autoimmune destruction of pancreatic β cells and chronic insulin resistance secondary to other endocrinopathies such as hyperadenocorticism and acromegaly.[3,4] In cats, DM is often a result of pancreatic islet amyloid deposition, which is suggested to be a hallmark of type 2 diabetes in humans.[3,5] Obesity is believed to increase the risk of DM in cats, but a clear link has not been established in dogs.[3,5,6]

Most dogs diagnosed with DM are females between 5 and 12 years of age (median 9 years); juvenile-onset DM is uncommon.[7] The dog breeds most at risk of developing DM are Miniature Poodles, Bichon Frisés, Keeshonds, Alaskan Malamutes, and Miniature Schnauzers.[3,7] Risk factors for the development of DM in cats include age, sex, neutering, and obesity.[3] Thus most cats diagnosed with DM are neutered males more than 10 years of age and obese. The clinical presentation for both dogs and cats is similar to that observed in people with DM. Clinical signs including polyuria/polydipsia and weight loss despite polyphagia are most common.[4,5] In addition, dogs may present with acute onset of blindness as a result of bilateral cataracts and cats may

The authors have nothing to disclose.
[a] Department of Veterinary Pathobiology, College of Veterinary Medicine, University of Missouri, 900 East Campus Drive, A345 Clydesdale Hall, Columbia, MO 65211, USA
[b] Department of Veterinary Medicine and Surgery, College of Veterinary Medicine, University of Missouri, 900 East Campus Drive, A376 Clydesdale Hall, Columbia, MO 65211, USA
* Corresponding author.
*E-mail address:* wiedmeyerc@missouri.edu

Clin Lab Med 31 (2011) 41–50
doi:10.1016/j.cll.2010.10.010
0272-2712/11/$ – see front matter © 2011 Elsevier Inc. All rights reserved.

labmed.theclinics.com

show nonspecific gastrointestinal abnormalities such as periodic vomiting or anorexia.[8] The diagnosis of DM in dogs and cats is straightforward and made based on clinical findings, persistent hyperglycemia, and glucosuria. However, the diagnosis in cats may be problematic as a result of often-encountered stress hyperglycemia.[5] Transient hyperglycemia induced by epinephrine in cats can exceed the renal threshold for glucose and result in hyperglycemia and glucosuria, 2 hallmarks for diagnosis of DM. It may be beneficial or necessary to sample the cat after several hours to determine whether the hyperglycemia is persistent, or use other available tests such as plasma levels of fructosamine (discussed later) and clinical signs.[5] Treatment options for dogs and cats with DM include insulin therapy, oral hypoglycemic agents, and dietary modifications.[9] Of these treatments, insulin therapy is the most effective means of maintaining glycemic control.[4,5,9] Although oral hypoglycemic drugs are often used in people with diabetes, they have limited effectiveness in dogs and cats and thus are not a reliable treatment option. Most insulin types available for use in people are commonly used in dogs and cats. The primary aims of therapy in diabetic dogs and cats are: (1) resolution of clinical signs, (2) avoidance of insulin-induced hypoglycemia, and (3) return to usual lifestyle.[4,5] Most dogs and cats require insulin to be administered twice per day to prevent complications from hyperglycemia and the development of ketosis.[5,9] Common complications from poor glycemic control include cataract formation in dogs, diabetic neuropathy in cats, chronic urinary tract infections, and ketosis.[2] The diabetic nephropathy and vascular abnormalities commonly observed in people are observed rarely in dogs and cats. As in people, proper management of glycemic control is necessary to avoid complications.

## CLINICAL AND LABORATORY METHODS FOR MONITORING GLYCEMIC CONTROL IN DOGS AND CATS

Several techniques can be used to monitor and maintain glycemic control in dogs and cats undergoing treatment of DM. One fundamental technique is to educate pet owners on the clinical signs associated with poor glycemic control (eg, polyuria, polyphagia, weight loss). Clinical monitoring by the pet owner directly engages them in the well-being of their pet and relies on good communication with the attending veterinarian.[1,2,5] For example, pet owners are asked to monitor water consumption and urination frequency and, if possible, keep a daily log.[1,2] This information can be reviewed by the veterinarian and provides useful in-home data to assist in making clinical judgments. Although changes in clinical signs can be the first indication of poor glycemic regulation in many animals, this method fails to provide detailed information pertaining to glucose homeostasis, may be complicated by concurrent diseases, and relies heavily on the observational skills of the pet owner.

Serial monitoring of blood glucose concentration (ie, a blood glucose curve) is considered the gold standard by which to gauge glycemic control in dogs and cats with DM.[1,2] When performed properly, blood glucose curves can be used to determine the proper insulin type, dosage, and frequency of administration necessary to maintain appropriate glycemic control and avoid the Somogyi phenomenon.[2,4,5] To obtain a blood glucose curve, blood samples are collected via repeated venipuncture or through use of an indwelling central venous catheter every 2 to 4 hours for 12 to 24 hours. Because of this time frame, hospitalization and handling or restraint of the animal are typically required and may result in epinephrine-induced hyperglycemia (especially in cats) and alterations in normal dietary habits and exercise, skewing individual blood glucose concentrations and altering the results of the blood glucose curve.[2,10,11] Also because of the invasive nature of sampling for a blood glucose curve, marked day-to-day variability in glucose curves has been documented in diabetic dogs[12] and cats.[13] For these reasons, blood glucose curves can be problematic, difficult to interpret, and may not correlate with real-life glycemic control. Overall, blood glucose curves are an important fine-tuning tool for monitoring diabetic dogs and cats, but are not practical for routine monitoring.

An alternative to the in-hospital serial blood glucose curve is in-home testing of blood glucose. Home monitoring of diabetic dogs and cats is made possible in part by the wide acceptance and success of disease management in human diabetic patients. In addition, complications that can occur with serial blood glucose curves performed in the hospital are avoided. Protocols that use sampling of capillary blood from the dog or cat and a handheld glucometer have been described.[14–16] The most common location for obtaining capillary blood from both dogs and cats is the ear. Using a lancet designed for finger-pricks in people or a small-gauge needle, a capillary blood sample of good quality and quantity can be easily obtained in a relatively painless manner. For glucose measurement, most portable blood glucose devices designed for use in people are acceptable for use in veterinary patients.[17,18] Because of the ease of sample acquisition and inexpensive equipment necessary, home monitoring can be performed by pet owners. Although this technique empowers the owner to closely monitor disease and avoid hospitalization, caution should be taken with owners with regard to making decisions on therapy (ie, insulin dose and frequency of administration). The best practice is for owners to consult with the treating veterinarian before decisions to change therapy are made.

If home monitoring of blood glucose is not desired by the pet owner, an inexpensive alternative is monitoring of urine glucose.[2] Because urine is technically easy to acquire and glucose can be semiquantitatively measured with urine dipsticks, it is a suitable substitute for home measurement of blood glucose in pets. Most adequately controlled diabetic dogs and cats maintain trace to 1+ (on a 3+ scale) amounts of urine glucose. Consistently high urine glucose levels signal the need for closer monitoring of blood glucose, and a negative urine glucose result may be useful for detecting hypoglycemia.[2] Regardless of the urine glucose results, pet owners should be warned not to make decisions regarding insulin therapy without consulting their veterinarian.

For routine assessment in small animals with good clinical control of their DM, measures of long-term glycemic control can be used.[19–21] The most common laboratory tests used to evaluate long-term glycemic control in diabetic dogs and cats are glycated hemoglobin and fructosamine.[1,2] Glycated hemoglobin results from an irreversible, nonenzymatic, insulin-independent binding of glucose to hemoglobin in red blood cells (RBCs).[20,22] Glycated hemoglobin can be measured using conventional assay systems similar to those used in people. Like in people, glycated hemoglobin measurements in dogs and cats provide information regarding long-term glycemic control.[22] However, based on differences in RBC life span between the species, the long-term glycemic control information varies. Dogs have an RBC life span of approximately 100 days and in cats it is approximately 70 days.[2] In contrast, RBC life span in people is 120 days.[23] Therefore, measurement of glycated hemoglobin provides glycemic control information over the previous 10 to 14 weeks in dogs and 6 to 9 weeks in cats, compared with weeks to months in people.[2,23] Fructosamines are glycated proteins found in blood that result from the irreversible, nonenzymatic, insulin-independent binding of glucose to serum proteins.[19,24] The glycemic information provided by measurement of fructosamines is dependent on the life span of proteins in the circulation. Unlike the differences observed in RBCs and glycated hemoglobin, the average life span of serum proteins in people, dogs, and presumably, cats (ie, ~14 days) is nearly equal.[2,23] Thus serum fructosamine offers information regarding average glucose concentration over the previous 2 to 3 weeks. Another laboratory test similar to fructosamine is glycated albumin. Glycated albumin provides the same information as fructosamine and is routinely used in some places (such as Japan) where the assay for fructosamine is unavailable.[25,26] Glycated hemoglobin, fructosamine, and glycated albumin have the advantage of not being affected by acute changes in blood glucose, such as the epinephrine-induced hyperglycemia that occurs frequently in cats.[2,25,27–30] However, serum fructosamine values can be falsely altered by marked hypoproteinemia, azotemia, and hyperlipidemia in dogs, and by hyperthyroidism in cats. Glycated hemoglobin values can be altered by decreased RBC survival and anemia.[22,31,32] Despite widespread use of glycated hemoglobin for monitoring glycemic control in diabetic people, it is infrequently used in veterinary medicine. Fructosamine is more commonly used to monitor diabetic dogs and cats, partly because of assay availability, and is believed to provide more useful information regarding changes in insulin therapy because it changes more rapidly than glycated hemoglobin. These assays do not provide information about glucose nadirs or acute change in glucose concentration in response to insulin administration.

## NEW TECHNOLOGY FOR MONITORING GLYCEMIC CONTROL

A continuous glucose monitoring system (CGMS) (CGMS Gold, Medtronic Minimed, Northridge, CA, USA) that uses novel technology has recently been introduced in veterinary medicine as a method for monitoring glycemic control in dogs and cats.[33,34] This system was designed for use in human diabetic patients in an attempt to alleviate the need for repeated finger-pricks and measurement of capillary blood glucose. Sensors that measure glucose continuously have been sought as an alternative to single-point capillary blood glucose measurement to achieve better overall glycemic control. The CGMS is designed to measure glucose in subcutaneous interstitial fluid (ISF) rather than in blood.[35] Subcutaneous ISF is ideal for measuring glucose concentration because it is easily and safely accessed and because ISF glucose rapidly equilibrates with blood and therefore correlates well with blood glucose concentration. The dynamic relationship between plasma and ISF glucose has been extensively studied.[35–37] The CGMS measures ISF glucose using a small, flexible amperometric sensor inserted through the skin into the subcutaneous space and attached to a recording device. The sensor consists of an electroenzymatic 3-electrode cell by which a constant potential is maintained between a working electrode and a reference electrode.[35] Glucose detection by the sensor is based on the generation of hydrogen peroxide from the reaction of glucose and oxygen catalyzed by glucose oxidase.[35,38–40] Oxidation of hydrogen peroxide results in the generation of an electrical signal that is translated into a glucose concentration by a recording device.[35,40] Using the CGMS, the ISF glucose concentration is recorded every 5 minutes (288 readings per 24 hours) by the sensor and stored in the recording device until the data are downloaded to a computer for analysis with specialized software.

The CGMS avoids several limitations of traditional blood glucose curves, including intermittent assessment of blood glucose concentration, hospitalization, animal restraint, and repeated phlebotomy. Because the CGMS provides 288 data points per 24 hours, it provides a detailed insight into daily changes in ISF glucose concentration. Once the CGMS is placed, the instrument is calibrated daily through measurement of blood glucose but more importantly, hospitalization is not necessary and the dog or cat can remain in its home environment. These advantages can minimize diagnostic confusion caused by epinephrine-induced hyperglycemia in cats. In addition, because the animal can be kept in its home environment and its normal daily routine maintained, a more natural state of ISF glucose can be assessed. Disadvantages of CGMS for monitoring diabetic dogs and cats include a limited dynamic range for ISF glucose (40–400 mg/dL), the requirement of 3 daily blood glucose determinations for proper calibration of the instrument, and animal/owner compliance in maintaining attachment and integrity of the unit.

Since being validated as a method for monitoring ISF glucose in dogs and cats, the CGMS has gained popularity among veterinarians as an additional tool for assessing glycemic control.[33,34] Evaluation of dogs and cats receiving insulin therapy for DM is the most common use of the CGMS[33,41]; however, other uses such as glucose monitoring during anesthesia have also been developed in veterinary medicine.[42,43]

Placement of the CGMS on a dog or cat has been described previously.[33,34,41,44,45] The duration of monitoring with the CGMS varies from 48 to 72 hours depending on the clinical needs of the animal; the CGMS also provides trends in daily glucose homeostasis. During the monitoring period, the animal should be returned to its home environment as soon as possible and pet owners instructed to maintain routine insulin administration times and dosages, feeding schedule, and exercise regimen. The instrument requires daily calibration according to the manufacturer's instructions; this can be done by the attending veterinarian or the pet owner using a valid handheld glucometer. After the monitoring period, the instrument is removed and the sensor attachment site examined for excessive redness or swelling. Attachment of the CGMS has been shown to result in minimal discomfort or irritation to the animal.[33]

## CLINICAL CASE EXAMPLES

This section describes 2 cases of client-owned animals presented to the University of Missouri–Columbia, College of Veterinary Medicine, Veterinary Medical Teaching Hospital. Both animals had been previously diagnosed with DM based on pertinent clinical signs and clinicopathologic findings and were referred to the Teaching Hospital for glycemic monitoring using the CGMS. Both owners consented to placement of the CGMS.

### Diabetic Dog: A 10-Year-old, Female, Spayed Toy Poodle

This dog was referred for persistent polyuria, polydipsia, and glucosuria, having been diagnosed with DM approximately 6 weeks before presentation. The dog was being managed with insulin therapy (NPH insulin [Novolin-N, Novo Nordisk Inc, Princeton, NJ, USA], 1.5 units every 12 hours, subcutaneously) and a high-fiber diet (Hills Pet Nutrition Inc, Topeka, KS, USA). Initial CGMS monitoring for 72 hours revealed a brief episode of ISF glucose concentration of 400 mg/dL or greater between 5:00 and 7:00 PM (**Fig. 1A**). This episode occurred shortly after instrument attachment and may have been a result of alteration in daily routine or stress; increases in ISF glucose concentration were not so dramatic for the remainder of the monitoring period. Insulin administration resulted in moderate decreases in ISF glucose, as expected. The ISF glucose concentration over the entire monitoring period (mean ± standard deviation = 240 ± 63 mg/dL; range = 88–400 mg/dL) was slightly higher than the clinically desired concentration (ie, 150–200 mg/dL) and most likely explained the dog's persistent clinical signs. Based on the results of this monitoring, the insulin dose was increased to 2.0 units every 12 hours, subcutaneously, and the diet was maintained. In addition, it was recommended that continued glycemic monitoring be achieved by owner observation (for changes in behavior or clinical signs) and by periodic measurement of serum fructosamine. Approximately 1 and 3 months after the initial CGMS monitoring, serum

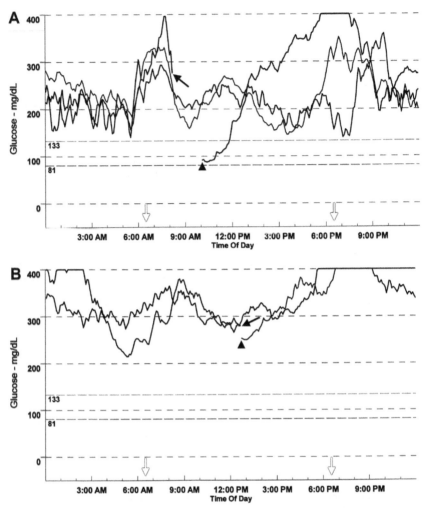

**Fig. 1.** Composite graphs of ISF glucose monitoring using a CGMS in a toy poodle with DM. (A) The initial monitoring period (~72 hours) and (B) a second monitoring period (~48 hours) approximately 11 months later are shown. The reference interval for canine serum glucose concentration is 81 to 133 mg/dL, as indicated by the closely dashed lines. The start of the monitoring is indicated by an arrowhead and the end of monitoring is indicated by a solid arrow. Times of insulin administration are indicated by the open arrows on the x-axis.

fructosamine levels were 584 mmol/L and 562 mmol/L, respectively (canine reference value <250 mmol/L), revealing poor glycemic control. After each fructosamine result, the insulin dose was increased by 0.5 units, every 12 hours, subcutaneously, and the same diet regimen maintained. Approximately 11 months after initial CGMS monitoring, a second period of monitoring was performed because of worsening polyuria and polydipsia as well as cataract formation. The monitoring revealed longer episodes, especially in the evening, of ISF glucose concentration of 400 mg/dL or greater (see **Fig. 1**B) Also, ISF baseline values throughout the second monitoring period (334 ± 48 mg/dL; range, 215–400 mg/dL) were higher than those during the initial monitoring period. Because of the worsening glycemic control, the insulin dose was again increased by 1.0 unit and the diet was modified. Shortly after the last monitoring, the dog experienced an episode of diabetic ketoacidosis and was killed.

This case shows the multiple methods that can be used to maintain glycemic control in a diabetic dog. Adequate glycemic control was not achieved in this case despite the methods used. In addition, this case offers a glimpse of the complex nature of diabetes in veterinary patients.

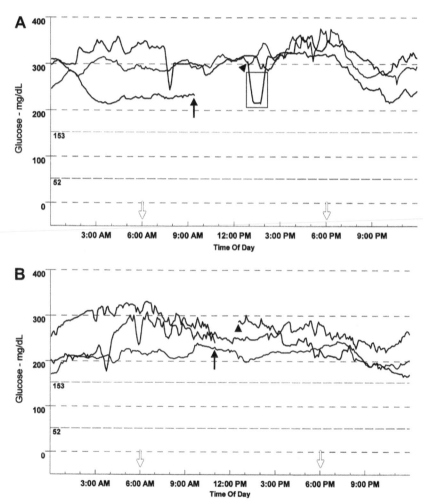

**Fig. 2.** Composite graphs of ISF glucose monitoring using a CGMS in a diabetic cat. (A) The initial monitoring period and (B) a second monitoring period approximately 6 weeks later, each ~72 hours long, are shown. The box in graph A indicates a slight dislodging of the CGMS probe; the problem was corrected by readjustment and recalibration. The reference interval for feline serum glucose concentration is 52 to 153 mg/dL, as indicated by the closely dashed lines. The start of monitoring is indicated by an arrowhead and the end of monitoring is indicated by a solid arrow. Times of insulin administration are indicated by the open arrows on the x-axis.

### Diabetic Cat: A 9-Year-old, Male, Castrated Domestic Longhair

This cat was diagnosed with DM approximately 18 months before presentation and was referred for hindlimb weakness (a plantigrade stance) and marked glucosuria. The cat had been treated with insulin (NPH, 3.0 units every 12 hours, subcutaneously) for 1 month after the initial diagnosis, and subsequently was managed solely with a weight-reduction diet. Insulin therapy was reinstituted using glargine (2 units, every 12 hours, subcutaneously [Lantus, Sanofi Aventis, Kansas City, MO, USA]), followed by CGMS monitoring 2 weeks later. The CGMS revealed moderate fluctuations in ISF glucose concentration during the 72-hour monitoring period (296 ± 38 mg/dL; range 214–376 mg/dL) (**Fig. 2**A). Based on the results, the owner was advised to increase the insulin dose by 0.5 units and to switch the cat's food to a prescription diabetes management diet (Nestlé Purina PetCare Company, St Louis, MO, USA). At a recheck approximately 6 weeks later the owner reported improvement in the plantigrade stance. Results of a second CGMS monitoring, after the changes in insulin dose and diet, revealed fluctuations similar to those in the first, but with an improved mean ISF glucose concentration (242 ± 37; range 166–331 mg/dL) (see **Fig. 2**B). The owner was advised to maintain the current insulin regimen and to continue to monitor the cat clinically.

Results from the use of CGMS in these cases show the effectiveness of therapy using long-acting insulin. In contrast to the dog, the fluctuations in interstitial glucose in the cat were not so profound. With proper case management, improved glycemic control and reduction in clinical signs can be improved in diabetic cats.

## SUMMARY

Numerous methods are available for monitoring diabetic dogs and cats. Most of these methods hinge on a watchful, dedicated pet owner working closely with their veterinarian. Because dogs and cats are dependent on their owner for glycemic control, it is important that the pet owner be educated about the disease, the clinical signs associated with poor glycemic control, and the effects of hypoglycemia. In addition, the veterinarian is responsible for educating the owner and making correct therapeutic choices in response to changes in the monitoring protocol. The monitoring protocol typically is chosen depending on the needs of the pet, the capabilities of the owner, the ease of the technique, and cost. As the clinical cases show, new CGMS technology recently introduced to veterinary medicine has made managing diabetic dogs and cats easier but still challenging. Continued advances in technology, diets, and ancillary methods along with broader use will assist greatly in the future management of diabetic animals in veterinary medicine.

## REFERENCES

1. Feldman E, Nelson RW. Canine and feline endocrinology and reproduction. 3rd edition. St Louis (MO): Saunders; 2004.
2. Bennett N. Monitoring techniques for diabetes mellitus in the dog and the cat. Clin Tech Small Anim Pract 2002;17(2):65–9.
3. Hoenig M. Comparative aspects of diabetes mellitus in dogs and cats. Mol Cell Endocrinol 2002;197(1–2):221–9.
4. Fleeman LM, Rand JS. Management of canine diabetes. Vet Clin North Am Small Anim Pract 2001;31(5):855–80, vi.
5. Rand JS, Martin GJ. Management of feline diabetes mellitus. Vet Clin North Am Small Anim Pract 2001;31(5):881–913.

6. Rand JS, Fleeman LM, Farrow HA, et al. Canine and feline diabetes mellitus: nature or nurture? J Nutr 2004;134(Suppl 8):2072S–80S.
7. Catchpole B, Ristic JM, Fleeman LM, et al. Canine diabetes mellitus: can old dogs teach us new tricks? Diabetologia 2005;48(10):1948–56.
8. Greco DS. Diagnosis of diabetes mellitus in cats and dogs. Vet Clin North Am Small Anim Pract 2001;31(5):845–53, v–vi.
9. Weaver KE, Rozanski EA, Mahony OM, et al. Use of glargine and lente insulins in cats with diabetes mellitus. J Vet Intern Med 2006;20(2):234–8.
10. Rand JS, Kinnaird E, Baglioni A, et al. Acute stress hyperglycemia in cats is associated with struggling and increased concentrations of lactate and norepinephrine. J Vet Intern Med 2002;16(2):123–32.
11. Nelson R. Stress hyperglycemia and diabetes mellitus in cats. J Vet Intern Med 2002;16(2):121–2.
12. Fleeman L, Rand J. Evaluation of day-to-day variability of serial blood glucose concentration curves in diabetic dogs. J Am Med Assoc 2003;222:317–21.
13. Alt N, Kley S, Haessig M, et al. Day-to-day variability of blood glucose concentration curves generated at home in cats with diabetes mellitus. J Am Vet Med Assoc 2007;230:1011–7.
14. Casella M, Wess G, Hassig M, et al. Home monitoring of blood glucose concentration by owners of diabetic dogs. J Small Anim Pract 2003;44(7):298–305.
15. Casella M, Wess G, Reusch CE. Measurement of capillary blood glucose concentrations by pet owners: a new tool in the management of diabetes mellitus. J Am Anim Hosp Assoc 2002;38(3):239–45.
16. Wess G, Reusch C. Capillary blood sampling from the ear of dogs and cats and use of portable meters to measure glucose concentration. J Small Anim Pract 2000;41(2):60–6.
17. Wess G, Reusch C. Assessment of five portable blood glucose meters for use in cats. Am J Vet Res 2000;61(12):1587–92.
18. Cohn LA, McCaw DL, Tate DJ, et al. Assessment of five portable blood glucose meters, a point-of-care analyzer, and color test strips for measuring blood glucose concentration in dogs. J Am Vet Med Assoc 2000;216(2):198–202.
19. Reusch CE, Liehs MR, Hoyer M, et al. Fructosamine. A new parameter for diagnosis and metabolic control in diabetic dogs and cats. J Vet Intern Med 1993;7(3):177–82.
20. Elliott DA, Nelson RW, Feldman EC, et al. Glycosylated hemoglobin concentration for assessment of glycemic control in diabetic cats. J Vet Intern Med 1997;11(3):161–5.
21. Jensen AL. Glycated blood proteins in canine diabetes mellitus. Vet Rec 1995;137(16):401–5.
22. Elliott DA, Nelson RW, Feldman EC, et al. Glycosylated hemoglobin concentrations in the blood of healthy dogs and dogs with naturally developing diabetes mellitus, pancreatic beta-cell neoplasia, hyperadrenocorticism, and anemia. J Am Vet Med Assoc 1997;211(6):723–7.
23. Goldstein DE, Little RR, Lorenz RA, et al. Tests of glycemia in diabetes. Diabetes Care 2004;27(Suppl 1):S91–3.
24. Crenshaw KL, Peterson ME, Heeb LA, et al. Serum fructosamine concentration as an index of glycemia in cats with diabetes mellitus and stress hyperglycemia. J Vet Intern Med 1996;10(6):360–4.
25. Sako T, Mori A, Lee P, et al. Serum glycated albumin: potential use as an index of glycemic control in diabetic dogs. Vet Res Commun 2009;33(5):473–9.
26. Sako T, Mori A, Lee P, et al. Diagnostic significance of serum glycated albumin in diabetic dogs. J Vet Diagn Invest 2008;20(5):634–8.

27. Loste A, Marca MC. Fructosamine and glycated hemoglobin in the assessment of glycaemic control in dogs. Vet Res 2001;32(1):55–62.
28. Lutz TA, Rand JS, Ryan E. Fructosamine concentrations in hyperglycemic cats. Can Vet J 1995;36(3):155–9.
29. Marca MC, Loste A, Ramos JJ. Effect of acute hyperglycaemia on the serum fructosamine and blood glycated haemoglobin concentrations in canine samples. Vet Res Commun 2000;24(1):11–6.
30. Goldstein DE, Little RR, Lorenz RA, et al. Tests of glycemia in diabetes. Diabetes Care 2004;27(7):1761–73.
31. Marca MC, Loste A, Unzueta A, et al. Blood glycated hemoglobin evaluation in sick dogs. Can J Vet Res 2000;64(2):141–4.
32. Reusch CE, Haberer B. Evaluation of fructosamine in dogs and cats with hypo- or hyperproteinaemia, azotaemia, hyperlipidaemia and hyperbilirubinaemia. Vet Rec 2001;148(12):370–6.
33. Wiedmeyer CE, Johnson PJ, Cohn LA, et al. Evaluation of a continuous glucose monitoring system for use in dogs, cats, and horses. J Am Vet Med Assoc 2003; 223(7):987–92.
34. Davison LJ, Slater LA, Herrtage ME, et al. Evaluation of a continuous glucose monitoring system in diabetic dogs. J Small Anim Pract 2003;44(10):435–42.
35. Rebrin K, Steil GM, van Antwerp WP, et al. Subcutaneous glucose predicts plasma glucose independent of insulin: implications for continuous monitoring. Am J Physiol 1999;277(3 Pt 1):E561–71.
36. Rebrin K, Steil GM. Can interstitial glucose assessment replace blood glucose measurements? Diabetes Technol Ther 2000;2(3):461–72.
37. Steil GM, Rebrin K, Hariri F, et al. Interstitial fluid glucose dynamics during insulin-induced hypoglycaemia. Diabetologia 2005;48(9):1833–40.
38. Abel P, Muller A, Fischer U. Experience with an implantable glucose sensor as a prerequisite of an artificial beta cell. Biomed Biochim Acta 1984;43(5):577–84.
39. Bindra DS, Zhang Y, Wilson GS, et al. Design and in vitro studies of a needle-type glucose sensor for subcutaneous monitoring. Anal Chem 1991;63(17):1692–6.
40. Poitout V, Moatti-Sirat D, Reach G. Development of a glucose sensor for glucose monitoring in man: the disposable implant concept. Clin Mater 1994;15(4):241–6.
41. Ristic JM, Herrtage ME, Walti-Lauger SM, et al. Evaluation of a continuous glucose monitoring system in cats with diabetes mellitus. J Feline Med Surg 2005;7(3):153–62.
42. Bilicki KL, Schermerhorn T, Klocke EE, et al. Evaluation of a real-time, continuous monitor of glucose concentration in healthy dogs during anesthesia. Am J Vet Res 2010;71(1):11–6.
43. Affenzeller N, Benesch T, Thalhammer JG, et al. A pilot study to evaluate a novel subcutaneous continuous glucose monitoring system in healthy Beagle dogs. Vet J 2010;184(1):105–10.
44. Wiedmeyer CE, Johnson PJ, Cohn LA, et al. Evaluation of a continuous glucose monitoring system for use in veterinary medicine. Diabetes Technol Ther 2005; 7(6):885–95.
45. DeClue AE, Cohn LA, Kerl ME, et al. Use of continuous blood glucose monitoring for animals with diabetes mellitus. J Am Anim Hosp Assoc 2004;40(3):171–3.

# Assay Validation and Diagnostic Applications of Major Acute-phase Protein Testing in Companion Animals

Mads Kjelgaard-Hansen, DVM, PhD[a],*, Stine Jacobsen, DVM, PhD[b]

## KEYWORDS

- Acute-phase proteins • Assay validation • C-reactive protein
- Serum amyloid A • Veterinary clinical pathology

## MAJOR ACUTE PHASE PROTEINS

Use of acute-phase proteins (APPs) for assessment of health and disease in animals has increased greatly within the last decade. This increase has been the result not only of increased knowledge in the field, which is needed for interpretation of measurement results, but also of the increased access to appropriate assay systems for detection of relevant APPs. In human medicine, the APP C-reactive protein (CRP) is included in all routine blood profiles for detection of inflammation, and several bedside assay systems for use in the doctor's office are available.[1,2] In veterinary medicine, few such near-patient test systems are available,[3–5] and progression in the field is hampered by the species specificity of APPs, because assay systems developed for one protein in one species may, for technical or biologic reasons, not be relevant for measurements in another species.

An APP is defined as a protein whose levels change by at least 25% during inflammation[6]; major APPs are those whose blood levels increase more than tenfold following infection or other inflammatory stimuli (**Fig. 1**).[6] Other common features of major APPs are (1) a short lag time (hours) from onset of inflammation to a measurable increase in blood concentration, (2) a short half-life (hours) causing plasma concentrations to decrease soon after inflammation has subsided, and (3) low plasma

---

The authors have nothing to disclose.

[a] Department of Small Animal Clinical Sciences, Faculty of LIFE Sciences, University of Copenhagen, Gronnegaardsvej 3, DK-1870 Frederiksberg C, Denmark

[b] Department of Large Animal Sciences, Faculty of LIFE Sciences, University of Copenhagen, Hoejbakkegaard Alle 5, DK-2630 Taastrup, Denmark

* Corresponding author.

*E-mail address:* mjkh@life.ku.dk

Clin Lab Med 31 (2011) 51–70
doi:10.1016/j.cll.2010.10.002
0272-2712/11/$ – see front matter © 2011 Elsevier Inc. All rights reserved.

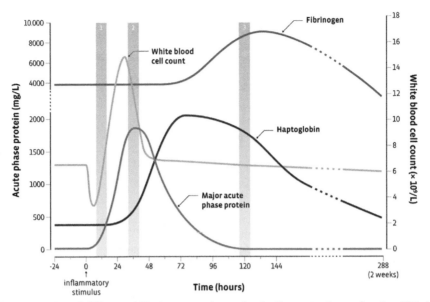

**Fig. 1.** Kinetics of different APPs in companion animals. Concentrations of major APPs in plasma are very low (often immeasurable) in healthy individuals and increase quickly by several hundredfold (sometimes thousandfold) after an inflammatory stimulus. Minor APPs such as fibrinogen and haptoglobin also are detectable in healthy individuals and only a gradual and small response is observed in response to inflammation, with peak values often only 2 to 4 times healthy levels. After resolution of disease, blood concentrations of major APPs decrease quickly, whereas minor acute-phase proteins can remain increased for several weeks. The leukocyte response is often sinoidal, with an initial decrease (caused by initial margination and adhesion to endothelial cells) and a subsequent cytokine-induced increase in WBC count. A decrease may also be observed in fibrinogen concentration immediately after a potent inflammatory stimulus because of consumption after activation of the coagulation cascade or extravasation after increases in vascular permeability (not shown in the figure). Measured levels of acute-phase reactants are thus dependent on the timing of sampling. Samples obtained during peracute inflammation (*gray bar 1*) could have decreased, normal or somewhat increased WBC counts and concentrations of minor APPs will be within (or even less than) reference limits, whereas concentrations of major APPs will be slightly increased. In acute inflammation (*gray bar 2*), WBC count and concentrations of major APPs are increased to more than the reference values, whereas concentrations of minor APPs may still be within reference limits because of the slower synthesis of these proteins. After inflammation has been resolved (*gray bar 3*), WBC count and concentrations of major APPs quickly return to baseline, but levels of minor APPs may still be increased, because these proteins have a long or very long half-life.

concentration in the healthy animal. These features make this group of proteins particularly well suited for diagnosing and monitoring disease. The dynamics of major APPs are such that concentrations rise and fall closely in parallel with increased and decreased disease activity, in contrast with the dynamics of minor APPs (which have longer half-lives), such as fibrinogen and haptoglobin, for which concentrations remain increased for several days even after a single inflammatory stimulus; this has been shown, for example, in surgical[7,8] and experimental infection[9] studies in horses. The low physiologic concentration of major APPs in combination with the marked increase during the acute-phase response gives a favorable signal-to-noise ratio, facilitating interpretation and limiting the clinical effect of interindividual variation in baseline concentrations, which can pose a problem for other inflammatory markers (**Fig. 2**).[8]

Acute-phase proteins are synthesized in the liver in response to release of proinflammatory cytokines in diseases such as bacterial and viral infections, immune-mediated disease, neoplasia, aseptic tissue injury (trauma, surgery), necrosis, and burns (**Fig. 3**). The reader is referred to other reviews for more detailed information on the APP response.[10] Studies have shown that several APPs, including CRP and serum amyloid A (SAA), are synthesized by extrahepatic tissues such as mammary gland epithelium,[11] articular chondro- and synoviocytes,[12,13] pulmonary tissue,[14] intestine,[15] adipocytes,[16] endometrium,[17] leukocytes,[18,19] and kidneys,[20] where they have been suggested to serve as an innate defense against invading pathogens and to modulate local inflammation. Locally synthesized APPs may serve as potential local markers of inflammatory activity, and their levels may be measured in body fluids other than blood.

Use of APPs for detection or monitoring of inflammation in companion animals bears many similarities to use of APP in humans, where measurements are performed with the purpose of diagnosing disease or tailoring treatment of 1 particular individual. Veterinarians also deal with disease diagnosis in larger populations, for example herds or flocks of animals at a farm, a production batch (a tank of milk or a group of animals for slaughter), or in disease surveillance programs, in which representative animals in a population are tested. Use of APPs in assessment of herd or flock health in food-producing animals such as cattle, swine, and poultry, or assessment of product quality, such as milk, has been described,[21–24] and the reader is referred to previous reviews for more information.[25,26]

This review focuses on so-called major APPs and their use in companion animal (canine, feline, and equine) medicine. The major APPs possess many desirable characteristics that make them well suited for use in patient management as diagnostic and prognostic markers and for monitoring purposes. Veterinary assay development and evaluation, now and in the future, are described.

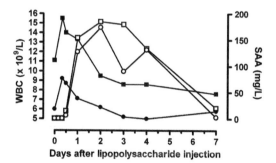

**Fig. 2.** WBC count (closed symbols) and serum amyloid A (SAA) concentration (open symbols) in 2 horses after intra-articular injection of 3 μg of *Escherichia coli* lipopolysaccharide. Both horses developed significant leukocytosis in response to the injection, but peak WBC counts depended on the preinjection WBC of the horse (the WBC count of the horse depicted by the circles stayed within reference limits at all times). In contrast, SAA concentrations increased in both horses, independently of baseline levels. (*From* Jacobsen S, Niewold TA, Halling-Thomsen M, et al. Serum amyloid A isoforms in serum and synovial fluid in horses with lipopolysaccharide-induced arthritis. Vet Immunol Immunopathol 2006; 110(3–4):328; with permission.)

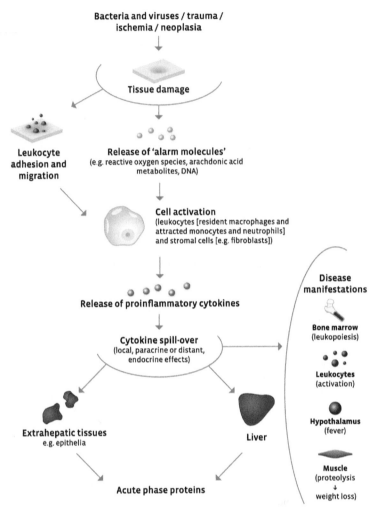

**Fig. 3.** Overview of the acute-phase response. Multiple inflammatory stimuli can elicit the acute-phase response, because any kind of tissue damage leads to activation of leukocytes (recruited neutrophils as well as resident macrophages) and stromal cells such as fibroblasts. On activation, cells secrete proinflammatory cytokines that have numerous effects on the body, including leukocytosis, fever, and weight loss. In the liver (and certain extrahepatic tissues), cytokines such as interleukin (IL)-6, IL-1 and tumor necrosis factor α result in synthesis of acute-phase proteins, which are subsequently released into the blood or other body fluids.

## PROBLEMS WITH SPECIES SPECIFICITY

Measuring APPs in different species is challenging, because APPs are species specific: some proteins with acute-phase properties in one species show no, or only very limited, acute-phase properties in another. For example, CRP is a major APP in dogs and humans, but is a minor APP in horses and constitutively expressed in cattle. One notable exception to the species specificity of APPs is SAA, which is a major APP in all mammalian species investigated thus far except the rat

(**Table 1**).[27] Species specificity requires that researchers or clinicians wanting to measure a new APP in a particular species must either develop a new assay (which can be time consuming as well as costly) or must validate an assay for measurement of the protein in another species (heterologous detection). Succesful examples of the latter approach is validation of human SAA and CRP assays for use in horses and dogs, respectively[28,29]; these assays are now used routinely in the authors' laboratory. Moreover, knowledge about an APP in one species cannot be readily extrapolated to another species, in which healthy levels, response to inflammation or infection, and diagnostic and prognostic potential may be different.

The diagnostic specificity of APPs in veterinary species can be increased by measuring their concentrations in biologic fluids other than blood, providing information on disease processes in the compartment of interest. For example, increased SAA concentrations have been shown in mastitic milk[30] and in synovial fluid from dogs and horses with joint inflammation.[31–33] Studies have shown that, in animals, SAA produced extrahepatically is of a different isoform (so-called SAA3) than that synthesized by hepatocytes[11,30,33]; therefore, assays specific for SAA3 may increase the specificity of compartment-specific testing. The human SAA3 gene is silent,[34] so humans do not produce this specific local isoform of SAA, unlike almost all other mammalian species studied.

## ROUTINE DETERMINATION AND AVAILABILITY OF ASSAY SYSTEMS

The general characteristics and apparent clinical benefits of major APPs in companion animals might suggest that they should be included widely for routine clinical purposes in veterinary medicine. However, this is not yet the case, as exemplified by CRP in dogs. Canine CRP was characterized and purified in the 1970s[35,36] and its kinetics and clinical applications were studied using locally developed, in-house, species-specific assays through the 1980s and 1990s.[37–39] Species-specific assays were made commercially available in ~2000, which greatly boosted the number of clinical research reports. Despite this long history and the resulting high level of

**Table 1**
Species specificity of major acute-phase proteins in veterinary species

| Species | Major Acute-phase Proteins | Other Proteins with Acute-phase Properties | Constitutively Expressed Proteins | References |
|---|---|---|---|---|
| Horse | Serum amyloid A | Fibrinogen, haptoglobin, CRP, ceruloplasmin, α1-acid glycoprotein | — | 76,122 |
| Dog | CRP, serum amyloid A | Fibrinogen, haptoglobin, ceruloplasmin, α1-acid glycoprotein | — | 74,75 |
| Cat | Serum amyloid A, α1-acid glycoprotein | Haptoglobin, ceruloplasmin | CRP | 74,77,81 |
| Cow | Serum amyloid A, haptoglobin | Fibrinogen, ceruloplasmin, α1-acid glycoprotein | CRP | 25,123 |
| Pig | Serum amyloid A, major acute-phase protein, haptoglobin | Fibrinogen, C-reactive protein | α1-Acid glycoprotein | 25,124,125 |

knowledge about canine CRP, routine application has spread only slowly and, until recently, was limited to certain laboratories with special interest in companion animal APPs. The main reason for this has been the limited practicability (see later discussion) of the formats of the species-specific assays available.[40] When lacking species-specific assays, veterinary clinical pathologists have a tradition of directly applying, or slightly modifying, assays developed for human purposes for companion animals (after thorough validation). Several attempts to establish heterologous measurement of canine CRP were also made, but cross-reactivity was insufficient for diagnostic purposes.[41–43] In 2003, a human-based automated assay with cross-reacting poly-clonal antibody was identified[29] that significantly improved practicability for canine CRP, which now is applicable for use on random-access analyzers. Despite this, use of the CRP assay was still limited to laboratories with special interest in CRP biochemistry because the cross-reactivity of the polyclonal heterologous antibodies was potentially unstable across production batches, requiring more quality control measures than were feasible in smaller laboratories. However, the demonstration of continuous acceptable cross-reactivity[44,45] over several years, increased application of internal species-specific quality control measures in veterinary laboratories,[46] and use of species-specific calibration material[45] has now seemingly facilitated the dissemination and routine clinical application of polyclonal CRP assays in canine medicine. A species-specific, low-throughput canine CRP assay relevant for clinical practice has been available on the Japanese market since 2000,[5] and has had a great effect on routine point-of-care diagnostics in Japan.[47] Other such commercially available, canine-specific, point-of-care CRP assays are emerging,[4] and are expected to have similar effects on routine diagnostic use where made available.

The story of routine measurement of major APPs in horse and cats is similar to that of canine CRP; until discovery of a heterologous cross-reacting human assay for SAA,[28,48] measurement of major APPs in these species was mainly done for research purposes. One important difference from the heterologous determination of canine CRP is that the SAA assay is based on monoclonal antibodies, which has facilitated its dissemination markedly because of the increased stability of the cross-reactivity; research and routine clinical applications in equine medicine have spread especially quickly. Because SAA is also a major APP in dogs, this assay had the potential to be a true cross-species major APP assay for companion animals. However, it did not cross-react with canine SAA (Kjelgaard-Hansen, unpublished data, 2006), despite the highly conserved nature of SAA among mammals.[49] Thus, although species-specific homologous measurement of major APPs is preferred,[50] the major APP assays used routinely in companion animals are heterologous: CRP in dogs[29,44] and SAA in horses and cats.[28,48,51]

Routine implementation of novel, potentially useful biomarkers in veterinary medicine is not solely dependent on availability of valid and practical assays. As in human medicine,[52] the theory of evidence-based clinical practices is established in veterinary medicine,[53] and thus evidence is needed before a novel marker can be expected to be widely accepted and routinely applied. In addition, as in human medicine,[54] medical conservatism exists in veterinary medicine, and as stated by Knottnerus and Dinant[55] in 1997, "Important new evidence from research often takes a long time to be implemented in daily care, while established practices persist even if they have been proved to be ineffective or harmful." This article outlines a procedural backbone that can be used to provide evidence that a novel biomarker has influence on patient treatment, and examines the current level of evidence (and where additional studies are needed) for the clinical application of major APPs in companion animals.

## EVIDENCE-BASED ASSAY VALIDATION: OBSTACLES AND ACHIEVEMENTS

When introducing a new biomarker for diagnostic purposes, the decision must consider that: "A laboratory test is clinically useful only if it successfully answers a question of consequence to patient management."[56] This statement is the benchmark when performing a full evaluation of a new biomarker for clinical use. However, achieving this benchmark encompasses many aspects and can form the basis of philosophic discussions within the community of clinical pathologists or between clinical pathologists and clinicians. Biomarker evaluation is best addressed in a stepwise manner, similar to how new treatment strategies or drugs are tested for clinical use.[56,57] The 4 phases (I–IV) of the full evaluation of a novel biomarker encompass all relevant steps, from assessing analytical performance to usefulness analysis of the effect on patient management (**Table 2**). When going from phase I to phase IV in the evaluation, there is an increasing demand on resources, and thus the biggest advantage of the stepwise approach is the chance of detecting critical flaws and deficiencies in the methodology or biomarker as early as possible, thus saving resources.

Application of new diagnostic markers in veterinary medicine, including major APP assays, seldom awaits the full 4-phase validation. Although aspects of all phases (I–IV) have been addressed, failure to completely do so may be the main reason that routine implementation of APP assays is progressing slower than expected. The major components of each phase are discussed to help identify possible obstacles hindering faster dissemination of APP assays for routine use in veterinary clinical settings.

### Phase I: Analytical Performance

In this step, the assay is not necessarily applied to clinical material, because the focus is on basic performance and validity of results. However, it is important that species-specific material be used, and that separate studies of analytical performance be performed for each species. The basic steps in this phase are evaluation of imprecision, inaccuracy, detection limit, and practicability; practicability has a focus on future clinical application.[58] Methodologies for estimation of imprecision and detection limit are well established and similar across human and veterinary clinical pathology.[58] However, because recognized standards are not established for companion animal acute-phase proteins, veterinary laboratories are limited to indirect or relative estimates of inaccuracy, for example through spiking-recovery and linearity studies[58]; where an APP assay already exists in another format, method comparison can be used.[59] An inherent result of this lack of recognized standard material is that direct comparison of results across laboratories and methodologies cannot readily be made, because absolute inaccuracy remains unassessed.

**Table 2**
The 4 phases of a complete assay validation for diagnostic purposes

| Phase | Test Performance Parameters | Description |
| --- | --- | --- |
| I | Analytical | Assessment of analytical and practicability characteristics |
| II | Overlap | Assessment of value in health and disease |
| III | Clinical | Evaluation of diagnostic sensitivity and specificity in clinical settings of interest |
| IV | Outcome and usefulness | Assessment of whether the individual (or community) gain advantage from the test |

To evaluate the acceptability of analytical performance estimates, clinically relevant quality specifications need to be established, which is as big a challenge in veterinary as in human clinical pathology. The different methods for establishing quality specifications are ranked hierarchically based on clinical relevance and objectivity.[60,61] For some canine APPs, top-ranked data on biologic variation are available.[62] However, in most cases, veterinary laboratories are left with data from lower-ranked methods that are of limited or undefined clinical relevance, making some of the more subjective expert-based methods relevant (see Ref.[63] for details). If basic performance is acceptable for future clinical application, continuous quality control must be established based on the validation data. In this regard, the biggest challenge for companion animal APP assays is the lack of commercially available control material, which needs to be species specific.[45] Although it is a laborious task, this issue can be, and often is, solved by establishing pooled patient material locally and using it as an internal control[46]; most companion animal major APPs have long-term stability when frozen. Thus, although most components of analytical performance of veterinary APP assays compare readily with those of human assays, the lack of recognized veterinary standards and control material leaves several aspects less well defined.

If the analyte is to be made available for routine clinical use, it is important to investigate practicability, which is best done in this early phase of test validation to ensure that the format of the methodology is relevant and preferred. Major components of practicability are:

- Commercial availability of the assay
- Necessary personnel to run the assay
- Necessary level of technical education of staff
- Turnaround time
- Accessibility during analysis (single test, batch runs, or randomly accessible)
- Throughput
- Cost
- Necessary technical level of equipment to run the assay
- Type of result (quantitative or qualitative).

Assay availability is crucial to dissemination and routine application of novel biomarkers, and, as described earlier, was an issue for the clinical use of canine CRP. The commercial availability of species-specific assays for canine CRP since 2000 has had a positive effect on the annual number of clinical research reports involving measurements of this marker in dogs.

The remaining components of practicability are tightly connected to the format of a given assay, and a schism exists in this regard. To assess acceptability of, for example, accessibility during analysis, cost, and type of result, it is necessary to know the typical clinical setting in which the marker will be applied, which often requires knowledge of clinical performance, the focus of phase III. Thus, a risk exists that critical shortcomings in the practicability of a given assay may not be revealed before phase III or even phase IV. The diagnostic characteristics of canine CRP and equine SAA made it relevant for them to be included in routine serum biochemistry panels for dogs and horses in the authors' laboratory. In large-scale laboratories, such application requires that certain practicability characteristics be met; short turnaround time, random access during analysis, high throughput, and low cost are desirable, whereas the necessary technical level of high-end equipment is often already present. Such requirements of practicability will often disqualify certain assay formats such as enzyme-linked immunosorbent assays because of lack of random-accessibility during analytical runs. Regarding type of result, quantification of major APPs in absolute (rather than qualitative) concentrations provides valuable diagnostic and prognostic information and can be used for monitoring purposes. This information is most likely the reason for the widespread use of the quantitative canine CRP point-of-care test in Japan, whereas the semiquantitative canine CRP point-of-care tests, despite worldwide availability, are used much less.[64,65]

## Phase II: Overlap Performance

The purpose of the second phase of test validation is to detect differences in analyte values between healthy and diseased individuals, and should be seen as a resource-sparing prelude to the resource-demanding third phase. In this phase, the analyte of interest typically is measured in 20 to 30 healthy individuals and 20 to 30 individuals having a well-defined disease of interest (for APPs these often comprise inflammatory/infectious and noninflammatory groups). Descriptive statistics are obtained and the observed concentrations are compared among groups by means of basic parametric or nonparametric statistics, and visualized by dot plots. Because this is meant to be a low-resource step, the material is often highly selected for individuals in advanced stages of disease, resulting in an unrealistically high prevalence of disease. Thus, if major overlap in analyte concentrations is observed between healthy and inflamed/infected groups, the diagnostic value of the test is questionable and it will most likely not pass phase III evaluation.

## Phase III: Clinical Performance

In evaluating true clinical performance it is necessary to focus on bias and relevance. Unlike in phase II, estimates of diagnostic capacity (diagnostic sensitivity and specificity) in phase III should be free from critical bias and reflect the performance in a population of clinical relevance. Creating this freedom is not a straightforward task, and it is discussed often within both human and veterinary clinical pathology communities. This task was the focus of the Standards for Reporting of Diagnostic Accuracy (STARD) initiative in 2003.[66] This initiative focused mainly on standardizing reports of investigations of the diagnostic accuracy of tests to ensure complete transparency, but the final recommendations also address how to appropriately conduct such studies to ensure the ability to generalize results and to avoid bias.[66,67] The recommendations include a list of 25 points that should be specifically addressed in studies on diagnostic accuracy, including an important prototypical flow diagram that provides transparency of possible bias in patient recruitment, execution of the test in question, and the reference standard.[66] The checklist has recently been recommended for veterinary use,[68] and examples now exist of veterinary application.[69] A wider adoption could be wished for in veterinary studies, including studies on diagnostic performance of APPs in companion animals. A wider application was also wished for in human studies in a 4-year follow-up of the STARD initiative.[70] It is hoped that the recent recommendation will have an effect on future veterinary studies.

At completion of phase III, valid estimates of diagnostic sensitivity and specificity should have been obtained and, if conducted at a relevant level of prevalence, estimates of positive and negative predictive values also should be available. These estimates can then be compared with the analytical performance of existing diagnostic systems to decide on the clinical value of the assay in question.

## Phase IV: Outcome and Usefulness Performance

The ultimate step in the evaluation of an assay is to assess whether the individual (or community) gains advantage from use of the test (ie, whether it has consequences to patient management).[56] It is difficult to set criteria for outcome and quality specifications for clinically useful information and is often costly to perform studies to prove that a novel test system will provide additional clinically useful information compared with existing systems. This difficulty is probably the reason this phase is performed seldom in veterinary diagnostics. Sometimes, specific aspects can be identified that argue for the superiority of a novel assay (eg, it provides equivalent clinically useful information faster or more cost-effectively than established parameters; or sample material is more easily obtained, or has better stability, than with established methods). For example, the superior storage and stability characteristics of major APPs in animals, compared with cellular markers of inflammation (eg, white blood cell [WBC] counts), have an important positive effect on their routine use in the authors' laboratory.

Data at this level of test validation can be obtained at various levels of evidence and can readily be ranked, using the well-known hierarchy of evidence-based medicine, according to bias and relevance.[52] Compared with human diagnostics, in which meta-analyses often exist, including on the use of APPs in various clinical settings,[71,72] evidence in companion animal diagnostics is frequently at the level of a case report or case series, although observational studies exist.[73] This lower level of evidence is most likely a result of the limited commercial potential of companion animal diagnostics, such that most studies are conducted without significant funding and are motivated mainly by academic interest.

## DIAGNOSTIC APPLICATIONS OF MAJOR ACUTE PHASE PROTEINS IN COMPANION ANIMAL MEDICINE

The dynamic characteristics of major APPs in companion animals make them potentially useful in several stages of patient management, especially (1) for establishing a diagnosis, because of their specific induction by proinflammatory mediators, their real-time reflection of inflammatory activity, and their large-amplitude response enhancing diagnostic sensitivity; (2) for evaluating prognosis at the time of diagnosis; and (3) for monitoring after the diagnosis has been made, because traditional treatment regimens do not seem to exert any significant direct effects on major APPs in companion animals, levels of which thus continue to reflect inflammatory activity during treatment.

### Establishing a Diagnosis

Major APPs reliably indicate systemic inflammation in cats, dogs, and horses, as reviewed by several active researchers.[74–77] First, measurement of major APPs aids in differentiation between diseases with and without an inflammatory component, in situations in which traditional markers of inflammation, such as WBC count and fibrinogen concentration, are of less value. The WBC response is a sinoidal curve, such that counts may decrease in the acute stage of inflammation or in severe inflammation (eg, sepsis), before leukocytosis develops; interpretation of WBC count is thus quite dependent on the timing of sampling (see **Fig. 1**). Plasma fibrinogen concentration is a commonly used, but minor, APP that can be influenced by factors other than inflammation. For example, decreased fibrinogen levels caused by consumptive coagulopathies or increased vascular permeability may mask inflammation-induced hyperfibrinogenemia and make interpretation of results difficult. Concentrations of major APPs only increase in response to an inflammatory stimulus, but measured concentrations are still dependent on timing of sampling because of the bell shape of the response curve. Repeated measurements are thus necessary to determine whether a sample was obtained in a pre- or postpeak situation (see **Fig. 1**).

Second, assessment of major APPs are of value in the peracute and acute stages of disease for ruling infection in or out, because bacteria and bacterial products, such as gram-negative lipopolysaccharide, seem to cause a more pronounced APP response than that seen in most viral infections or in aseptic/traumatic inflammation.[78] Moreover, major APPs start to increase within hours after the inflammatory stimulus,[33,79–81] serving as first-line indicators of inflammatory activity and, in the case of bacterial infections, allowing antibiotic treatment to be initiated early, with benefits to outcome.

In equine medicine, SAA has been used in a limited number of studies for diagnosing the presence of infection in foals.[82–85] Sepsis has been shown to produce particularly high serum SAA concentrations,[83,84] but local infections also can increase blood levels of SAA[82,84]; SAA may thus aid in deciding whether to treat with antibiotics. Diagnosing infections in neonatal foals can be a challenge, because the clinical signs are nonspecific, and diseases with a noninfectious cause, such as prematurity, failure of passive transfer, neonatal maladjustment syndrome, and isoerythrolysis, can manifest similarly to infectious diseases such as sepsis. Moreover, the WBC response in the neonatal foal has been shown to be sluggish, and may thus not reflect current disease status. SAA was found to discriminate infectious from noninfectious disease in foals more specifically than WBC count and fibrinogen,[83] and significantly higher SAA concentrations were observed in foals with high versus low sepsis scores.[85] In contrast, serum SAA concentrations were normal in young foals with umbilical abscesses,[84] a fairly common local infection. The investigators suggested that the apparent lack of acute-phase response was caused by walling-off of the abscess, dampening the stimulus for hepatic SAA synthesis.

Potential use of SAA for diagnosis of *Rhodococcus equi* pneumonia, a chronic infection that is difficult to treat, with a high prevalence and case-fatality rate in older foals, also has been investigated.[86] The study showed that SAA concentration measured at 7 to 14 and 21 to 28 days of age in approximately 200 foals from 2 farms endemically infected with *R equi* did not predict development of *R equi* pneumonia, nor did SAA levels differ between foals diagnosed with *R equi* pneumonia and age-matched controls. As a possible explanation for this surprising negative finding, the investigators suggested that the sampling interval of 2 weeks may have been too long given the rapid kinetics of the SAA response. An APP with a slower pattern of increase and decrease (eg, fibrinogen) may be more relevant for screening purposes.

In adult horses, SAA has been used to differentiate infectious (enteritis, colitis, peritonitis, and abdominal abscesses) from noninfectious causes of acute abdominal pain.[87] Similarly, horses with infectious joint disease had higher serum and synovial fluid concentrations of SAA than horses with noninfectious joint disease (osteoarthritis, osteochondrosis).[31]

In canine medicine, several studies on CRP support its routine diagnostic use as a complementary marker of inflammation to traditional markers, such as WBC count,[47] and for specific indications, such as pancreatitis,[88] inflammatory bowel disease,[89] and steroid-responsive meningitis-arteritis.[90,91] Studies on the diagnostic potential of major APPs in cats are limited to reports on their concentrations in hospitalized cats with various diseases (eg, urinary tract infection, renal disease, and feline infectious peritonitis) compared with healthy individuals.[81,92] Rare examples of more advanced attempts to estimate true diagnostic values in specific feline diseases are available.[93]

Thus, few studies exist on the routine diagnostic use of major APPs in companion animals that provide state-of-the-art estimates of diagnostic performance in specific clinical indications. However, the cumulative mass of knowledge leaves little doubt that concentrations of major APPs are reliably increased in diseases with systemic inflammatory activity.

### Prognostication

In equine medicine only 1 large study on the use of SAA for prognostic purposes is available.[87] This study involved 718 horses with acute abdominal pain admitted to 1 of 2 centers; serum SAA was measured at admission and compared between subsets of horses. In survivors, serum SAA concentration was significantly lower (median 1.4 mg/L) than in horses that died or were euthanized (median 10.8 mg/L), and, when a cutoff value of 50 mg/L was applied, a significantly larger proportion of non-survivors than survivors had serum SAA concentrations greater than the cutoff. Despite the large sample size of this retrospective study, details on inclusion and exclusion criteria were not provided, leaving it as a large and advanced phase II evaluation of the use of SAA for diagnosis of acute abdominal disease.

In horses undergoing castration, postoperative infectious complications occurred more frequently in horses with preoperatively increased serum SAA levels than in horses with normal SAA levels,[94] and SAA may thus be an indicator of surgical risk in horses undergoing elective surgery, as shown for CRP in humans.[95–97] In a study involving Standardbred trotters with reduced racing performance mainly caused by respiratory disease, serum SAA concentrations had no clear predictive value on performance.[98]

In canine medicine, the prognostic significance of CRP concentration at the time of admission to the hospital has been investigated for several diseases, often by means of well-designed prospective studies. CRP did not have prognostic significance in dogs with primary immune-mediated hemolytic anemia[99,100] in a population of critically ill dogs admitted to an intensive care unit,[101] or in dogs with systemic inflammatory response syndrome (SIRS),[102] and had only a weak association with outcome (survival) in dogs naturally infected with *Babesia rossi*.[103] These observations are highly relevant because most of them involved clinical settings in which a high fraction of patients have marked inflammation and high mortality. In dogs with SIRS[102] or pancreatitis,[88] the lack of decline in CRP concentrations within 2 to 3 days after treatment seemed to be relevant to outcome (survival).

### Monitoring

Major APPs have been used for monitoring response to treatment and development of infectious complications in companion animals. When using APPs for this purpose, the concept of a dose-response relationship between the magnitude of the underlying inflammation and serum concentrations of major APPs is important, because APP concentrations used for monitoring must reflect parallel changes in inflammatory activity. Strong indications of such a relationship have been shown in horses and dogs subjected to surgery of varying intensity,[8,104] in dogs with experimentally induced stomach ulcers,[105] in dogs with *Trypanosoma brucei* infection,[106] and in a study of 4 horses receiving 1 or 3 μg of lipopolysaccharide by intra-articular injection (see **Fig. 2**).[33] In all of these studies, the larger the inflammatory stimulus (surgical trauma, parasite burden, severity of ulceration, amount of lipopolysaccharide), the higher the serum concentrations of major APPs.

Response to treatment has been investigated in 2 studies on equine joint disease. Levels of SAA in synovial fluid decreased throughout the course of treatment in 3 horses with infectious joint disease[31] and were found to be lower after intra-articular (rather than intravenous) administration of morphine in horses with experimentally induced arthritis.[79] In the study of *R equi* pneumonia in foals,[83] a decrease in serum SAA concentrations paralleled successful treatment in 1 foal. Similar evidence at a case report level exists in canine medicine, in which a major APP was used successfully to monitor disease activity relevant to clinical decision making in a dog with type II immune-mediated polyarthritis[107] or with a pyogranuloma.[108] Potential clinical usefulness of canine CRP as a marker of treatment efficacy was also identified in a randomized-controlled clinical trial of novel treatment of inflammatory bowel disease in dogs.[109]

When APPs are used for monitoring occurrence of infectious complications in animals, it is important to first characterize the normal or expected APP response for the existing or underlying disease, so deviations from the expected response, such as sustained increases or further increases in APP concentrations, can be assessed. This characterization has been done in both dogs and horses, for which the bell-shaped response curves of several major and minor APPs were described in patients recovering uneventfully from surgery.[8,78,104,110–116] A study of horses undergoing castration showed that, in those classified clinically as having excessive postoperative inflammation, SAA levels remained increased for at least 8 days after surgery, whereas in horses classified as having an expected amount of postoperative inflammation, SAA levels returned to preoperative levels by day 8.[7] In dogs ovariohysterectomized for treatment of pyometra, the expected postoperative dynamics of CRP and SAA were shown.[117]

Even though some studies have reported very low or undetectable SAA levels in both neonatal (0–3 days old) and older foals,[82,116] several studies have shown slightly increased serum SAA levels (up to 120 mg/L) in healthy foals within the first 7 days of life.[84,115,118,119] The finding for healthy foals suggests that parturition is an inflammatory event, in which increased SAA concentration may be the result of trauma occurring during passage through the birth canal or caused by intestinal absorption of SAA (the protein has been found in colostrum).[11,120] However, in diseased foals, significant and sustained increases in serum SAA levels were found,[84,118,119] suggesting that SAA can be used to monitor the occurrence of disease complications even in the presence of physiologic inflammation during parturition.

In a study of experimental influenza infection, SAA concentrations were increased in the convalescent period in a subset of horses, but had returned to baseline levels in most horses. Some of the horses with persistently high SAA had clinical signs of secondary bacterial infection, suggesting that bacterial superinfection was the cause of the sustained SAA response.[121]

## SUMMARY

It is evident from review of the available literature on current clinical use and potential future use of major APPs in companion animals that, despite evidence being restricted almost solely to solidly proven excellent overlap performance (phase II) of these markers in detecting inflammatory activity, clinically relevant studies at higher evidence levels do exist. The available body of literature shows a clear, yet seemingly untapped, potential for more extended routine clinical use of major APP testing in companion animal medicine, as soon as practicability aspects of assays and medical conservatism are overcome. For research groups having extensive knowledge of major APPs in various clinical settings, these markers of inflammation already are a routine part of the diagnosis and monitoring of inflammatory diseases.

## REFERENCES

1. Esposito S, Tremolati E, Begliatti E, et al. Evaluation of a rapid bedside test for the quantitative determination of C-reactive protein. Clin Chem Lab Med 2005; 43(4):438–40.
2. Zecca E, Barone G, Corsello M, et al. Reliability of two different bedside assays for C-reactive protein in newborn infants. Clin Chem Lab Med 2009;47(9): 1081–4.
3. Jacobsen S, Kjelgaard-Hansen M. Evaluation of a commercially available apparatus for measuring the acute phase protein serum amyloid A in horses. Vet Rec 2008;163:327–30.
4. Kjelgaard-Hansen M. Clinical applicability of a point-of-care patient-side canine-specific commercially available quantitative assay for determination of C-reactive protein [abstract]. Vet Clin Pathol 2009;38(s1):E22.
5. Onishi T, Inokuma H, Ohno K, et al. C-reactive protein concentrations in normal and diseased dogs - measured by laser nephelometric immunoassay [in Japanese]. Nippon Juishikai Zasshi 2000;53(9):595–601.
6. Kushner I. The phenomenon of the acute phase response. Ann N Y Acad Sci 1982;38:939–48.
7. Jacobsen S, Jensen JC, Frei S, et al. Using serum amyloid A and other acute phase reactants to monitor the inflammatory response after castration in horses – a field study. Eq Vet J 2005;37(6):552–6.
8. Jacobsen S, Nielsen JV, Kjelgaard-Hansen M, et al. Acute phase response to surgery of varying intensity in horses: a preliminary study. Vet Surg 2009;38: 762–9.
9. Hobo S, Niwa H, Anzai T. Evaluation of serum amyloid A and surfactant protein D in sera for identification of the clinical condition in horses with bacterial pneumonia. J Vet Med Sci 2007;69(8):827–30.
10. Gabay C, Kushner I. Acute-phase proteins and other systemic response to inflammation. N Engl J Med 1999;340(6):448–54.
11. McDonald TL, Larson MA, Mack DR, et al. Elevated extrahepatic expression and secretion of mammary-associated serum amyloid A 3 (M-SAA3) into colostrum. Vet Immunol Immunopathol 2001;83:203–11.
12. Kumon Y, Suehiro T, Hashimoto K, et al. Local expression of acute phase serum amyloid A mRNA in rheumatoid arthritis synovial tissue and cells. J Rheumatol 1999;26:785–90.
13. Zerega B, Pagano A, Pianezzi A, et al. Expression of serum amyloid A in chondrocytes and myoblasts differentiation and inflammation: possible role in cholesterol homeostasis. Matrix Biol 2004;23:35–46.
14. Ramage L, Proudfoot L, Guy K. Expression of C-reactive protein in human lung epithelial cells and upregulation by cytokines and carbon particles. Inhal Toxicol 2004;16(9):607–13.
15. Vreugdenhil AC, Dentener MA, Snoek AM, et al. Lipopolysaccharide binding protein and serum amyloid A secretion by human intestinal epithelial cells during the acute phase response. J Immunol 1999;163:2792–8.
16. Benditt EP, Meek RL. Expression of the third member of the serum amyloid A gene family in mouse adipocytes. J Exp Med 1989;169:1841–6.
17. Christoffersen M, Baagoe CD, Jacobsen S, et al. Evaluation of the systemic acute phase response and endometrial gene expression of serum amyloid A and pro- and anti-inflammatory cytokines in mares with experimentally induced endometritis. Vet Immunol Immunopathol 2010;138(1–2):95–105.

18. Meek RL, Eriksen N, Benditt EP. Murine serum amyloid A$_3$ is a high density lipoprotein and is secreted by macrophages. Proc Natl Acad Sci U S A 1992;89:7949–52.

19. Urieli-Shoval S, Meek RL, Hanson RH, et al. Human serum amyloid A genes are expressed in monocyte/macrophage cell lines. Am J Pathol 1994;145(3): 650–60.

20. Jabs WJ, Lögering BA, Gerke P, et al. The kidney as a second site of human C-reactive protein formation in vivo. Eur J Immunol 2003;33(1):152–61.

21. Toussaint MJ, van Ederen AM, Gruys E. Implication of clinical pathology in assessment of animal health and in animal production and meat inspection. Comp Haematol Int 1995;5:149–57.

22. Gånheim C, Alenius S, Persson-Waller K. Acute phase proteins as indicators of calf herd health. Vet J 2007;173(3):645–51.

23. Petersen HH, Ersbøll AK, Jensen CS, et al. Serum haptoglobin concentration in Danish slaughter pigs of different health status. Prev Vet Med 2002;54:325–35.

24. Akerstedt M, Waller KP, Sternesjö A. Haptoglobin and serum amyloid A in bulk tank milk in relation to raw milk quality. J Dairy Res 2009;76(4):483–9.

25. Petersen HH, Nielsen JP, Heegaard PM. Application of acute phase protein measurements in veterinary clinical chemistry. Vet Res 2004;35:163–87.

26. Chamanza R, van Veen L, Tivapasi MT, et al. Acute phase proteins in the domestic fowl. Worlds Poult Sci J 1999;55:61–71.

27. Uhlar CM, Whitehead AS. Serum amyloid A, the major vertebrate acute-phase reactant. Eur J Biochem 1999;265:501–23.

28. Jacobsen S, Kjelgaard-Hansen M, Petersen HH, et al. Evaluation of a commercially available human serum amyloid A (SAA) turbidometric immunoassay for determination of equine SAA concentrations. Vet J 2006;172:315–9.

29. Kjelgaard-Hansen M, Jensen AL, Kristensen AT. Evaluation of a commercially available human C-reactive protein (CRP) turbidometric immunoassay for determination of canine serum CRP concentration. Vet Clin Pathol 2003;32(2):81–7.

30. Jacobsen S, Niewold TA, Kornalijnslijper E, et al. Kinetics of local and systemic isoforms of serum amyloid A in bovine mastitic milk. Vet Immunol Immunopathol 2005;104(1-2):21–31.

31. Jacobsen S, Halling-Thomsen M, Nanni S. Concentrations of serum amyloid A in serum and synovial fluid from healthy horses and horses with joint disease. Am J Vet Res 2006;67(10):1738–42.

32. Kjelgaard-Hansen M, Christensen MB, Lee MH, et al. Serum amyloid A isoforms in serum and synovial fluid from spontaneously diseased dogs with joint diseases or other conditions. Vet Immunol Immunopathol 2007;117(3–4): 296–301.

33. Jacobsen S, Niewold TA, Halling-Thomsen M, et al. Serum amyloid A isoforms in serum and synovial fluid in horses with lipopolysaccharide-induced arthritis. Vet Immunol Immunopathol 2005;110(3–4):325–30.

34. Kluve-Beckerman B, Drumm ML, Benson MD. Nonexpression of the human serum amyloid A three (SAA3) gene. DNA Cell Biol 1991;10(9):651–61.

35. Riley RF, Coleman MK. Isolation of C-reactive proteins of man monkey, rabbit and dog by affinity chromatography on phosphorylated cellulose. Clin Chim Acta 1970;30:483–96.

36. Riley RF, Zontine W. Further observations on the properties of dog C-reactive protein and the C-reactive protein response in the dog. J Lab Clin Med 1972; 80(5):698–703.

37. Caspi D, Baltz ML, Snel F, et al. Isolation and characterization of C-reactive protein from the dog. Immunology 1984;53(2):307–13.

38. Conner JG, Eckersall PD, Ferguson J, et al. Acute phase response in the dog following surgical trauma. Res Vet Sci 1988;45(1):107–10.
39. Yamamoto S, Tagata K, Nagahata H, et al. Isolation of canine C-reactive protein and characterization of its properties. Vet Immunol Immunopathol 1992;30(4):329–39.
40. Eckersall PD. Acute phase proteins: from research laboratory to clinic. Vet Clin Pathol 2010;39(1):1–2.
41. Yamamoto M, Miyaji S, Abe N, et al. Canine C-reactive protein (CRP) does not share common antigenicity with human CRP. Vet Res Commun 1993;17(4):258–66.
42. Yamamoto S, Tagata K, Otabbe K, et al. Serum levels of C-reactive protein in dogs and simple techniques for its measurement. Nippon Juishikai Zasshi 1993;46(10):870–3.
43. Concannon PW, Gimpel T, Newton L, et al. Postimplantation increase in plasma fibrinogen concentration with increase in relaxin concentration in pregnant dogs. Am J Vet Res 1996;57(9):1382–5.
44. Klenner S, Bauer N, Moritz A. Evaluation of three automated human immunotur-bidimetric assays for the detection of C-reactive protein in dogs. J Vet Diagn Invest 2010;22:544–52.
45. Kjelgaard-Hansen M. Comments on measurement of C-reactive protein in dogs [letter]. Vet Clin Pathol 2010;39:402–3.
46. Kjelgaard-Hansen M, Jensen AL, Kristensen AT. Internal quality control of a turbi-dimetric immunoassay for canine serum C-reactive protein based on pooled patient samples. Vet Clin Pathol 2004;33(3):139–44.
47. Nakamura M, Takahashi M, Ohno K, et al. C-reactive protein concentration in dogs with various diseases. J Vet Med Sci 2008;70(2):127–31.
48. Hansen AE, Schaap MK, Kjelgaard-Hansen M. Evaluation of a commercially available human serum amyloid A (SAA) turbidimetric immunoassay for determination of feline SAA concentration. Vet Res Commun 2006;30(8):863–72.
49. Woo P, Edbrooke M, Betts J, et al. Serum amyloid A gene regulation. In: Mackiewicz A, Kushner I, Baumann H, editors. Acute phase proteins. Molecular biology, biochemistry and clinical application. 1st edition. Boca Raton (FL): CRC Press; 1993. p. 397–408.
50. Ceron JJ, Martinez-Subiela S, Ohno K, et al. A seven-point plan for acute phase protein interpretation in companion animals. Vet J 2008;177(1):6–7.
51. Tamamoto T, Ohno K, Ohmi A, et al. Verification of measurement of the feline serum amyloid A (SAA) concentration by human SAA turbidimetric immuno-assay and its clinical application. J Vet Med Sci 2008;70(11):1247–52.
52. Evidence-based Medicine Working Group. Evidence-based medicine: a new approach to teaching the practice of medicine. JAMA 1992;268:2420–5.
53. Aragon CL, Budsberg SC. Applications of evidence-based medicine: cranial cruciate ligament injury repair in the dog. Vet Surg 2005;34(2):93–8.
54. Martensen RL. The effect of medical conservatism on the acceptance of impor-tant medical discoveries. JAMA 1996;276(24):1933.
55. Knottnerus JA, Dinant GJ. Medicine based evidence, a prerequisite for evidence based medicine. BMJ 1997;315(7116):1109–10.
56. Zweig MH, Robertson EA. Why we need better test evaluations. Clin Chem 1982;28(6):1272–6.
57. Fraser CG. Biological variation: from principles to practice. Washington, DC: AACC Press; 2001. p. 1–151.

58. Jensen AL, Kjelgaard-Hansen M. Diagnostic test validation. In: Weiss DJ, Wardrop KJ, editors. Schalm's veterinary hematology. 6th edition. Ames (IA): Blackwell; 2010. p. 1027–33.
59. Jensen AL, Kjelgaard-Hansen M. Method comparison in the clinical laboratory. Vet Clin Pathol 2006;35(3):276–86.
60. Fraser CG, Petersen PH. Analytical performance characteristics should be judged against objective quality specifications. Clin Chem 1999;45(3):321–3.
61. Kenny D, Fraser CG, Petersen PH, et al. Consensus agreement. Scand J Clin Lab Invest 1999;59:585.
62. Kjelgaard-Hansen M, Mikkelsen LF, Kristensen AT, et al. Study on biological variability of five acute phase reactants in dogs. Comp Clin Path 2003;12(2):69–74.
63. Kjelgaard-Hansen M, Jensen AL. Subjectivity in defining quality specifications for quality control and test validation. Vet Clin Pathol 2010;39(2):134–5.
64. McGrotty YL, Knottenbelt CM, Ramsey IK, et al. Evaluation of a rapid assay for canine C-reactive protein. Vet Rec 2004;154(6):175–6.
65. Kjelgaard-Hansen M, Stadler M, Jensen AL. Canine serum C-reactive protein detected by means of a near-patient test for human C-reactive protein. J Small Anim Pract 2008;49(6):282–6.
66. Bossuyt PM, Reitsma JB, Bruns DE, et al. Towards complete and accurate reporting of studies of diagnostic accuracy: the STARD initiative. Standards for reporting of diagnostic accuracy. Clin Chem 2003;49(1):1–6.
67. Bossuyt PM, Reitsma JB, Bruns DE, et al. The STARD statement for reporting studies of diagnostic accuracy: explanation and elaboration. Clin Chem 2003; 49(1):7–18.
68. Christopher MM. Improving the quality of reporting of studies of diagnostic accuracy: let's STARD now. Vet Clin Pathol 2007;36(1):6.
69. Wiinberg B, Jensen AL, Johansson PI, et al. Development of a model based scoring system for diagnosis of canine disseminated intravascular coagulation with independent assessment of sensitivity and specificity. Vet J 2010;185(3): 292–8.
70. Smidt N, Overbeke J, de Vet H, et al. Endorsement of the STARD Statement by biomedical journals: survey of instructions for authors. Clin Chem 2007;63(11): 1983–5.
71. Uzzan B, Cohen R, Nicolas P, et al. Procalcitonin as a diagnostic test for sepsis in critically ill adults and after surgery or trauma: a systematic review and meta-analysis. Crit Care Med 2006;34(7):1996–2003.
72. He LP, Tang XY, Ling WH, et al. Early C-reactive protein in the prediction of long-term outcomes after acute coronary syndromes: a meta-analysis of longitudinal studies. Heart 2010;96(5):339–46.
73. Jergens AE, Schreiner CA, Frank DE, et al. A scoring index for disease activity in canine inflammatory bowel disease. J Vet Intern Med 2003;17(3):291–7.
74. Ceron JJ, Eckersall PD, Martynez-Subiela S. Acute phase proteins in dogs and cats: current knowledge and future perspectives. Vet Clin Pathol 2005;34(2): 85–99.
75. Murata H, Shimada N, Yoshioka M. Current research on acute phase proteins in veterinary diagnosis: an overview. Vet J 2004;168(1):28–40.
76. Jacobsen S, Andersen PH. The acute phase protein serum amyloid A (SAA) as a marker of inflammation in horses. Eq Vet Edu 2007;19(1):38–46.
77. Paltrinieri S. The feline acute phase reaction. Vet J 2008;177:26–35.
78. Pepys MB, Baltz ML, Tennent GA. Serum amyloid A (SAA) in horses: objective measurement of the acute phase response. Eq Vet J 1989;21(2):106–9.

79. Lindegaard C, Bech-Gleerup KC, Thomsen MH, et al. Anti-inflammatory effect of intra-articular morphine in a model of induced equine arthritis. Am J Vet Res 2010;71(1):69–75.
80. Higgins MA, Berridge BR, Mills BJ, et al. Gene expression analysis of the acute phase response using a canine microarray. Toxicol Sci 2003;74(2):470–84.
81. Kajikawa T, Furuta A, Onishi T, et al. Changes in concentrations of serum amyloid A protein, alpha 1-acid glycoprotein, haptoglobin, and C-reactive protein in feline sera due to induced inflammation and surgery. Vet Immunol Immunopathol 1999;68(1):91–8.
82. Chavatte PM, Pepys MB, Roberts B, et al. Measurement of serum amyloid A protein (SAA) as an aid to differential diagnosis of infection in newborn foals. In: Plowright W, Rossdale PD, Wade JF, editors. Proceedings of the 6th International Conference on Infectious Diseases. Newmarket (UK): R&W Publications; 1991. p. 33–8.
83. Hultén C, Demmers S. Serum amyloid A (SAA) as an aid in the management of infectious disease in the foal: comparison with total leukocyte count, neutrofil count and fibrinogen. Eq Vet J 2002;34(7):693–8.
84. Stoneham SJ, Palmer L, Cash R, et al. Measurement of serum amyloid A in the neonatal foal using a latex agglutination immunoturbidometric assay: determination of the normal range, variation with age and response to disease. Eq Vet J 2001;33(6):599–603.
85. Gardner RB, Nydam DV, Luna JA, et al. Serum opsonization capacity, phagocytosis, and oxidative burst activity in neonatal foals in the intensive care unit. J Vet Intern Med 2007;21:797–805.
86. Cohen ND, Chaffin MK, Vandenplas ML, et al. Study of serum amyloid A concentrations as a means of achieving early diagnosis of Rhodococcus equi pneumonia. Eq Vet J 2005;37(3):212–6.
87. Vandenplas ML, Moore JN, Barton MH, et al. Concentrations of serum amyloid A and lipopolysaccharide-binding protein in horses with colic. Am J Vet Res 2005; 66(9):1509–16.
88. Mansfield CS, James FE, Robertson ID. Development of a clinical severity index for dogs with acute pancreatitis. J Am Vet Med Assoc 2008;233(6):936–44.
89. Jergens AE. Clinical assessment of disease activity for canine inflammatory bowel disease. J Am Anim Hosp Assoc 2004;40(6):437–45.
90. Bathen-Noethen A, Carlson R, Menzel D, et al. Concentrations of acute-phase proteins in dogs with steroid responsive meningitis-arteritis. J Vet Intern Med 2008;22(5):1149–56.
91. Lowrie M, Penderis J, McLaughlin M, et al. Steroid responsive meningitis-arteritis: a prospective study of potential disease markers, prednisolone treatment, and long-term outcome in 20 dogs (2006–2008). J Vet Intern Med 2009;23(4): 862–70.
92. Sasaki K, Ma Z, Khatlani TS, et al. Evaluation of feline serum amyloid A (SAA) as an inflammatory marker. J Vet Med Sci 2003;65(4):545–8.
93. Paltrinieri S, Giordano A, Tranquillo V, et al. Critical assessment of the diagnostic value of feline alpha1-acid glycoprotein for feline infectious peritonitis using the likelihood ratios approach. J Vet Diagn Invest 2007;19(3):266–72.
94. Busk P, Jacobsen S, Martinussen T. Administration of perioperative penicillin reduces postoperative serum amyloid A response in horses being castrated standing. Vet Surg 2010;39:628–43.
95. Amar D, Zhang H, Park B, et al. Inflammation and outcome after general thoracic surgery. Eur J Cardiothorac Surg 2008;32:431–4.

96. Hashimoto K, Ikeda Y, Korenaga D, et al. The impact of preoperative serum C-reactive protein on the prognosis of patients with hepatocellular carcinoma. Cancer 2005;103:1856–64.

97. Shiu YC, Lin JK, Huang CJ, et al. Is C-reactive protein a prognostic factor of colorectal cancer? Dis Colon Rectum 2008;51:443–9.

98. Richard EA, Fortier GD, Pitel P-H, et al. Sub-clinical diseases affecting performance in Standardbred trotters: Diagnostic methods and predictive parameters. Vet J 2010;184:282–9.

99. Griebsch C, Arndt G, Raila J, et al. C-reactive protein concentration in dogs with primary immune-mediated hemolytic anemia. Vet Clin Pathol 2009;38(4):421–5.

100. Mitchell KD, Kruth SA, Wood RD, et al. Serum acute phase protein concentrations in dogs with autoimmune hemolytic anemia. J Vet Intern Med 2009; 23(3):585–91.

101. Chan DL, Rozanski EA, Freeman LM. Relationship among plasma amino acids, C-reactive protein, illness severity, and outcome in critically ill dogs. J Vet Intern Med 2009;23(3):559–63.

102. Gebhardt C, Hirschberger J, Rau S, et al. Use of C-reactive protein to predict outcome in dogs with systemic inflammatory response syndrome or sepsis. J Vet Emerg Crit Care (San Antonio) 2009;19(5):450–8.

103. Koster LS, Van SM, Goddard A, et al. C-reactive protein in canine babesiosis caused by *Babesia rossi* and its association with outcome. J S Afr Vet Assoc 2009;80(2):87–91.

104. Kjelgaard-Hansen M, Strom H, Mikkelsen LF, et al. Grading of surgical trauma by means of canine C-reactive protein measurements. Vet Clin Pathol 2008; 37(s1):6.

105. Otabe K, Ito T, Sugimoto T, et al. C-reactive protein (CRP) measurement in canine serum following experimentally-induced acute gastric mucosal injury. Lab Anim 2000;34:434–8.

106. Ndung'u JM, Eckersall PD, Jennings FW. Elevation of the concentration of acute phase proteins in dogs infected with *Trypanosoma brucei*. Acta Trop 1991; 49(2):77–86.

107. Kjelgaard-Hansen M, Jensen AL, Houser GA, et al. Use of serum C-reactive protein as an early marker of inflammatory activity in canine type II immune-mediated polyarthritis: case report. Acta Vet Scand 2006;48(1):9–12.

108. Yuki M, Hirano T. Use of a combination of prednisolone and rosuvastatin for treatment of a pyogranuloma in a dog. J Am Vet Med Assoc 2010;236(7):767–9.

109. Jergens AE, Crandell J, Morrison JA, et al. Comparison of oral prednisone and prednisone combined with metronidazole for induction therapy of canine inflammatory bowel disease: a randomized-controlled trial. J Vet Intern Med 2010;24: 269–77.

110. Serin G, Ulutas PA. Measurement of serum acute phase proteins to monitor postoperative recovery in anoestrous bitches after ovariohysterectomy. Vet Rec 2010;166(1):20–2.

111. Allen BV, Kold SE. Fibrinogen response to surgical tissue trauma in the horse. Eq Vet J 1988;20(6):441–3.

112. Dabrowski R, Wawron W, Kostro K. Changes in CRP, SAA and haptoglobin produced in response to ovariohysterectomy in healthy bitches and those with pyometra. Theriogenology 2007;67(2):321–7.

113. Eurell TE, Wilson DA, Baker GJ. The effect of exploratory laparotomy on the serum and peritoneal haptoglobin concentrations of the pony. Can J Vet Res 1993;57:42–4.

114. Miller MS, Moritz A, Röcken M, et al. Bestimmung von Serum-Amyloid A, Hapto-globin und Fibrinogen als Entzündungsparameter nach Kastration von Hengsten [Evaluation of serum amyloid A, haptoglobin and Fibrinogen as inflammatory markers after castration of stallions]. Tierärztl Prax 2007;35(G):69–74.

115. Nunokawa Y, Fujinaga T, Taira T, et al. Evaluation of serum amyloid A protein as an acute-phase reactive protein in horses. J Vet Med Sci 1993;55(6):1011–6.

116. Pollock PJ, Prendergast M, Schumacher J, et al. Effects of surgery on the acute phase response in clinically normal and diseased horses. Vet Rec 2005;156: 538–42.

117. Dabrowski R, Kostro K, Lisiecka U, et al. Usefulness of C-reactive protein, serum amyloid A component, and haptoglobin determinations in bitches with pyometra for monitoring early post-ovariohysterectomy complications. Theriogenology 2009;72(4):471–6.

118. Duggan VE, Holyoak GR, MacAllister CG, et al. Influence of induction of partu-rition on the neonatal acute phase response in foals. Theriogenology 2007;67: 372–81.

119. Paltrinieri S, Giordano A, Villani M, et al. Influence of age and foaling on plasma protein electrophoresis and serum amyloid A and their possible role as markers of neonatal septicaemia. Vet J 2008;176:393–6.

120. Duggan VE, Holyoak GR, MacAllister CG, et al. Amyloid A in equine colostrum and early milk. Vet Immunol Immunopathol 2008;121:150–5.

121. Hultén C, Sandgren B, Skioldebrand E, et al. The acute phase protein serum amyloid A (SAA) as an inflammatory marker in equine influenza virus infection. Acta Vet Scand 1999;40(4):323–33.

122. Crisman MV, Scarratt WK, Zimmerman KL. Blood proteins and inflammation in the horse. Vet Clin North Am Equine Pract 2008;24(2):285–97.

123. Jacobsen S, Andersen PH, Toelboell T, et al. Dose dependency and individual variability of the lipopolysaccharide-induced bovine acute phase protein response. J Dairy Sci 2004;87(10):3330–9.

124. Heegaard PM, Klausen J, Nielsen JP, et al. The porcine acute phase response to infection with *Actinobacillus pleuropneumoniae*. Haptoglobin, C-reactive protein, major acute phase protein and serum amyloid A protein are sensitive indicators of infection. Comp Biochem Physiol B Biochem Mol Biol 1998; 119(2):365–73.

125. Skovgaard K, Mortensen S, Boye M, et al. Rapid and widely disseminated acute phase protein response after experimental bacterial infection of pigs. Vet Res 2009;40(3):23.

# Infectious and Zoonotic Disease Testing in Pet Birds

Carolyn Cray, PhD

**KEYWORDS**

• Aspergillosis • Avian • Bird • Bornavirus • Chlamydophilosis
• Mycobacteriosis

Market research statistics place pet bird ownership at 11 to 16 million birds in the United States, with the average annual visits to a veterinarian at less than 1 and an average annual visit expenditure of $25.[1] New pet owners, especially those purchasing their first bird, are often uninformed as to how to care for them properly and what potential health problems these special pets may present.[2] Little attention may be given to potential zoonotic diseases, which are increasingly recognized to be carried and transmitted by exotic pets and wildlife species.[3] Pet birds have been famously noted for the transmission of psittacosis, or parrot fever.[4] The diagnosis of this and other infectious diseases continues to be problematic. Although the true effect of the major avian infectious diseases on public health cannot be completely assessed, it is notable that veterinary diagnostic laboratories struggle to diagnose infectious agents similar to those diagnosed by their medical laboratory counterparts, including mycobacteria and *Aspergillus* spp. Unlike in domestic animals, diagnostic testing in avian species remains in the early stages of development with little validation or standardization,which is a major complication in the diagnosis of avian disease and, in turn, in understanding the possible zoonotic potential of the clinically ill bird.

This article describes the current status of laboratory diagnostic testing for aspergillosis, mycobacteriosis, chlamydophilosis (psittacosis), and bornavirus infection, the major infectious diseases affecting pet birds. The special challenges involved in the diagnostic testing of pet birds are emphasized. By drawing attention to both the importance and often difficulty of diagnosing these serious and potentially zoonotic infectious diseases, it is hoped that future efforts and collaborations can be maximized to optimize and improve testing.

The author has nothing to disclose.
Division of Comparative Pathology, Department of Pathology, University of Miami Miller School of Medicine, PO Box 016960 R-46, Miami, FL 33101, USA
*E-mail address:* c.cray@miami.edu

## SPECIAL CHALLENGES IN AVIAN DIAGNOSTIC TESTING

Avian species present special challenges to veterinary diagnostic laboratories. First is the frequent acquisition of very–low volume samples. Heparinized plasma is commonly used in avian medicine for serologic and biochemical determinations because the collection of serum often results in large fibrin clots and latent fibrin formation that can affect test results and further decrease sample volume, thus reducing the number of tests that may be performed.[5,6] Many veterinary practitioners prefer heparinized samples because they can also be used for a complete blood cell count, so heparinized whole blood and plasma are common specimens for infectious disease testing. In some cases, veterinarians may resort to diluting samples to obtain sufficient volume for the desired panel of diagnostic tests, which can adversely affect results.[7]

Lack of species-specific reagents also can be especially problematic when working with avian, exotic, and wildlife species. This problem often requires laboratories to use less sensitive and sometimes more laborious methods for infectious disease testing, such as immunodiffusion, agglutination, complement fixation (CF), and neutralization testing. Species-specific polyclonal and monoclonal antibodies would be preferred reagents so that more sensitive techniques such as enzyme-linked immunosorbent assay (ELISA) could be used, but the number of different avian species defies the production of such materials.[8–10] Anti–chicken IgG has been used with variable success depending on the commercial vendor.[11,12] One anti–chicken IgG reagent was found to cross-react with IgG in 47 species from 21 different avian orders, although a second anti–chicken IgG and an anti–macaw IgG preparation had no reactivity.[11] It is notable that several studies have been published without prevalidation of the anti–avian immunoglobulin reagents.[13,14]

Finally, infectious disease testing in pet birds lacks the standardization necessary to ensure consistency and accuracy of results across laboratories and methods partly due to the lack of commercially available reagents and partly due to the lack of published methods. Many antigens cannot be purchased and require production at the laboratory level, resulting in considerable variations in serologic methods and results. In avian diagnostics, only the ELISA kits for antigen detection developed for the human clinical pathology market have allowed for some degree of reproducible testing between laboratories (see sections on aspergillosis and chlamydophilosis later).

## INFECTIOUS DISEASE TESTING
### Aspergillosis

Although aspergillosis is uncommon in humans except for severely immunocompromised patients, it has been reported in several mammalian species including dogs, horses, cows, and dolphins.[15] In birds, aspergillosis is a major cause of morbidity and mortality with a wide species range.[16] Although perhaps more prevalent in captive waterfowl and penguins, aspergillosis has been well documented in pet birds. Both acute and chronic forms have been recognized. Whereas acute infection can result in severe respiratory compromise because of a large exposure to fungal spores, chronic infection, in which the disease develops slowly over a long period, is a more frequent cause of death in pet birds. Infection may be focal or generalized. In some cases, respiratory distress is readily evident along with lethargy and changes in vocalization. Hematologic changes may include leukocytosis and anemia, and plasma liver enzyme and creatine kinase activities may be increased.[17] Radiography and endoscopy are common testing options, although the latter is problematic in severely ill birds.

In veterinary medicine, serologic testing for aspergillosis has been reported in horses, dogs, and birds.[18–26] Methodologies have included agarose gel immunodiffusion (AGID) and ELISA. AGID offers the ability to test any animal species because a species-specific conjugating antibody is not needed, but it is relatively insensitive when compared with ELISA.[18] Antemortem diagnostic testing of avian species was first used in the early 1990s with the description of an antibody ELISA.[19] ELISA methods have also been used to describe the high incidence of anti-Aspergillus antibody in captive and wild penguin species.[22,27,28] Antibody production in immunized and experimentally infected birds was studied using this method, in which it was generally concluded that the value of antibody detection in some avian species was low.[23,26]

In the United States, anti-Aspergillus antibody ELISA is currently available at the author's laboratory (Division of Comparative Pathology, University of Miami, Miami, FL, USA) where the results of this technique are reported as index of reactivity (sample absorbance/absorbance of a pool of negative control samples). Recently, a multiyear study of the antibody ELISA reactivity in more than 1300 avian samples was reported.[20] The samples were categorized into 4 groups: psittaciform (ie, parrot/pet bird), raptor (ie, hawk, eagle, and owl), penguin, and zoo species (ie, land and water-fowl). Significantly higher levels of antibody were observed in the raptor, penguin, and zoo species groups compared with a mean negative antibody index in the pet bird group. These data indicate that anti-Aspergillus antibody can be found normally in some species of birds. A smaller study was further conducted using approximately 300 cases for which clinical information was available, allowing them to be categorized as presumptive normal or confirmed infected.[20] There was no statistical difference in the mean antibody indices in those groups, although the confirmed infected birds were more likely to be positive for aspergillosis than the presumptive normal birds. The findings of this study were consistent with those of a smaller study of 7 parrots with confirmed aspergillosis.[29] In summary, although ELISA seems to have limited value as a single test for detecting avian aspergillosis, it might have applicability in parrots because most parrot species are seronegative such that the presence of antibody would be considered unusual and possibly clinically relevant.

In mammals, it has been proposed that $T_H1$ or macrophage modulation rather than antibody production is more important in managing fungal infection.[30] Antibody levels may also be affected by the release of mycotoxins secreted during fungal replication.[31] Additional studies are underway in the author's laboratory to broaden the database of confirmed results to include different avian species and different types of infection. The value of this type of testing may be further refined with modifications to the ELISA to increase its sensitivity as well as with testing for specific antigens (rather than the present method of testing for bulk antigen) via ELISA or Western blot.

New assays for the diagnosis of avian aspergillosis have been adapted from advancements made in human clinical pathology testing through the use of the commercial antigen detection ELISA kit, Platelia Aspergillus (Bio-Rad Laboratories, Redmond, WA, USA), which detects circulating galactomannan. This test has been widely applied for the diagnosis of invasive aspergillosis in immunocompromised human patients.[32,33] The test detects β-galactofuranose, which is secreted into the blood during replication of the organism.[1–5] The assay uses a pretreatment step to unlock antigen-antibody complexes, and the result is reported as an index rather than as a titer. Through 2006, the manufacturer recommended using a positive cutoff value of 1.5 or 1.0, but this was later changed to 0.5 to improve the sensitivity of the assay with human specimens.[32] Studies using this assay have been conducted in many animal species. In dogs, a high incidence of antibody to *Aspergillus* sp was reported, but with a variable presence (index) of galactomannan.[21] Horses also often tested positive for the antibody, but in the absence of galactomannan.[25] However, dogs and horses with systemic aspergillosis had a higher incidence of galactomannan positivity. In cows with experimental or natural aspergillus infection that resulted in systemic disease, galactomannan was frequently detected.[34,35]

In an early study of experimental infection in ducks with a research-based galactomannan ELISA, the high predictive value of this type of assay in birds was first noted.[23] Using a high cutoff value of 1.0, a study was conducted on parrot samples using the commercial ELISA kit.[24,36] The investigators reported a sensitivity of 30% and a specificity of 86%. Birds in the poorest clinical condition had the highest galactomannan indices. This observation is consistent with that in other species and laboratory animal models in which galactomannan values were suggested to be associated with the level of fungal burden.[32,35] The ELISA kit was also used to study a large colony of falcons.[37] Using the high cutoff value of 1.0, the assay had a sensitivity of 12% and a specificity of 85%. Recently, the author's group published a large avian study using the Platelia kit and a cutoff index of 0.5.[38] Specimens from many parrot species had weakly positive results, whereas mostly negative results were obtained in penguin, raptor, and zoo species. The author's group proposed that this might be caused by the presence of high levels of circulating antibody in the latter groups of species, which may effectively clear galactomannan from the circulation. In an extension of this study, more than 2.4-fold higher mean galactomannan indices were found in birds with confirmed aspergillosis in contrast to presumptive normal birds. The overall test sensitivity and specificity were 67% and 73%, respectively. When the cutoff was increased to 1.0, the reanalyzed results were consistent with those of other published avian studies.

Based on the overall study data, the current positive cutoff for the diagnosis of aspergillosis has been raised to 0.7 for avian samples, although this may be refined with future studies in which larger sample sizes from different avian species can be obtained and analyzed. The galactomannan ELISA has been recognized in human medicine to be an imperfect test, with some cross-reactivity with other microbial antigens, potential for environmental contamination of patients through food and air, and interference by certain medications and treatments.[32,39] In addition, the sensitivity of the assay can be complicated by the site of infection, the antifungal treatments, and the phase of replication of the organism.[32,39] These issues are likely complicating factors in avian patients also. To this point, negative galactomannan levels were reported in birds with tracheal granulomas caused by *Aspergillus* sp in contrast to birds having air sac and lung involvement, which had quite high indices.[40] The presence of antibody in avian patients is also likely a complicating factor because most birds with a high antibody titer have a negative galactomannan index.

Protein electrophoresis (EPH) has been used as an adjunct test for avian aspergillosis to detect the presence of an ongoing acute phase response.[38,40] In the serosurvey described earlier,[38] samples from most pet birds had normal electrophoretograms. EPH results from presumptive normal birds, however, were significantly different from those of birds with confirmed infection; 30% of normal birds had abnormal EPH results, whereas 72% of birds with confirmed aspergillosis had abnormal results. A moderate to marked increase in β-globulin concentration was the predominant change and the test had a sensitivity of 73% and specificity of 70% for infection. These results were consistent with those in 2 smaller studies of aspergillosis in parrot species.[29,40]

Other testing options are also being drawn from the human medical laboratory including antigen testing for β-glucan, a major cell wall component in many fungal species including *Aspergillus*. Recently, a commercial assay has been developed to detect 1, 3-β-D glucan.[41] Although the use of β-glucan in laboratory animal models of aspergillosis has been documented, its application in veterinary medicine remains unpublished.[42] In a large study of chickens with confirmed *Aspergillus flavus* infection, the value of this test seemed limited because high levels of β-glucan were found in all birds, including those that were confirmed to not be infected (H.L. Shivaprasad, BVSc, MS, PhD, California Animal Health and Food Safety Laboratory, Tulare, CA, personal communication, March 2010). The same study showed significantly higher galacto-mannan and antibody levels in infected birds. In contrast, a study of 13 confirmed aspergillosis positive and 42 aspergillosis-negative seabirds from a rehabilitation center showed significantly higher levels of both galactomannan and β-glucan as well as abnormal EPH results (Julia Burco, DVM, MPVM, PhD, Oregon Department of Fish and Wildlife, Corvallis, OR, personal communication, May 2010).

Polymerase chain reaction (PCR) has also been used for the diagnosis of aspergil-losis in avian species and is offered at some veterinary diagnostic laboratories. However, testing is not standardized, a problem that also currently plagues the imple-mentation of this test in medical laboratories.[43] PCR is perhaps best applied to biopsy and necropsy tissues and to swab specimens of the trachea or air sac; testing of blood samples has yielded variable results. Negative PCR results in a blood sample should not be used to rule out the possibility of infection (Bob Dahlhausen, DVM, Veterinary Molecular Diagnostics, Inc, Milford, OH, personal communication, May 2010).

Because no single test offers 100% sensitivity and specificity and infection may occur in different forms, a test panel may be the most beneficial to the avian patient as it is to the human patient with aspergillosis (**Table 1**). When the serodiagnostic panel of antibody, galactomannan, and EPH were combined, sensitivity was increased over that of individual tests (C.Cray, unpublished observations, 2010). Several novel technologies and investigations are underway in medical clinical pathology, which will likely benefit avian aspergillosis diagnostics in the future. This advancement will aid the current multidimensional approach using routine clinical pathology testing, radiography, biopsy, and serologic testing to make a diagnosis.

### Chlamydophilosis

Psittacosis or parrot fever (chlamydophilosis) is caused by *Chlamydophila psittaci*. The disease was first recognized in the United States in the early 1900s and has been linked to a few large outbreaks in humans including one pandemic caused by expo-sure to infected pet birds. The severity of the disease in humans may range from subclinical infection to mild illness to systemic illness with severe pneumonia. Infection more commonly occurs with domiciliary or occupational contact. In 1995, a large group of birds was shipped to a pet store chain in Georgia.[44] One of these birds subse-quently died and was determined to have chlamydophilosis. Local health officials

| Table 1 |
| --- |
| Summary of antemortem diagnostic testing options for avian infectious diseases within the United States |

| Disease | Testing Options |
| --- | --- |
| Aspergillosis | Antibody (ELISA, AGID), antigen (ELISA), PCR, culture |
| Chlamydophilosis | Antibody (CF, IFA), antigen (ELISA, MIF), PCR, culture |
| Mycobacteriosis | Antibody (Western blot, research), PCR, culture |
| Bornavirus infection | Antibody (Western blot, research), PCR |

*Abbreviations:* AGID, agarose gel immunodiffusion; CF, complement fixation; ELISA, enzyme-linked immunosorbent assay; IFA, indirect immunofluorescence assay; MIF, microimmunofluores-cence; PCR, polymerase chain reaction.

conducted an extensive follow-up of all individuals who had purchased birds from the same shipment. They found an attack rate of acute respiratory illness of 10.7% and clinical illness or seroconversion in 31% of exposed households. The effect of psittacosis on public health is difficult to determine, even though this is a reportable disease in many countries.[45] Awareness of the disease by physicians is often low, and symptoms in humans can be highly variable. In the United States, the National Association of State Public Health Veterinarians issues a compendium of measures to control infection among birds and humans.[46] This compendium can serve as a key reference point for available diagnostic testing options.

As with other chlamydial organisms, C psittaci is an obligate intracellular bacterium. Although perhaps more known for infecting parrots (psittacine birds), a high infection rate has also been documented in pigeons.[47] In total, more than 460 bird species in 30 orders have been shown to be susceptible to infection, including several wild bird species.[47,48] Transmission occurs with close proximity because the agent is excreted in feces and nasal discharges. Infection may be subclinical, acute, or chronic. Acute infection is characterized by fever, lethargy, anorexia, and bright green fecal droppings (the latter because of biliverdin, the main breakdown product of heme in birds).[47,49] Birds with chronic infection may not show clinical signs until stressed; infections often manifest as conjunctivitis, enteritis, pneumonitis, and hepatitis.[47] Clinical signs may vary with species, age, and presence of environmental stressors, which can confound diagnosis.[50,51] Leukocytosis, increased liver enzyme activities, and increased bile acids concentrations are usually observed.[51]

The diagnosis of chlamydophilosis remains a problem in avian medicine. During the past 20 years, numerous attempts have been made to develop a sensitive and specific test for the causative agent. Diagnostic options at present in the United States include 2 serologic assays, PCR on blood or on swabs from the choana (the avian nasopharynx) or the cloaca (the common cavity in birds through which feces, urine, and reproductive discharges pass), antigen capture ELISA, and culture (see **Table 1**). Culture has been considered for several years as the gold standard, although false-negative results caused by intermittent shedding and organism lability have undermined this assertion.

Early antemortem diagnostic tests were based on traditional means of detecting a humoral immune response. Serologic assays include elementary body agglutination (EBA), latex agglutination (LA), CF, indirect immunofluorescence assay (IFA), and blocking ELISA. Results of EBA, LA, and CF were compared as part of a retrospective study of 119 cases.[52] The EBA assay had the highest specificity for IgM, making it a more appropriate test for diagnosis of acute infection. Using single sample analysis of each case, the EBA test had a sensitivity of 94% and a specificity of 61%. When paired samples were analyzed for increasing titers using the IgG-specific LA and CF tests, 61% of infected birds had a significant change in titer compared with 5% of clinically normal birds. An IFA using anti–chicken IgG with broad avian reactivity was developed based on a previously reported method.[11,53,54] Using this method, 9% of pet birds were found to be positive for the infection (C.Cray, unpublished observations, 2010). The method also was applied in an outbreak at a pet store during which 16 birds were evaluated within 1 month after the histologic confirmation of infection in 1 bird.[54] Of the 16 birds, 7 had negative EBA results and positive IFA results while 2 had positive EBA results and positive IFA results. The discrepancy of results between EBA and IFA likely reflect the differential measurement of IgM and IgG in EBA and IFA, respectively, and the period after infection at which testing occurred. Of note, 2 of the birds seroconverted in the absence of clinical signs. This observation may reflect a possible carrier state or exposure resulting in antibody production, both of which have been proposed as particular diagnostic dilemmas for IgG-based serologic tests.[54,55] An ELISA using recombinant chlamydial proteins has also been described and has apparent high sensitivity and specificity.[56] At the time of writing, only CF and IFA are available at veterinary diagnostic laboratories in the United States.

Antigen-based assays for birds originated with the use of microimmunofluorescence (MIF) of smears made from the conjunctiva, cloaca, or choana. In the 1990s, lateral flow ELISAs for the detection of *Chlamydia trachomatis* were developed and found to be useful because they did cross-react with *C psittaci*. In a study of 246 birds with positive rates of infection of 4% to 9%, the sensitivity was 75% and specificity ranged from 85% to 96% depending on the source of the sample for ELISA.[57] The diagnostic accuracy of lateral flow ELISA is impaired by intermittent shedding of the organism and antigen degradation as well as potential false-positive results caused by the presence other bacterial flora. Although not commonly used, the test is offered at veterinary diagnostic laboratories, primarily as a rapid (screening) test option.

More recent advances in the diagnosis of chlamydophilosis in pet birds have included PCR detection methods, which have mostly supplanted the use of the antigen detection assays. PCR methods have been developed for the detection of *C psittaci*–specific DNA and are reported to be valid with both fecal and tissue samples.[58,59] PCR and antigen ELISA were found to be superior to cell culture, and PCR assays seemed to be useful to exclude potential false-positive ELISA results. The higher sensitivity of PCR as compared with culture was reported in studies of wild birds.[60] Similarly, the higher sensitivity of PCR compared with embryonated egg culture and MIF was reported in studies of pet birds.[61] One report found poor comparative performance between tissue and fecal specimens.[62]

PCR testing for chlamydophilosis has become prevalent in the avian veterinary community, although it was first regarded with suspicion.[63] To the author's knowledge, no epidemiologic investigations have been published regarding the incidence of PCR-positive results in avian populations. At the time of writing, PCR is readily available at many veterinary diagnostic laboratories, but there has been no standardization of methodologies. Many practitioners use it both as a diagnostic test for clinically ill birds as well as a screening test for apparently normal birds. The latter may be especially problematic, given the intermittent shedding of the organism in chronically infected birds. With potential differences among avian species and among individual patients, including other concurrent diseases and previous treatment, there may be no best test for this condition. Therefore, it is still recommended that a combination of test methods be used to screen and test for chlamydophilosis.[46]

### Mycobacteriosis

As with chlamydophilosis, mycobacteriosis is a potential zoonotic disease for humans who own pet birds. In one case, an Amazon parrot was presented with proliferative skin lesions and was euthanized because of general poor health.[64] Histologic examination revealed acid-fast bacteria in the skin lesions and several granulomas throughout the carcass. The owners had pulmonary tuberculosis and had recently completed treatment. *Mycobacterium tuberculosis* was identified through culture, and restriction fragment length polymorphism analysis and mycobacterial interspersed repetitive units subtyping indicated that isolates from both the owner and pet bird were the same. Other studies have suggested that pet birds have contracted the disease from their infected owners.[65] Although the overall public health implications of avian mycobacteriosis remain to be assessed, it is notable that mycobacterial infection in pet birds and other exotic animals has zoonotic potential.[66]

Mycobacterial infections have been recognized in both captive and wild avian species with a worldwide distribution.[65] Species differences in susceptibility to infection may be because of immunogenetics and the presence of stressors related to poor husbandry practices.[65,67] Clinical signs vary widely, with the most consistent finding being weight loss. Outbreaks are not common—the disease usually affects only individual birds within a collection or household.[68] A recent report of mycobacteriosis in zoo birds found a very low disease incidence of 3.5% and concluded that the infection was not easily transmitted.[69] Using molecular fingerprinting methods, a diversity of strain types was observed in the same collection of birds, indicating that infection was likely acquired independently.[70] In a large multiyear study of more than 5000 birds that underwent necropsy, the incidence of mycobacteriosis was reported as 3.8%.[71] Studies using the more recent applications of molecular techniques have noted a predominance of *Mycobacterium genavense*.[72,73]

Antemortem diagnosis of mycobacteriosis is problematic because of variation in disease presentation, lack of adequate diagnostic tests, and difficulty obtaining positive cultures (see **Table 1**).[67] Intradermal testing is especially problematic in avian species because of the presence of feathers and has been described to have low sensitivity for mycobacteriosis.[65,68] Lymphocytosis and anemia can be present in infected birds but are also commonly observed with other inflammatory conditions.[65,68] Increased liver enzyme activities may also be present depending on the extent of tissue involvement.[67,68] Fecal smears can be stained to examine for acid-fast bacteria; however, negative results are commonly observed in birds positive for the infection. Routine cultures of all mycobacterial species are difficult, although culture techniques have been greatly aided by new molecular methodologies developed for human isolates; however, the latter technology is not readily available in most veterinary diagnostic laboratories.[68] Radiography, endoscopy, and biopsy remain the standard tests for diagnosis.[67,68]

Antemortem and postmortem diagnoses of mycobacteriosis in birds has been aided by the development of PCR methods for the detection of *Mycobacterium sp*. In a study on experimentally infected quail, the sensitivity of different techniques was compared using fecal samples.[74] Of 130 samples, acid-fast staining gave positive results in 7% to 30%, PCR in 20%, and culture in 53%. Intermittent shedding of the organism may play a key role in potential false-negative results.[65] PCR testing of fecal specimens, cloacal swabs, and biopsy specimens is currently available at veterinary diagnostic laboratories but has not been further validated or standardized. An early report suggested that PCR had low specificity but high sensitivity, with possible identification of subclinical or early stages of infection.[75] However, many retrospective studies using formalin-fixed tissues have used PCR as the gold standard.[69,72,73,76]

The immune response of birds to *Mycobacterium sp* has been well studied in a captive collection of wildfowl through the use of ELISA and agglutination methods.[77–79] Using postmortem findings as the gold standard, the ELISA was found to have a sensitivity of 77% and specificity of 56%.[79] High antibody titers were frequently observed in association with increased morbidity and mortality.[77] In a recent study, a Western blot assay was used to detect seroconversion in a flock of ringneck doves with a known high incidence of mycobacterial infection.[80] Of the 34 doves in the study, 17 were infected with *Mycobacterium avium* as confirmed by acid-fast staining, culture, or PCR analysis. Of the infected doves 88% were seropositive. This result was in contrast to that in 11 seronegative doves that were confirmed to be negative for *M avium* by necropsy. The investigators noted differences in the level of antibody production depending on the species of dove. While it seems that the Western blot offers high specificity and sensitivity for the diagnosis of mycobacteriosis in dove species, further investigations are warranted to judge its applicability to other avian species and to birds in various stages of infection. Serologic tests for avian mycobacteriosis are not commercially available.

### Avian Bornavirus Infection

Borna disease virus (BDV) was recognized more than 100 years ago in horses and sheep in which it induces a dehabilitating meningoencephalitis.[81] A member of the Bornaviridae family, BDV was later described as an RNA virus that could infect a wide variety of other species including rabbits, cats, nonhuman primates, and some avian species.[81] Clinical signs ranged from severe neurologic changes to asymptomatic infection. In recent years, BDV has been associated, although with much contention, with mental disorders in humans.[82]

Proventricular dilation disease (PDD), an often-fatal disease in birds, is considered a major threat to aviculture and the maintenance of endangered avian species.[83,84] First described in the 1970s, the syndrome is associated with inflammation of the nervous system and gastrointestinal dysfunction as well as emaciation, seizures, and other neurologic changes.[85,86] The cause has long been proposed to be infectious, but only recently was it described to be associated with a novel avian bornavirus (ABV).[87] Pyrosequencing of brain tissues from affected parrots resulted in the identification of 2 strains of this virus; subsequent PCR amplification methods determined that the virus was present not only in the brain but also in the proventriculus and adrenal gland.[87] Work by other investigators demonstrated the transfer of PDD in cockatiels inoculated with homogenates of brain tissue that was positive for ABV.[88] This potential causative organism was further demonstrated in an outbreak of PDD in a population of psittacine birds.[89] After exposure to a bird that later succumbed to fatal confirmed PDD, additional 10 birds developed clinical signs and died; ABV RNA was detected in necropsy tissues.[89]

Investigations using serologic testing have demonstrated a high association of PDD with the presence of antibody to ABV. In one report, 90% of birds confirmed to have PDD were seropositive versus only 16% of presumptive normal birds.[90] In additional studies by the same investigators, some antibody-positive birds were observed to shed ABV in feces.[90] In another study, 32% of clinically normal birds were found to shed ABV.[91] Similarly, a study of healthy macaws demonstrated both seroconversion and shedding of the agent.[92] These findings raise questions as to whether ABV is the causative agent of PDD or whether the cause may be multifactorial and perhaps relate to immunogenetics or other resistance factors.

Diagnostic testing options for the detection of ABV have been rapidly changing since the recent description of this infectious agent (see **Table 1**). Necropsy and biopsy tissues can be examined for the presence of ABV as described in several publications.[87–92] Noninvasive antemortem testing would be preferable; to this point, testing of fecal specimens has been reported.[90] However, PCR methods have not been standardized and likely among between veterinary diagnostic laboratories. Western blot assays have also been described.[90–92] Antigen stock has included both tissue culture lysate and recombinant proteins. Although both PCR and Western blot assays show promise, larger groups of affected birds should be examined and the results compared with those obtained by biopsy to best determine the relative sensitivity and specificity of these test options.

### SUMMARY

Given the increasing ownership of pet birds, the potential for zoonotic infection, and opportunities to gain more knowledge about these infections and their causative agents, standardization of infectious disease testing for avian species must be a major focus of future diagnostic studies. Although new technologies including PCR have been widely applied, there is considerable variability among laboratories that is not adequately addressed by quality assurance programs, performance parameters, or disease-defining criteria. However, the lack of standardization has not limited the acceptance and use of these assays as diagnostic tools by veterinary practitioners, in part because better alternatives do not yet exist. In addition, lack of species-specific reagents and preanalytical errors resulting from small sample size and sample quality may affect test results. Future research and potential collaborations with the medical diagnostic community are essential to help meet quality goals within the veterinary diagnostic community and ensure that accurate methods are developed and validated for infectious disease testing in pet birds. While this goal may be optimistic, wider recognition of the public health value and importance of comparative avian laboratory medicine will help move us in the right direction.

## REFERENCES

1. U.S. Pet ownership & demographics sourcebook (2007 edition). Schaumburg (IL): AVMA; 2007.
2. Hess L. The do's and dont's of selecting an avian/exotic pet. J Avian Med Surg 2008;22(3):260–6.
3. Chomel BB, Belotto A, Meslin FX. Wildlife, exotic pets, and emerging zoonoses. Emerg Infect Dis 2007;13(1):6–11.
4. Stewardson AJ, Grayson ML. Psittacosis. Infect Dis Clin North Am 2010;24(1): 7–25.
5. Hawkins MG, Kass PH, Zinkl JG, et al. Comparison of biochemical values in serum and plasma, fresh and frozen plasma, and hemolyzed samples from orange-winged Amazon parrots (Amazona amazonica). Vet Clin Pathol 2006; 35(2):219–25.
6. Harr KE. Clinical chemistry of companion avian species: a review. Vet Clin Pathol 2002;31(3):140–51.
7. Waldoch J, Wack R, Christopher MA. Avian plasma chemistry analysis using diluted samples. J Zoo Wildl Med 2009;40(4):667–74.
8. Graczyk TK, Cranfield MR, Skjoldager ML, et al. An ELISA for detecting anti-Plasmodium spp. antibodies in African black-footed penguins (Spheniscus demersus). J Parasitol 1994;80(1):60–6.
9. Lung NP, Thompson JP, Kollias GV Jr, et al. Development of monoclonal antibodies for measurement of immunoglobulin G antibody responses in blue and gold macaws (Ara ararauna). Am J Vet Res 1996;57(8):1157–61.
10. Baghian A, Reyes CV, Mendoza A, et al. Production of a rabbit anti-cockatiel immunoglobulin G and characterization of its cross-reactivities with immunoglobulin G of other psittacine species. Avian Dis 1999;43(1):48–54.
11. Cray C, Villar D. Cross-reactivity of anti-chicken IgY antibody with immunoglobulins of exotic avian species. Vet Clin Pathol 2008;37(3):328–31.
12. Martinez J, Tomas G, Merino S, et al. Detection of serum immunoglobulins in wild birds by direct ELISA: a methodological study to validate the technique in different species using antichicken antibodies. Funct Ecol 2003;17:700–6.
13. Chiles RE, Reisen WK. A new enzyme immunoassay to detect antibodies to arboviruses in the blood of wild birds. J Vector Ecol 1998;23(2):123–35.

14. Ebel GD, Dupuis AP 2nd, Nicholas D, et al. Detection by enzyme-linked immuno-sorbent assay of antibodies to West Nile virus in birds. Emerg Infect Dis 2002; 8(9):979–82.

15. Tell LA. Aspergillosis in mammals and birds: impact on veterinary medicine. Med Mycol Suppl 2005;43:571–3.

16. Converse KA. Aspergillosis. In: Thomas NJ, Hunter BD, Atkinson CA, editors. Infectious diseases of wild birds. 1st edition. Hoboken (NJ): Blackwell Publishing; 2007. p. 360–74.

17. Jones MR, Orosz SE. The diagnosis of aspergillosis in birds. Sem Av Exot Pet Med 2000;9:52–8.

18. Billen F, Peeters D, Peters IR, et al. Comparison of the value of measurement of serum galactomannan and Aspergillus-specific antibodies in the diagnosis of canine sino-nasal aspergillosis. Vet Microbiol 2009;133(4):358–65.

19. Brown PA, Redig PT. Aspergillus ELISA: a tool for detection and management. Proceedings of the Annual Conference of Association of Avian Veterinarians. 1994. p. 295–7.

20. Cray C, Watson T, Arheart KL. Serosurvey and diagnostic application of antibody titers to Aspergillus in avian species. Avian Dis 2009;53:491–4.

21. Garcia ME, Caballero J, Cruzado M, et al. The value of the determination of anti-Aspergillus IgG in the serodiagnosis of canine aspergillosis: comparison with gal-actomannan detection. J Vet Med B Infect Dis Vet Public Health 2001;48(10): 743–50.

22. German AC, Shankland GS, Edwards J, et al. Development of an indirect ELISA for the detection of serum antibodies to Aspergillus fumigatus in captive penguins. Vet Rec 2002;150(16):513–8.

23. Graczyk TK, Cranfield MR, Klein PN. Value of antigen and antibody detection, and blood evaluation parameters in diagnosis of avian invasive aspergillosis. Mycopathologia 1998;140:121–7.

24. Le Loc'h G, Deville M, Risi E, et al. Evaluation of the serological test Platelia Aspergillus for the diagnosis of aspergillosis. Proceedings of European Associa-tion of Avian Veterinarians. 2005. p. 260–6.

25. Guillot J, Sarfati J, de Barros M, et al. Comparative study of serological tests for the diagnosis of equine aspergillosis. Vet Rec 1999;145(12):348–9.

26. Martinez-Quesada J, Nieto-Cadenazzi A, Torres-Rodriguez JM. Humoral immunoresponse of pigeons to Aspergillus fumigatus antigens. Mycopathologia 1993;124(3):131–7.

27. Reidardson TH, McBain JF. Diagnosis and treatment of aspergillosis in temperate penguins. Erkrankungen der Zootiere 1992;34:155–8.

28. Graczyk TK, Cockrem JF. Aspergillus spp. seropositivity in New Zealand penguins. Mycopathologia 1995;131(3):179–84.

29. Ivey ES. Serologic and plasma protein electrophoretic findings in 7 psittacine birds with aspergillosis. J Avian Med Surg 2000;14:103–6.

30. Blanco JL, Garcia ME. Immune response to fungal infections. Vet Immunol Immu-nopathol 2008;125(1–2):47–70.

31. Richard JL, Peden WM, Williams PP. Gliotoxin inhibits transformation and its cyto-toxic to turkey peripheral blood lymphocytes. Mycopathologia 1994;126(2):109–14.

32. Mennink-Kersten MA, Donnelly JP, Verweij PE. Detection of circulating galacto-mannan for the diagnosis and management of invasive aspergillosis. Lancet Infect Dis 2004;4(6):349–57.

33. Miceli MH, Grazziutti ML, Woods G, et al. Strong correlation between serum Aspergillus galactomannan index and outcome of aspergillosis in patients with

hematological cancer: clinical and research implications. Clin Infect Dis 2008; 46(9):1412–22.

34. Jensen AL, Kjelgaard-Hansen M. Method comparison in the clinical laboratory. Vet Clin Pathol 2006;35(3):276–86.

35. Jensen HE, Stynen D, Sarfati J, et al. Detection of galactomannan and the 18 kDa antigen from Aspergillus fumigatus in serum and urine from cattle with systemic aspergillosis. J Vet Med B 1993;40(6):397–408.

36. Le Loc'h G, Arne P, Bourgerol C, et al. Detection of circulating serum galactomannan for the diagnosis of avian aspergillosis. Proceedings of the 16th Annual Congress of the International Society for Human and Animal Mycology. 2006. p. P-0020.

37. Arca-Ruibal B, Wernery U, Zachariah R, et al. Assessment of a commercial sandwich ELISA in the diagnosis of aspergillosis in falcons. Vet Rec 2006;158(13): 442–4.

38. Cray C, Watson T, Rodriguez M, Arheart K. Application of galactomannan analysis and protein electrophoresis in the diagnosis of aspergillosis in avian species. J Zoo Wildl Med 2009;40(1).64–70.

39. Wheat LJ, Walsh TJ. Diagnosis of invasive aspergillosis by galactomannan antigenemia detection using an enzyme immunoassay. Eur J Clin Microbiol Infect Dis 2008;27(4):245–51.

40. Cray C, Reavill DR, Romagnano A, et al. Galactomannan assay and protein electrophoresis findings in psittacine birds with aspergillosis. J Avian Med Surg 2009;23(2):125–35.

41. Marty FM, Koo S. Role of (1–>3)-beta-D-glucan in the diagnosis of invasive aspergillosis. Med Mycol 2009;47(Suppl 1):S233–40.

42. Ahmad S, Khan ZU, Theyyathel AM. Diagnostic value of DNA, (1–3)-beta-d-glucan, and galactomannan detection in serum and bronchoalveolar lavage of mice experimentally infected with Aspergillus terreus. Diagn Microbiol Infect Dis 2007;59(2):165–71.

43. White PL, Bretagne S, Klingspor L, et al. Aspergillus PCR: one step closer to standardization. J Clin Microbiol 2010;48(4):1231–40.

44. Moroney JF, Guevara R, Iverson C, et al. Detection of chlamydiosis in a shipment of pet birds, leading to recognition of an outbreak of clinically mild psittacosis in humans. Clin Infect Dis 1998;26(6):1425–9.

45. Beeckman DS, Vanrompay DC. Zoonotic Chlamydophila psittaci infections from a clinical perspective. Clin Microbiol Infect 2009;15(1):11–7.

46. Smith KA. Compendium of measures to control Chlamydophila psittaci infection among humans (psittacosis) and pet birds (avian chlamydiosis). 2010. Available at: http://www.nasphv.org/documents/psittacosis.pdf. Accessed May 14, 2010.

47. Harkinezhad T, Geens T, Vanrompay D. Chlamydophila psittaci infections in birds: a review with emphasis on zoonotic consequences. Vet Microbiol 2009; 135(1–2):68–77.

48. Kaleta EF, Taday EM. Avian host range of Chlamydophila spp. based on isolation, antigen detection and serology. Avian Pathol 2003;32(5):435–61.

49. Harkinezhad T, Verminnen K, Van Droogenbroeck C, et al. Chlamydophila psittaci genotype E/B transmission from African grey parrots to humans. J Med Microbiol 2007;56(Pt 8):1097–100.

50. Vanrompay D, Ducatelle R, Haesebrouck F. Chlamydia psittaci infections: a review with emphasis on avian chlamydiosis. Vet Microbiol 1995;45(2–3):93–119.

51. Fudge AM. A review of methods to detect Chlamydia psittaci in avian patients. J Avian Med Surg 1997;11(3):153–65.

52. Grimes J. Evaluation and interpretation of serologic responses in psittacine bird chlamydiosis and suggested complementary diagnostic procedures. J Avian Med Surg 1996;10(2):75–83.
53. Salinas J, Caro MR, Cuello F. Comparison of different serological methods for the determination of antibodies to Chlamydia psittaci in pigeon sera. Zentralbl Veterinarmed B 1993;40(4):239–44.
54. Cray C, Bonda M. Application of IFA serology to the diagnosis of chlamydophilosis in a pet store. Association of Avian Veterinarians Clinical Forum. 2005. p. 7–9.
55. Grimes JE, Arizmendi F. Usefulness and limitations of three serologic methods for diagnosing or excluding chlamydiosis in birds. J Am Vet Med Assoc 1996;209(4):747–50.
56. Vanrompay D, Lublin A, Vanloock M, et al. Serology of Chlamydiaceae psittaci infections in psittaciformes by use of a recombinant enzyme-linked immunosorbent assay: recombinant DNA technology at work. Sem Avian Exot Pet Med 2000;9(1):43–9.
57. Ley DH, Flammer K, Cowen P, et al. Performance characteristics of diagnostic tests for avian chlamydiosis. J Assoc Avian Vet 1993;7(4):203–7.
58. Hewinson RG, Griffiths PC, Bevan BJ, et al. Detection of Chlamydia psittaci DNA in avian clinical samples by polymerase chain reaction. Vet Microbiol 1997;54(2):155–66.
59. Messmer T, Tully TN, Ritchie BW, et al. A tale of discrimination: differentiation of chlamydiaceae by polymerase chain reaction. Sem Avian Exot Pet Med 2000;9(1):36–42.
60. McElnea CL, Cross GM. Methods of detection of Chlamydia psittaci in domesticated and wild birds. Aust Vet J 1999;77(8):516–21.
61. Celebi B, Ak S. A comparative study of detecting Chlamydophila psittaci in pet birds using isolation in embryonated egg and polymerase chain reaction. Avian Dis 2006;50:489–93.
62. Trevejo RT, Chomel BB, Kass PH. Evaluation of the polymerase chain reaction in comparison with other diagnostic methods for the detection of Chlamydia psittaci. J Vet Diagn Invest 1999;11(6):491–6.
63. Isaza R. Use of PCR testing in diagnosing chlamydiosis. J Avian Med Surg 2000;14(2):122–7.
64. Peters M, Prodinger WM, Gummer H, et al. Mycobacterium tuberculosis infection in a blue-fronted Amazon parrot (Amazona aestiva aestiva). Vet Microbiol 2007;122(3–4):381–3.
65. Tell LA, Woods L, Cromie RL. Mycobacteriosis in birds. Rev Sci Tech 2001;20(1):180–203.
66. Hoop RK. Public health implications of exotic pet mycobacteriosis. Sem Avian Exot Pet Med 1997;6(1):3–8.
67. VanDerHeyden N. Clinical manifestations of mycobacteriosis in pet birds. Sem Avian Exot Pet Med 1997;6(1):18–24.
68. Lennox AM. Mycobacteriosis in companion psittacine birds: a review. J Avian Med Surg 2007;21(3):181–7.
69. Witte CL, Hungerford LL, Papendick R, et al. Investigation of factors predicting disease among zoo birds exposed to avian mycobacteriosis. J Am Vet Med Assoc 2010;236(2):211–8.
70. Schrenzel M, Nicolas M, Witte C, et al. Molecular epidemiology of Mycobacterium avium subsp. avium and Mycobacterium intracellulare in captive birds. Vet Microbiol 2008;126(1–3):122–31.

71. Hoop RK, Bottger EC, Pfyffer GE. Etiological agents of mycobacterioses in pet birds between 1986 and 1995. J Clin Microbiol 1996;34(4):991–2.

72. Tell LA, Leutenegger CM, Larsen RS, et al. Real-time polymerase chain reaction testing for the detection of Mycobacterium genavense and Mycobacterium avium complex species in avian samples. Avian Dis 2003;47(4):1406–15.

73. Manarolla G, Liandris E, Pisoni G, et al. Avian mycobacteriosis in companion birds: 20-year survey. Vet Microbiol 2009;133(4):323–7.

74. Tell LA, Foley J, Needham ML, et al. Diagnosis of avian mycobacteriosis: comparison of culture, acid-fast stains, and polymerase chain reaction for the identification of Mycobacterium avium in experimentally inoculated Japanese quail (Coturnix coturnix japonica). Avian Dis 2003;47(2):444–52.

75. Thornton CG, Cranfield MR, MacLellan KM, et al. Processing postmortem specimens with C18-carboxypropylbetaine and analysis by PCR to develop an antemortem test for Mycobacterium avium infections in ducks. J Zoo Wildl Med 1999; 30(1):11–24.

76. Gyimesi ZS, Stalis IH, Miller JM, et al. Detection of Mycobacterium avium subspecies avium in formalin-fixed, paraffin-embedded tissues of captive exotic birds using polymerase chain reaction. J Zoo Wildl Med 1999;30(3):348–53.

77. Cromie RL, Ash NJ, Brown MJ, et al. Avian immune responses to Mycobacterium avium: the wildfowl example. Dev Comp Immunol 2000;24(2–3):169–85.

78. Cromie RL, Brown MJ, Forbes NA, et al. A comparison and evaluation of techniques for diagnosis of avian tuberculosis in wildfowl. Avian Pathol 1993;22:617–30.

79. Zsivanovits HP, Neumann U, Brown MJ, et al. Use of an enzyme-linked immunosorbent assay to diagnose avian tuberculosis in a captive collection of wildfowl. Avian Pathol 2004;33(6):571–5.

80. Gray PL, Saggese MD, Phalen DN, et al. Humoral response to Mycobacterium avium subsp. avium in naturally infected ring-neck doves (Streptopelia risoria). Vet Immunol Immunopathol 2008;125(3–4):216–24.

81. Ludwig H. The biology of bornavirus. APMIS Suppl 2008;124:14–20.

82. Bode L. Human bornavirus infection– towards a valid diagnostic system. APMIS Suppl 2008;124:21–39.

83. Doneley RJ, Miller RI, Fanning TE. Proventricular dilatation disease: an emerging exotic disease of parrots in Australia. Aust Vet J 2007;85(3):119–23.

84. Gregory C, Latimer KS, Niagro F, et al. A review of proventricular dilation syndrome. J Assoc Avian Vet 1994;8:69–75.

85. Berhane YSD, Newman S, Taylor M, et al. Peripheral neuritis in psittacine birds with proventricular dilatation disease. Avian Pathol 2001;30:563–70.

86. Manni A, Gerlach H. Neuropathic gastric dilation in psittaciformes. Avian Dis 1987;31:214–21.

87. Honkavuori KS, Shivaprasad HL, Williams BL, et al. Novel borna virus in psittacine birds with proventricular dilatation disease. Emerg Infect Dis 2008;14(12): 1883–6.

88. Gancz AY, Kistler AL, Greninger AL, et al. Experimental induction of proventricular dilatation disease in cockatiels (Nymphicus hollandicus) inoculated with brain homogenates containing avian bornavirus 4. Virol J 2009;6:100.

89. Kistler AL, Smith JM, Greninger AL, et al. Analysis of naturally occurring avian bornavirus infection and transmission during an outbreak of proventricular dilatation disease among captive psittacine birds. J Virol 2010;84(4):2176–9.

90. Villanueva I, Gray P, Mirhosseini N, et al. The diagnosis of proventricular dilatation disease: use of a western blot assay to detect antibodies against avian borna virus. Vet Microbiol 2010;143(2–4):196–201.

91. Lierz M, Hafez HM, Honkavuori KS, et al. Anatomical distribution of avian bornavirus in parrots, its occurrence in clinically healthy birds and ABV-antibody detection. Avian Pathol 2009;38(6):491–6.
92. De Kloet SR, Dorrestein GM. Presence of avian bornavirus RNA and anti-avian bornavirus antibodies in apparently healthy macaws. Avian Dis 2009;53(4): 568–73.

# Diagnostic Hematology of Reptiles

Nicole I. Stacy, DrMedVet[a],*, A. Rick Alleman, DMV, PhD[b],
Katherine A. Sayler, MEd[b]

**KEYWORDS**

• Blood cell morphology • Hematology • Reptiles • Hemogram

Microscopic evaluation of the peripheral blood film is a powerful diagnostic tool and an essential part of the complete blood count in human and veterinary medicine. Blood cell counts and morphology vary greatly among the more than 8000 species of reptiles described, even among species within the same genus. In addition, many intrinsic and extrinsic factors complicate the evaluation of hematologic data in reptiles; thus, published reference intervals provide only a baseline for interpretation, and veterinarians need to be aware of these factors to accurately interpret and correlate hematologic and clinical findings in the reptile patient. Reptiles have become increasingly popular as pets and are frequently found in settings such as zoos and wildlife parks. Wild reptile populations often are subjects of health assessment studies and investigations of naturally occurring disease. For example, the recently discovered novel siadenovirus of Sulawesi tortoises (genus: *Siadenovirus*; species: *Sulawesi tortoise AdV1*) was associated with severe systemic disease; bone marrow myeloid necrosis was observed in 20 of 33 tortoises, and intranuclear inclusions were observed in myeloid and stromal cells of hematopoietic tissue in 19 of 20 tortoises. Several hematologic abnormalities also were observed, including anemia, leukopenia or leukocytosis, heteropenia or heterophilia, lymphopenia or lymphocytosis, and monocytosis, all of which are nonspecific indicators of a chronic inflammatory response.[1] This is just one example of how systemic disease can manifest in the hemogram of reptiles, alerting the veterinarian to the need for further (molecular) diagnostics, if clinically warranted.

Routine hematologic evaluation of reptiles includes determination of packed cell volume (PCV), hemoglobin (Hb) concentration, red blood cell (RBC) count, RBC indices, total white blood cell (WBC) count, leukocyte differential counts, and assessment of blood cell morphology. In small reptile patients, when only a limited amount of

Disclosure: The authors have nothing to disclose.
[a] Department of Large Animal Clinical Sciences, Aquatic Animal Health, University of Florida College of Veterinary Medicine, 2015 SW 16th Avenue, Gainesville, FL 32608, USA
[b] Department of Physiological Sciences, University of Florida College of Veterinary Medicine, 2015 SW 16th Avenue, Gainesville, FL 32608, USA
* Corresponding author.
*E-mail address:* stacyn@vetmed.ufl.edu

Clin Lab Med 31 (2011) 87–108
doi:10.1016/j.cll.2010.10.006
0272-2712/11/$ – see front matter © 2011 Elsevier Inc. All rights reserved.

blood can safely be withdrawn, a properly prepared blood film has priority, because microscopic evaluation alone can provide clinically relevant diagnostic information. Morphologic changes in peripheral blood cells can indicate specific disease processes, help to establish a list of differential diagnoses, and help monitor the health status of a patient during the course of disease or response to therapy. Annual or biannual health checks with blood analysis can help establish baseline values within individuals, which can be valuable for detecting hematologic abnormalities that develop with disease later in life. Because of their unique physiology and behavior, many chronic disease states in reptiles are not detected until in the advanced stages.[2]

This article describes the normal morphologic and functional features of reptilian blood cells and discusses the manifestation of physiologic and pathologic changes in the reptilian hemogram. The morphology of reptilian blood cells is based on their staining characteristics with Romanowsky-type stains. There are significant differences in the physiology of reptiles compared with common domestic animals; hematologic evaluation starts with blood sample collection, sample-handling techniques, and laboratory procedures, details of which are well documented elsewhere in the literature.[3,4]

One of the most challenging aspects of diagnostic hematology of reptiles is the accuracy of cell counts. Because reptiles have nucleated RBCs, manual methods must be used to quantify leukocytes. The Natt-Herrick method for obtaining total WBC counts has multiple sources of errors, including inadequate mixing or dilution of blood and stains, incorrect charging of the hemocytometer chamber, and errors in differentiating leukocytes from thrombocytes (which also are nucleated in reptiles). Therefore, total leukocyte estimates with designated formulas are useful during blood film evaluation to verify the manual counts. Erroneous manual counts can lead to misinterpretation of the leukogram, with potentially serious effect on the individual or study population. Manual counts are necessary, however, for determining absolute leukocyte counts (the concentration of cells per microliter of blood), which should be used (rather than percentages) for accurate interpretation of the leukogram. Cautious and consistent use of sampling techniques, specimen handling, and laboratory methods provide the most reliable laboratory results. With these aspects in mind, the validity of abnormalities observed in the hemogram must be interpreted in relation to the clinical presentation of the individual reptile.

Despite the availability of peer-reviewed information and recent advances in reptile medicine, there is an abundance of misinformation and speculations in the literature. The information in this article is based on the authors' collective experience with extensive clinical case material from the Zoological Medicine Service and department of Aquatic Animal Health at the College of Veterinary Medicine, University of Florida, as well as through multiple collaborative institutions. All of the information cited from textbooks and conference proceedings has been confirmed as accurate to the best of the authors' abilities.

## BLOOD CELL MORPHOLOGY AND FUNCTION IN REPTILES
### Erythrocytes

Erythrocytes of reptiles are similar in microscopic and ultrastructural morphology to those of other nonmammalian vertebrates. Reptilian, avian, amphibian, and fish erythrocytes are nucleated and therefore larger than their mammalian counterparts. When stained with Romanowsky-type stains, the mature erythrocyte of reptiles is elliptical and has abundant orange-pink cytoplasm. The nucleus is centrally positioned, is irregular to elliptical, and has condensed, deeply basophilic chromatin (**Fig. 1**).

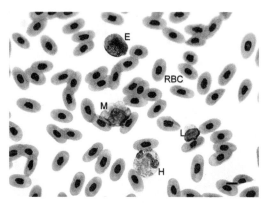

**Fig. 1.** Peripheral blood from a clinically healthy green iguana (*Iguana iguana*). E, green eosinophil; H, bilobed heterophil; L, lymphocyte; M, monocyte; RBC, mature erythrocytes. Wright-Giemsa, bar = 10 μm.

Erythroplastids (anucleated erythrocytes) are also occasionally observed in healthy reptiles (<0.5%), mostly snakes; they do not seem to have any clinical significance.[5–8] Aged erythrocytes with small round pyknotic nuclei can be identified in the circulation in low numbers in healthy reptiles. A low number of teardrop-shaped or fusiform erythrocytes may be observed in healthy reptiles and must be differentiated from erythrocytes deformed during the smearing process (personal observation of authors).[9]

The PCV of most clinically healthy reptiles ranges from 20% to 40%, lower than that of mammals and birds and indicating less oxygen-carrying capacity.[9–12] Hb concentration is similarly lower (5.5–12 g/dL).[2] Mean cell volume (MCV) is higher than that of mammals and varies with species. Because of the inverse relationship between erythrocyte number and size, species with higher MCV, such as turtles and snakes, have lower RBC counts than lizards, which have a lower MCV and higher RBC count.[10,13] The average erythrocyte lifespan ranges from 600 to 800 days in reptiles. This extremely slow turnover of erythrocytes (relative to human erythrocytes, which have a 120-day lifespan) is thought to be associated with the slow metabolic rate of reptiles.[9,10,13,14]

It is common to find a low percentage (<1%) of polychromatophils in the blood of healthy reptiles, particularly in young animals or animals in ecdysis (periodic skin shedding that can be complete [snakes and some lizards] or partial [chelonians and other species]).[3] Unlike polychromatophils in mammals, those in reptiles are smaller than mature erythrocytes and gradually enlarge (rather than decrease in size) during maturation. Reptilian polychromatophils are also rounder and more basophilic and have larger round, oval, or irregular nuclei than mature erythrocytes, with higher nuclear to cytoplasmic (N:C) ratios (**Fig. 2**). The nuclei of immature erythrocytes contain areas of less-densely packed euchromatin, indicating active Hb production. Earlier stages of immature erythrocytes also may be seen in reptile blood, in particular rubricytes, which have darker basophilic cytoplasm, larger round to oval nuclei, and coarser chromatin than polychromatophils. Rubricytes resemble lymphocytes and must be correctly identified during the leukocyte differential count (see **Fig. 2**). Mitotic erythroid precursors also are occasionally observed in the peripheral blood of healthy reptiles, but are more frequently observed in patients with active erythroid regeneration (see **Fig. 2**).

Reticulocyte stains such as new methylene blue can be used to quantify immature erythrocytes, in which residual RNA precipitates to form a distinct ring of basophilic aggregates surrounding the nucleus. Most healthy reptiles have less than 5%

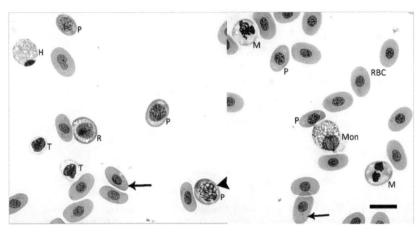

**Fig. 2.** Peripheral blood from a green sea turtle (*Chelonia mydas*) with anemia (PCV = 12%) and evidence of erythroid regeneration. Mature erythrocytes (RBC) with mild basophilic stippling (*arrows*). Polychromatophil undergoing mitosis (*arrowhead*). H, heterophil; M, mitotic figures in erythroid cell line; Mon, reactive monocyte; P, polychromatophils; R, rubriblast; T, thrombocytes. Wright-Giemsa, bar = 10 μm.

reticulocytes.[15] Absolute reticulocyte counts are not routinely evaluated. Assessment of the degree of polychromasia and quantitation of immature erythroid precursors are critical in determining whether an anemia is regenerative.

A low number of small punctate, basophilic inclusions and/or clear, distinct vacuoles are frequently observed in erythrocytes from healthy Chelonians (turtles and tortoises) and other reptile species.[3,9] These inclusions have been identified by electron microscopy as degenerated organelles; their clinical significance is unknown, but they must be differentiated from drying artifacts.[16] Similar single basophilic irregular inclusions have been identified ultrastructurally as aggregates of endoplasmic reticulum in erythrocytes of Eastern water dragons.[17] Symmetric; pale; and square, rectangular, or hexagonal inclusions resembling Hb crystals are frequently identified in erythrocytes of healthy iguanas (**Fig. 3**); the cause and clinical significance are unknown.[18,19]

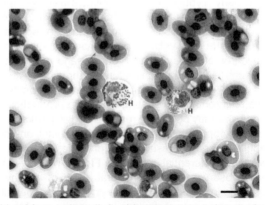

**Fig. 3.** Peripheral blood from a clinically healthy green iguana (*Iguana iguana*). Erythrocytes contain variably sized, pale rectangular to square cytoplasmic inclusions of unknown origin. H, bilobed heterophils. Wright-Giemsa, bar = 10 μm.

## Leukocytes

Reptilian leukocytes can be classified as granulocytes (heterophils, eosinophils, basophils) and mononuclear cells (lymphocytes, monocytes, azurophils). Leukocytes vary greatly in number and morphology of granules, cytochemical staining patterns, and relative concentration in the peripheral blood depending on species and genera.[20] In general, heterophils (named as such because of their prominent bright pink-orange cytoplasmic granules) are the equivalent of mammalian neutrophils, whereas monocytes and lymphocytes of reptiles have similar morphology and function as those of mammals, birds, and fish. Azurophils are unique to reptile species.

## Heterophils

Reptilian heterophils are large (10–23 μm) round cells with clear cytoplasm filled with bright pink-orange granules.[10,21] Crocodilians (alligators and crocodiles) and Chelonians have distinct fusiform granules, whereas Squamatans (lizards and snakes) have angular, pleomorphic, and densely packed granules (see **Figs. 1–3**).[3,22] Heterophil nuclei are eccentric and vary from round to oval (in most snakes, Chelonians, and Crocodilians) to bi- or multilobed (in lizards) (see **Figs. 1–3**).[21,22]

Heterophils in most species of reptiles compose 30% to 45% of leukocytes in the peripheral blood [9,10,13,23]; in chelonian and crocodilian species, they account for more than 50%.[16,22,24,25] Based on cytochemical and ultrastructural studies, heterophils appear similar to mammalian neutrophils, likely functioning to phagocytose bacteria and foreign material. They play a significant role in innate immunity in response to various inflammatory stimuli.[10,13,16,22,24,26] Toxic heterophils can be observed in reptiles with bacterial infections, severe inflammation, or necrosis; the degree of toxicity reflects the severity of disease. Morphologic findings in mild toxicity include cytoplasmic basophilia and degranulation; severe toxicity is characterized by cytoplasmic vacuolation, aberrant (pleomorphic) cytoplasmic granules, and excessive nuclear lobulation (**Figs. 4** and **5**).[3,4] As in mammals, quantitative and qualitative assessment of toxicity is important as a prognostic indicator.[3,4,27] Degranulation without basophilia can be an artifact of inappropriate sample handling, prolonged

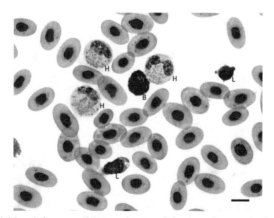

**Fig. 4.** Peripheral blood from a Chinese dragon (*Physignathus cocincinus*) with multiple subcutaneous abscesses and heterophilia. Heterophils (H) are mildly toxic (degranulation and cytoplasmic basophilia). Erythrocytes are mature and contain small, pale basophilic inclusions consistent with degenerate organelles. B, basophil; L, small lymphocytes. Wright-Giemsa, bar = 10 μm.

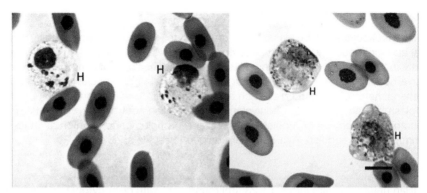

**Fig. 5.** Peripheral blood from (*left*) an American crocodile (*Crocodylus acutus*) and (*right*) a spectacled caiman (*Caiman crocodylus*). Heterophils (H) are severely toxic, with degranulation, indistinct cytoplasmic vacuolation, and abnormal granules. The caiman heterophils also have increased cytoplasmic basophilia and immature nuclei. Wright-Giemsa, bar = 10 μm.

storage, or inappropriate fixation of the blood film.[3,20,28] As in mammals, the presence of immature heterophils (left shift) is generally associated with inflammation. Compared with mature heterophils, immature heterophils have larger, occasionally pleomorphic nuclei; higher N:C ratios; and increased cytoplasmic basophilia and can contain a low number of small, dark purple primary granules.[4]

### Eosinophils

Eosinophil morphology in reptiles is similar to that of mammals. Eosinophils vary from 9 to 20 μm in diameter both between and within species. Eosinophils have a clear cytoplasm and round pink granules. Nuclei are central or eccentric and round, oval, elongated, or bilobed (**Fig. 6**).[3,22] Eosinophils are absent in most snake species but have been identified in king cobras (*Ophiophagus hannah*).[20,28,29] Eosinophil granules in iguanas, tegus, and rainbow lizards uniquely stain pale blue-green and are referred to as green eosinophils (see **Fig. 1**).[3–5] The authors have observed immature eosinophils in blood from a box turtle, based on the presence of dark blue primary granules

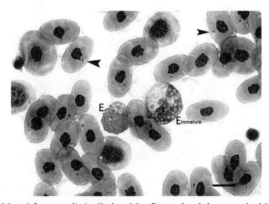

**Fig. 6.** Peripheral blood from a clinically healthy flowerback box turtle (*Cuora galbinifrons*). A mature eosinophil (E) and an immature eosinophil (E$_{immature}$). A few of the mature erythrocytes contain small, basophilic inclusions consistent with degenerate organelles (*arrowheads*). P, polychromatophils. Wright-Giemsa, bar = 10 μm.

admixed with the bright eosinophilic secondary granules (see **Fig. 6**) and by their larger and more pleomorphic nuclei.

Eosinophils compose 7% to 20% of leukocytes in healthy reptiles, with lower percentages in lizards and higher percentages in turtles. Although eosinophil function in reptiles has not been well studied, abnormally high eosinophil numbers have been associated with parasitic infections (eg, protozoa, helminths) and other types of antigenic stimulation.[3,30] Lower eosinophil percentages in free-ranging nesting leatherback turtles compared with loggerhead and green sea turtles were attributed to differences in diet and parasite load. Only a few helminth species have been found in leatherbacks, and because they mainly prefer jellyfish, the omnivorous loggerheads and green turtles are frequently infected with spirorchids and other parasites.[31,32] Eosinophils from infected snapping turtles have been reported to be able to phagocytize immune complexes,[30] and eosinophils from a healthy young American alligator had phagocytic and microbicidal capacity against *Staphylococcus aureus*.[24]

### Basophils

Basophils in reptiles are usually small cells (7–12 µm) but may reach 20 µm in some species. As in other species, basophils contain numerous small, round, dark purple (metachromatic) granules that frequently obscure the round nucleus (see **Fig. 4**).[9,22] Basophils with pale purple cytoplasm and clear, distinct vacuoles rather than granules can result from degranulation or lack of metachromatic staining (**Fig. 7**). Basophils of reptiles may degranulate during blood collection, delayed sample processing, or slide preparation. A lack of metachromatic staining of basophils and mast cells has been associated with the use of aqueous stains on blood films and cytologic preparations.[33]

The percentage of basophils varies greatly among reptile species.[34] Healthy turtles and tortoises have up to 40% basophils,[10,16] whereas healthy freshwater turtles (eg, Northern red-bellied cooters) have up to 65% basophils.[10,35–41] The percentage of basophils is reported to increase with certain hemoparasitic (eg, hemogregarines and trypanosomes) and viral (eg, iridovirus) infections.[10] The function of basophils in reptiles is not well understood. Basophils of snapping turtles express surface immunoglobulin and release histamine.[10,35,42]

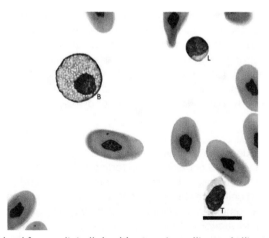

**Fig. 7.** Peripheral blood from a clinically healthy American alligator (*Alligator mississippiensis*). B, degranulated basophil; L, small lymphocyte; T, thrombocyte. Wright-Giemsa, bar = 10 µm.

### Lymphocytes

Reptilian lymphocytes are similar in their morphology to those of mammals and birds and vary in size from 5 to 15 μm (see **Figs. 1, 4** and **7**).[10] It can be challenging to differentiate small lymphocytes from thrombocytes when performing a total WBC count using a hemocytometer or during blood film evaluation (see **Fig. 7**). Large lymphocytes, reactive lymphocytes, and lymphoblasts may be observed occasionally, especially in disease conditions that cause immune stimulation. Plasmacytoid lymphocytes and granular lymphocytes can also be observed during immune stimulation. Plasma cells are rarely observed in the peripheral blood of reptiles with inflammatory or infectious diseases.[9] Similar to the lymphocytes of birds and mammals, reptilian lymphocytes are categorized as B cells and T cells with corresponding functions, including immunoglobulin production and cell-mediated immune responses, respectively.[10]

In most reptile species, lymphocytes are the predominant leukocyte and compose up to 80% of leukocytes.[10,20,34,43–45] Causes of lymphocytosis include inflammation or infection, wound healing, parasitism (eg, anisakiasis, spirorchidiasis, hematozoa), and viral diseases.[3] Lymphopenia can be associated with malnutrition and excess endogenous and exogenous corticosteroids.[3]

### Monocytes

Monocytes in reptiles are variable in size (8–25 μm) and shape (round or oval) and have distinct cytoplasmic borders and abundant pale blue-gray cytoplasm. Nuclei are round, oval, reniform, or multilobed and have smooth to slightly clumped chromatin (see **Fig. 1**).[10] Reactive monocytes can contain cytoplasmic vacuoles (see **Fig. 2**).

Monocytes usually compose 0% to 10% of leukocytes[10,13]; however, some reptile species have up to 20% monocytes.[46] Monocytes develop into macrophages after leaving the peripheral blood to enter into tissues. They are essential for granuloma and giant cell formation, a common response to microbial infections in reptiles.[47] The percentage of monocytes increases during chronic antigenic stimulation, chronic inflammation, and bacterial or parasitic diseases.[48]

Unique to reptiles, circulating monocytes and macrophages that contain melanin pigment (melanomacrophages), nucleoproteinaceous debris, or lipid vacuoles (**Fig. 8**) can be observed, all of which must be differentiated from intracellular organisms.[47] Erythrophagocytic macrophages can also be found in the peripheral blood. Potential causes include delayed sample processing and immune-mediated, infectious, or neoplastic disease.[27] The authors observed marked erythrophagia in an emerald tree boa that had a positive blood culture for *Corynebacterium* sp (**Fig. 9**); the erythrophagocytic macrophages disappeared shortly after the initiation of antimicrobial therapy (Stacy NI, DrMedVet, Alleman AR, DMV, PhD, unpublished data, 2009). Siderophagocytes and erythrophagocytes without anemia were identified in blood films of a corn snake 20 to 79 days after ovariosalpingectomy.[49]

### Azurophils

The azurophil is unique to reptile species. Azurophils are commonly observed in squamates and crocodilians, and occasionally in tortoises and turtles, and are morphologically (and possibly functionally) similar to both granulocytes and monocytes.[5,20,22,28] Azurophils are round cells with distinct cytoplasmic borders and pale blue-gray cytoplasm that contains numerous dustlike azurophilic to purple granules and sometimes a few clear, punctuate vacuoles. Nuclei are usually round or oval, eccentric, and have clumped chromatin (**Fig. 10**).[3] Immature azurophils have higher N:C ratios and more pleomorphic nuclei. Cytochemically, azurophils in snakes are similar to mammalian

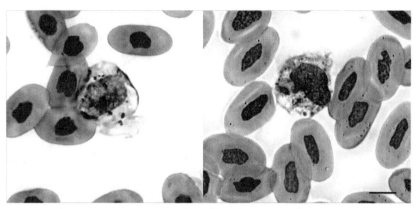

**Fig. 8.** Macrophages in peripheral blood. (*Left*) Melanomacrophage in a clinically healthy loggerhead sea turtle (*Caretta caretta*). (*Right*) Macrophage with intracytoplasmic nucleoproteinaceous debris in a common boa constrictor (*Boa constrictor imperator*). Macrophages are occasionally observed in the blood of clinically normal reptiles. Wright-Giemsa, bar = 10 μm.

neutrophils (positive for benzidine peroxidase, sudan black B (SBB), and periodic acid-Schiff), whereas azurophils of lizards are similar to mammalian monocytes (positive for acid phosphatase, negative for benzidine peroxidase and SBB).[15,18,20,22] Therefore, the authors recommend counting azurophils separately in snakes, but grouping them with monocytes in other reptile species. Azurophils are the second most common leukocyte type in snakes and may normally represent up to 35% of circulating leukocytes in some species.[20,29,45] Increased numbers are frequently

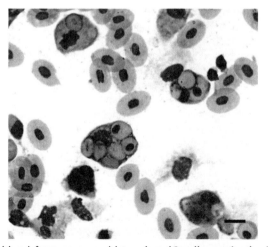

**Fig. 9.** Peripheral blood from an emerald tree boa (*Corallus caninus*) with positive blood culture for *Corynebacterium* sp Several monocytes (macrophages) contain phagocytized erythrocytes and greenish black hemosiderin pigment. Cell in the upper left appears mitotic. Wright-Giemsa, bar = 10 μm.

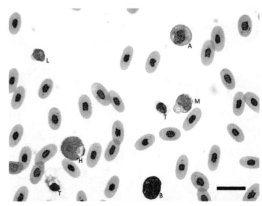

**Fig. 10.** Peripheral blood from a blood python (*Python brongersmai*) with chronic constipation. A, azurophil; B, basophil; H, heterophil; L, small lymphocyte; M, mildly vacuolated monocyte; T, thrombocytes, and mature erythrocytes. Wright-Giemsa, bar = 10 μm.

associated with inflammatory and infectious (ie, bacterial) diseases, particularly in acute stages.[50] Azurophils in reptile species other than snakes are found in low percentages, and increased numbers are considered to occur more frequently in chronic disease states, similar to monocytes.

### Thrombocytes

Unlike mammalian platelets, which are cytoplasmic fragments of megakaryocytes,[27] thrombocytes of reptiles, birds, amphibians, and fish are nucleated and represent a distinct cell line that most likely originates from the thromboblast in hematopoietic tissue, hence their name. Morphologic features of thrombocytes are similar to those of small lymphocytes, and their differentiation may be challenging. Thrombocytes are ellipsoid to oval, are approximately 8 to 16 × 5 to 9 μm, and have distinct cytoplasmic borders and scant, clear cytoplasm that may contain a few fine, dustlike, pink granules. Nuclei are round to oval, central, and have dense, dark chromatin (see **Figs. 2, 7,** and **10**).[4,10] During blood collection and/or blood film preparation, thrombocytes often become activated or rupture. Activated thrombocytes often clump and can have pseudopods or contain a few cytoplasmic vacuoles (see **Fig. 2**).[4] When thrombocytes are ruptured, they appear as free nuclei with smooth chromatin. Blood samples of reptiles are usually collected in lithium-heparin, which often causes thrombocytes and possibly leukocytes to clump.[5] Thrombocyte clumps can be helpful in identifying thrombocyte morphology of a particular species and aid in differentiating them from lymphocytes. Compared with lymphocytes, thrombocytes are slightly smaller; are round, oval, or elliptic; and have distinct cytoplasmic borders and central round or oval nuclei with denser, darker chromatin.

Thrombocytes function similar to mammalian platelets, including involvement in hemostasis and wound healing.[10] Thrombocytes may also have phagocytic capabilities.[51] Activated thrombocytes can phagocytize bacteria, nucleoproteinaceous debris, erythrocytes, hemosiderin, and melanin (personal observation of authors).[9] Immature thrombocytes are larger than mature cells and have higher N:C ratios and slightly basophilic cytoplasm.

Because thrombocytes frequently clump in heparinized blood samples, hemocytometer counts and blood film estimates can vary greatly and cannot be considered accurate. Thrombocyte numbers can be subjectively assessed by the examiner as normal, decreased, or increased. When thrombocytopenia is observed, difficult or slow blood withdrawal, delay in sample processing, clotted samples, and laboratory error need to be ruled out. As in thrombocytopenic mammals, there are numerous differentials for thrombocytopenia in reptiles.

## INTRINSIC AND EXTRINSIC FACTORS AFFECTING THE HEMOGRAM OF REPTILES

Age, sex, environment, and diet can dramatically affect the reptile hemogram with regard to both cell morphology and cell concentration in the peripheral blood.

### Age

Captive adult mugger crocodiles had higher RBC counts and significantly lower percentages of lymphocytes compared with juveniles and subadults.[52] Other described age-related hemogram changes include higher lymphocyte percentages and lower heterophil percentages in juvenile loggerhead turtles between the ages 1 month to 3 years, compared with adult turtles.[53]

### Sex

Hb and PCV values in captive New Guinea snapping turtles and in free-ranging desert tortoises were significantly higher in males compared with females.[25,39] However, PCVs in free-ranging juvenile green sea turtles, African pancake tortoises, and Gopher tortoises did not differ significantly based on sex.[54–56] Both gravid and nongravid female captive green iguanas had higher PCV and mean corpuscular hemoglobin concentration (MCHC) values than did males.[18] Male free-ranging radiated tortoises had higher RBC counts and PCVs than females,[57] similar to free-ranging desert tortoises, in which significantly higher RBC mass was documented in males than in females throughout the year.[25]

Higher heterophil counts were observed in adult male captive mugger crocodiles than in adult females.[52] Females reportedly have higher percentages of lymphocytes than males of the same species and age, under identical environmental conditions.[10,13,37]

### Ambient Environment and Season

Several components of the hemogram can be significantly affected by seasonal variation in temperature and other environmental factors and by hibernation status. Seasonal effects are multifactorial and can be influenced by rainfall, food availability, and temperature extremes.[25] Thus, it is difficult to apply broad patterns of changes across species, and any inferences drawn should be limited to a particular species and geographic area.

Reptiles have been reported to have higher RBC counts posthibernation (spring) than prehibernation (fall).[9,10,13,21] Free-ranging radiated tortoises had higher RBC counts and PCVs in summer than in winter (the hibernation period).[57] Captive South American rattlesnakes had significantly higher RBC count, PCV, Hb level, MCV, mean corpuscular hemoglobin (MCH), and MCHC and lower total WBC and thrombocyte counts in winter than in summer.[45] In contrast, a long-term health assessment study of alligator snapping turtles in Georgia and Florida revealed higher PCVs and basophil percentages in summer than in spring.[58] Gopher tortoises had lower total WBC counts and monocyte percentages in spring than in fall.[56] Higher heterophil counts[13] and fewer eosinophils[9,10,13,59] were observed in summer months than in hibernation periods. Lymphocyte percentages reportedly are lower in animals during ecdysis and winter than during summer months.[10,11,13,25] Monocyte numbers are not significantly affected by seasonal factors,[10,13] although high percentages of mono-cytes were reported in hibernating desert tortoises and dystocic chameleons.[25,60] Compared with other leukocytes, seasonal variation in basophil concentration is mild, with fewer basophils in desert tortoises during hibernation and higher numbers during active periods.[21,25] The percentage of basophils is rather affected by age and geographic region.[34]

In one study involving a large number of free-ranging desert tortoises, hibernating tortoises had lower lymphocyte and basophil percentages and higher monocyte and azurophil percentages than nonhibernating animals.[25] However, there were no significant seasonal, geographic, or sexual differences in total WBC and heterophil counts. In a group of 31 captive viperid snakes, no differences were observed in pre- and posthibernation samples in PCV or total and differential WBC counts.[61]

### Captive Versus Wild Reptiles

Differences in hemogram results from healthy captive reptiles compared with wild-caught reptiles of the same species have been attributed to ectoparasites and hemo-parasites in free-ranging animals and stress and husbandry in captive animals. Higher RBC and lymphocyte counts and lower heterophil and azurophil counts were reported in captive-bred king cobras than in wild-caught king cobras.[29] Similarly, estimated total WBC counts were higher and percentage of heterophils was lower in captive bog turtles compared with wild bog turtles.[37]

### Contamination of Blood Samples with Lymph

Many venipuncture sites in reptiles are in close proximity to lymph vessels such that hematologic (and biochemical) values can vary significantly depending on the collection site and potential dilution of the blood sample with extravascular fluid, lymph, or both.[62] Lymph contamination resulted in a significantly lower PCV and Hb concentration and a significantly higher lymphocyte count in samples from the dorsal coccygeal vein, subcarapacial venipuncture site, or postoccipital venous plexus of chelonian species.[62–64] When a blood sample from a reptile has a low PCV without evidence of erythroid regeneration and a high number of small lymphocytes, contamination with lymph should be suspected and another sample from a different site should be collected.

## DIAGNOSIS AND CAUSES OF ANEMIA IN REPTILES

In addition to an increase in polychromasia and earlier erythroid precursors, erythro-cyte morphologic findings associated with regenerative anemia in reptiles include basophilic stippling, binucleation, increased anisocytosis and anisokaryosis, and an increased number of mitotic figures. However, the nuclear changes also can be observed in erythrocytes of reptiles with severe inflammatory disease, malnutrition, or starvation or posthibernation, all of which usually are associated with nonregener-ative anemia.[5,65] Posthibernating reptiles can have a marked regenerative erythroid response with basophilic stippling.[65] Basophilic stippling also can be observed in reptiles with lead toxicosis.[3] An increased number of fusiform or teardrop-shaped erythrocytes has been associated with septicemia or chronic infectious disease (personal observation of authors).[9] RBC indices may help to characterize the erythroid response to disease, similar to their use in mammals.[2] A regenerative response in reptiles is typically associated with a decrease in MCV and MCHC.

Given the long life span of erythrocytes in reptiles, the duration and degree of anemia needs to be considered when evaluating the individual patient. Anemic reptiles with evidence of erythroid regeneration generally have a better prognosis than patients having no or a mild regenerative response. Anemia of chronic disease associated with decreased erythrocyte production (nonregenerative anemia) develops slowly and has been described as the most frequent type of anemia in reptile patients.[2,66] Commonly reported causes include systemic infectious disease; chronic degenerative or inflammatory diseases of the liver, kidney, spleen, or lungs; gastrointestinal disease; inappropriate husbandry; starvation; and hematopoietic neoplasia.[2,3,66] Most stranded, debilitated loggerhead turtles have nonregenerative anemia, which probably is multifactorial in origin.[31]

Erythrocytes from reptiles with iron-deficiency anemia often appear hypochromic in blood films and MCH and MCHC are lower. Causes for iron deficiency in reptiles include chronic inflammatory disease, iron-deficient diets, and malabsorption due to gastrointestinal disease.[2,3] Causes of hemorrhagic anemia in reptiles include trauma, ectoparasite infections (eg, ticks, mites, leeches), coagulopathies, gastrointestinal ulceration, and neoplasia.[2,3,66] Hemolysis can be associated with bacterial and parasitic infections, such as heavy *Plasmodium* sp infection, drugs, or toxins such as lead and zinc.[2]

## DIAGNOSIS AND CAUSES OF INFLAMMATION IN REPTILES

Heterophilia is frequently associated with inflammatory conditions, including infectious diseases (bacterial, parasitic), tissue injury, and necrosis. Other causes include neoplasia, gravidity, excess exogenous or endogenous glucocorticoids, and, rarely, granulocytic leukemia.[3,13,67] Acute, overwhelming infections in reptiles may result in heteropenia with a left shift and toxicity.[4] Severe heteropenia has been associated with fenbendazole administration in Hermann tortoises.[68]

In snakes, increased numbers of azurophils, with or without a left shift, are frequently associated with inflammatory or infectious (ie, bacterial) diseases, particularly in the acute stages.[50] As with monocytes, increased azurophil percentages in reptile species other than snakes are considered to occur more frequently in chronic disease states.

Inflammation in reptiles often results in granuloma formation, depending on the underlying cause of the lesion.[22,47] Although heterophils are among the first inflammatory cells involved in inflammatory reactions of reptiles, granulomas form within days, with densely packed necrotic heterophils in the center and monocytes, macrophages, and multinucleated giant cells at the periphery.[47,69] The presence of lymphocytes and plasma cells may indicate chronicity of the lesion. The reptilian inflammatory response is modulated by a variety of intrinsic and extrinsic factors, with temperature, season, and hormonal effects among the most extensively investigated.[47,69] The efficacy and duration of the inflammatory response in ectothermic reptiles can be influenced by ambient temperatures, with higher temperatures stimulating the host response and resulting in earlier resolution of inflammatory lesions.[47] These tissue reactions are typically reflected in the peripheral blood by heterophilia with or without a toxic left shift, monocytosis, and azurophilia. The main cause of leukocytosis in reptiles is infectious disease.[47,66]

A hallmark of bacterial infection is the presence of a toxic left shift, together with heterophilia or heteropenia. Bacteremia rarely is diagnosed microscopically by observation of intracytoplasmic bacteria within leukocytes in peripheral blood smears. Case reports of bacteremia include the description of a spirilliform bacterium in the peripheral blood and bone marrow of a rhinoceros iguana, *Chlamydia* sp inclusions in peripheral monocytes of flap-necked chameleons, and *Chlamydophila* inclusions in peripheral monocytes of emerald tree boas with pneumonia (as observed by the authors and confirmed by PCR).[4,70,71] When bacterial infection is suspected, further diagnostic testing is indicated (eg, blood culture or molecular diagnostics). Serial hemogram evaluations can help to monitor the progress of disease and response to treatment and to establish a prognosis.

## VIRAL INFECTIONS IN THE PERIPHERAL BLOOD

Some viral infections of reptiles may be diagnosed by observing characteristic cytoplasmic viral inclusions in blood cells. Viral inclusions in erythrocytes must be differentiated from Hb crystals, drying artifacts, and degenerated organelles. Viral inclusions in leukocytes must be differentiated from phagocytized cellular debris, hemosiderin, and melanin granules.

Inclusion body disease (IBD) of boas and pythons can result in mild to marked lymphocytosis and characteristic intracytoplasmic inclusions in lymphocytes (rarely in thrombocytes and basophils).[4] The cause of IBD is still unknown; a retrovirus has been suspected to be the causative agent but has yet to be confirmed by future research.[72] In Romanowsky-stained blood films, IBD inclusions are smooth, homogenous, pale, basophilic structures that often fill the cytoplasm and can displace the nucleus (**Fig. 11**). All body systems are affected by IBD, but inclusions can mostly be found in the neurons and glial cells of the central nervous system, epithelial cells of the mucosa of the alimentary tract, hepatocytes, renal tubular epithelial cells, and pancreas.[72] Identification of IBD inclusions in peripheral blood (buffy coat preparations are recommended) can help to confirm a clinical suspicion and establish an antemortem diagnosis. If inclusions are absent in peripheral blood from an animal with suspected IBD, histopathologic examination of biopsies of the liver, stomach, or esophageal tonsils is indicated to make a diagnosis.[73]

Iridoviral inclusions have been reported in blood cells of snakes, lizards, and turtles.[74–77] Iridoviral infections, formerly termed pirhemocytonosis, were correctly identified by using transmission electron microscopy to demonstrate viral particles

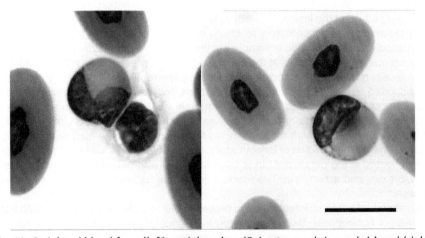

**Fig. 11.** Peripheral blood from (*left*) a rainbow boa (*Epicrates senchria senchria*) and (*right*) a common boa constrictor (*Boa constrictor imperator*) with inclusion body disease. Lymphocytes contain homogenous basophilic inclusions that displace the nucleus. A partially lysed thrombocyte is also seen in the image on the left. Wright-Giemsa, bar = 10 μm.

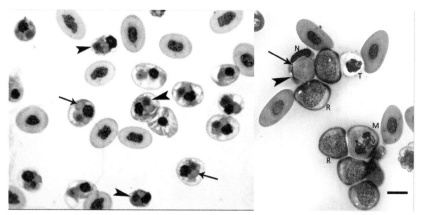

**Fig. 12.** Peripheral blood from a peninsula ribbon snake (*Thamnophis sauritus sackenii*) (*left*) and terciopelo (*Bothrops asper*) (*right*) with SEV infections. The erythrocytes contain crystalline inclusions (*arrows*) and granular eosinophilic viral inclusions (*arrowheads*) characteristic of SEV. Nucleus (N) of an erythroid precursor that contains a viral inclusion. M, mitotic figure; R, rubricyte; T, thrombocyte. Wright-Giemsa, bar = 10 μm.

consistent with *Iridoviridae*.[76,78] Iridoviral inclusions are seen in a variety of target cells, and their morphology varies in different reptile species. Infections have been reported as pathogens in reptiles, but inclusions in circulating erythrocytes have been noted without any apparent adverse effects. In lizards, the virus is termed lizard erythrocyte virus (LEV); inclusions appear in the cytoplasm of erythrocytes as small, punctuate to oval, dark pink amorphous structures, sometimes associated with rectangular albuminoid vacuoles.[76] Natural LEV infections have not been associated with clinical disease,[76] whereas experimental infections can induce systemic disease.[79] In snakes, the virus is termed snake erythrocyte virus (SEV) and inclusions are of 2 types. One type of inclusion is viral in origin and appears as punctuate aggregates of granular pink to dark purple material. The other type of inclusion is pale orange to pink, round to hexagonal, and crystalline and is thought to be composed of cellular and viral byproducts of lipids and proteins (**Fig. 12**).[77,80] SEV infection often is associated with severe anemia.[77,78,80] Iridoviral inclusions (frog virus 3; genus *Ranavirus*) have also been identified in monocytes, azurophils, and heterophils of an eastern box turtle. These cytoplasmic inclusions were 3 to 7 μm in diameter, round to oval, pink, and granular; this viral infection can also cause systemic illness.[75]

Poxviral inclusions were first described in a blood smear from a flap-necked chameleon as pleomorphic, basophilic to purple inclusions within monocytes.[71] Poxvirus infection has been reported in crocodilians, tegu lizards, and tortoises and can cause generalized skin disease with pustular lesions or benign skin tumors.[81]

## HEMOPARASITES

Most hemoparasites of reptiles are nonpathogenic; they are observed often in the blood of healthy, wild-caught animals. Pathogenic hemoparasites are associated with hemolytic anemia and other clinical disease, particularly when stress is a factor. This section briefly describes the morphology of the most common hemoparasites in reptiles. Detailed information can be found in a recent textbook.[82]

The term hemogregarine is used to describe a variety of morphologically similar organisms from 4 different genera. They can be found in most reptile species and

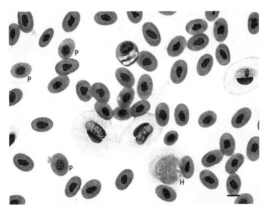

**Fig. 13.** Peripheral blood from an eastern indigo snake (*Drymarchon corais couperi*) with *Hepatozoon* sp infection. Gametocytes can be seen in 3 highly swollen erythrocytes and 1 rubricyte. H, heterophil; P, polychromatophils. Wright-Giemsa, bar = 10 μm.

cannot be differentiated based on morphology alone.[82] Hemogregarine gametocytes are readily identified within the cytoplasm of erythrocytes of infected animals. They are oblong organisms with a pale basophilic cytoplasm and central round to oval nuclei with dark purple chromatin. The organism may displace or wrap itself around the nucleus of the host cell (**Fig. 13**). Hemogregarines are generally considered nonpathogenic but have the ability to provoke a significant inflammatory response in unnatural or aberrant host species.[29,83,84]

More than 90 species and subspecies of *Plasmodium* have been described in reptiles.[82] Gametocytes of *Plasmodium* are morphologically similar to those of hemogregarines, with the difference that most malarial parasites typically contain refractile, golden-brown pigment granules (hemozoin). In addition, meronts and trophozoites (small, signet-ring structures) may also be identified in the peripheral blood of infected animals. Most *Plasmodium* spp are nonpathogenic in reptiles, but cases of mild to severe anemia have been reported.[9,85]

Trypanosomes of reptiles are morphologically similar to those infecting mammals and birds. They are extracellular, flagellate protozoa with a kinetoplast and an undulating membrane. Trypanosome infections have been reported in many reptile species; they generally result in lifelong subclinical infections and rarely cause clinical disease.[9,85,86]

Microfilarial infections have been described in many reptile species.[85] Although generally considered subclinical and an incidental finding, heavy infestations may result in clinical disease.[85,87] Filarid worms are readily identified in blood films of infected animals.

## HEMATOPOIETIC NEOPLASIA

As with other chronic diseases, hematopoietic neoplasms are not usually detected in reptiles until an advanced stage of disease has developed.[2] Diagnosis and differentiation of hematopoietic neoplasia in reptiles is based on the leukocyte differential and morphology (eg, atypical blast cells),[88,89] bone marrow evaluation, and cytochemical, immunocytochemical, or immunohistochemical staining.[89,90] Lymphoid malignancies with or without leukemia are among the most commonly described hematopoietic neoplasms in reptiles, particularly in snakes and lizards (**Fig. 14**), and also have

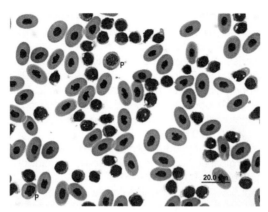

**Fig. 14.** Peripheral blood from an Asian cobra (*Naja naja kaouthia*) with marked leukocytosis (388,000/µL) diagnosed as a chronic lymphocytic leukemia. Neoplastic lymphocytes (L), polychromatophils (P). Lymphocytes were identified as T cell in origin by using immunocytochemistry. Wright-Giemsa, ×100 objective.

been rarely reported in chelonians and crocodilians.[88,91–94] Reported cases of lymphoid malignancies are sporadic, but a high incidence of multicentric lymphoma was documented in a colony of Egyptian spiny-tailed lizards.[95] Other hematopoietic neoplasms reported in reptile species include myelogenous leukemia,[90,96] chronic monocytic leukemia,[48] other myeloproliferative disorders,[91,97] and leukemia of undetermined origin in a desert spiny lizard.[98]

## SUMMARY

There have been significant advancements in the understanding of reptile hematology in recent years. Much work has been done to identify blood cell types and function in many species of reptiles using cytochemical and ultrastructural methods. Baseline data and reference intervals have been established for many species, and many of the infectious, environmental, and neoplastic processes affecting the hemogram of reptiles have been documented. However, given the vast number of species of reptiles and the increasing recognition of new disease processes using molecular techniques, continued investigations are needed in the future, especially evidence-based studies of disease and associated hematologic abnormalities.

## REFERENCES

1. Rivera S, Wellehan JFX, McManamon R, et al. Systemic adenovirus infection in Sulawesi tortoises (*Indotestudo forsteni*) caused by a novel siadenovirus. J Vet Diagn Invest 2009;21:415–26.
2. Saggese M. Clinical approach to the anemic reptile. J Exotic Pet Med 2009;18: 98–111.
3. Campbell TW. Hematology of reptiles. In: Thrall MA, editor. Veterinary hematology and clinical chemistry. Philadelphia: Lippincott Williams & Wilkins; 2004. p. 259–76.
4. Strik NI, Alleman AR, Harr KE. Circulating inflammatory cells. In: Jacobson ER, editor. Infectious diseases and pathology of reptiles. Boca Raton (FL): CRC Press; 2007. p. 167–218.

5. Hawkey CM, Dennett TB. Color atlas of comparative veterinary hematology: normal and abnormal blood cells in mammals, birds and reptiles. Ames (IA): Iowa State University Press; 1989.

6. Verma GK, Banerjee V. Intergeneric haematological studies in three selected reptiles: erythrocytes. Indian Journal of Animal Research 1982;16:49–53.

7. Desser SS. Morphological, cytochemical and biochemical observations on the blood of tuatara, *Sphenodon punctatus*. N Z J Zool 1978;5:503–8.

8. Desser SS. Haematological observations on a hibernating tuatara, *Sphenodon punctatus*. N Z J Zool 1979;6:77–8.

9. Frye FL. Hematology as applied to clinical reptile medicine. In: Frye FL, editor. Biomedical and surgical aspects of captive reptile husbandry, vol. 1. 2nd edition. Melbourne (FL): Kreiger; 1991. p. 209–77.

10. Sypek J, Borysenko M. Reptiles. In: Rowley AF, Ratcliffe NA, editors. Vertebrate blood cells. Cambridge (UK): Cambridge University Press; 1988. p. 211–56.

11. Wallach JD, Boever WJ. Diseases of exotic animals, medical and surgical management. Philadelphia: WB Saunders Co; 1983. p. 983–7.

12. Hawkey CM, Bennett PM, Gascoyne SC, et al. Erythrocyte size, number and hemoglobin content in vertebrates. Br J Haematol 1991;77:392–7.

13. Duguy R. Numbers of blood cells and their variations. In: Gans C, Parsons TC, editors. Biology of the reptilia, vol. 3. San Diego (CA): Academic Press; 1970. p. 93–109.

14. Altland PD, Brace KC. Red cell life span in the turtle and toad. Am J Physiol 1962;203:1188–90.

15. Heard D, Harr K, Wellehan J. Diagnostic sampling and laboratory tests. In: Girling SJ, Raiti P, editors. BSAVA manual of reptiles. 2nd edition. United Kingdom: Blackwell Publishing; 2004. p. 78–9.

16. Alleman AR, Raskin RE, Jacobson ER. Morphologic and cytochemical characteristics of blood cells from the desert tortoise, *Gopherus agasizzi*. Am J Vet Res 1992;53:1645–51.

17. Clark P, Johnstone AS, Ellison R, et al. Inclusions in the erythrocytes of eastern water dragons (*Physignathus lesueurii*). Aust Vet J 2001;79(1):61–2.

18. Harr KE, Alleman AR, Dennis PM, et al. Morphologic and cytochemical characteristics of blood cells and hematologic and plasma biochemical reference ranges in green iguanas. J Am Vet Med Assoc 2001;218:915–21.

19. Simpson CF, Jacobson ER, Harvey JW. Noncrystalline inclusions in erythrocytes of a rhinoceros iguana. Vet Clin Pathol 1980;9:24–6.

20. Alleman AR, Jacobson ER, Raskin RE. Morphologic, cytochemical staining and ultrastructural characteristics of blood from eastern diamondback rattlesnakes (*Crotalus adamanteus*). Am J Vet Res 1999;60:507–14.

21. Saint Girons MC. Morphology of the circulating blood cell. In: Gans C, Parsons TC, editors. Biology of the reptilia, vol. 3. New York: Academic Press; 1970.

22. Montali RJ. Comparative pathology of inflammation on the higher vertebrates (reptiles, birds and mammals). J Comp Pathol 1988;99:1–26.

23. Wright KM, Skeba S. Hematology and plasma chemistries of captive prehensile-tailed skinks (*Corucia zebrata*). J Zoo Wildl Med 1992;23:429–32.

24. Mateo MR, Roberts ED, Enright FM. Morphologic, cytochemical and functional studies of peripheral blood cells of young healthy American alligators (*Alligator mississippiensis*). Am J Vet Res 1984;45:1046–53.

25. Christopher MM, Berry KH, Wallis IR, et al. Reference intervals and physiologic alterations in hematologic and biochemical values of free-ranging desert tortoises in the Mojave desert. J Wildl Dis 1999;35:212–38.

26. Azevedo A, Lunardi LO. Cytochemical characterization of eosinophilic leukocytes circulating in the blood of the turtle (*Chrysemys dorbignih*). Acta Histochem 2003; 105(1):99–105.

27. Harvey JW. Atlas of veterinary hematology. Philadelphia: WB Saunders; 2001. p. 13.

28. Dotson TK, Ramsay EC, Bounous DI. A color atlas of the blood cells of the yellow rat snake. Compend Contin Educ Pract Vet 1995;17:1013–26.

29. Salakij C, Salakij J, Apibal S, et al. Hematology, morphology and ultrastructural characteristics of blood cells in king cobras (*Ophiophagus hannah*). Vet Clin Pathol 2002;31:116–26.

30. Mead KF, Borysenko M. Surface immunoglobulin on granular and agranular leukocytes in the thymus and spleen of the snapping turtle, *Chelydra serpentina*. Dev Comp Immunol 1984;8:109–20.

31. Deem SL, Dierenfeld ES, Sounget GP, et al. Blood values in free-ranging nesting leatherback sea turtles (*Dermochelys coriacea*) on the coast of the Republic of Gabon. J Zoo Wildl Med 2006;37:464–71.

32. Manfredi MT, Piccolo G, Prato F, et al. Parasites in Italian sea turtles I. The leatherback turtle *Dermochelys coriacea* (Linnaeus, 1766). Parassitologia 1996;38:581–3.

33. Allison RW, Velguth KE. Appearance of granulated cells in blood films stained by aqueous versus methanolic Romanowsky methods. Vet Clin Pathol 2009;39: 99–104.

34. Work TM, Raskin RE, Balazs GH, et al. Morphologic and cytochemical characteristics of blood cells from Hawaiian green turtles. Am J Vet Res 1998;59:1252–7.

35. Mead KF, Borysenko M, Findlay SR. Naturally abundant basophils in the snapping turtle, *Chyledra serpentina*, possesses surface antibody with reaginic function. J Immunol 1983;130:334.

36. Cannon MS. The morphology and cytochemistry of the blood leukocytes of Kemp's ridley sea turtles (*Lepidochelys kempi*). Can J Zool 1992;70:1336–40.

37. Brenner D, Lewbart G, Stebbins M, et al. Health survey of wild and captive bog turtles (*Clemmys muhlenbergii*) in North Carolina and Virginia. J Zoo Wildl Med 2002;33(4):311–6.

38. Innis CJ, Tlusty M, Wunn D. Hematologic and plasma biochemical analysis of juvenile head-started northern red-bellied cooters (*Pseudemys rubriventris*). J Zoo Wildl Med 2007;38(3):425–32.

39. Anderson NL, Wack RF, Hatcher R. Hematology and clinical chemistry reference ranges for clinically normal, captive New Guinea snapping turtle (*Elseya novaguineae*) and the effects of temperature, sex and sample type. J Zoo Wildl Med 1997;28:394–403.

40. Kumar De T, Maiti BR. Differential leukocyte count in both sexes of an Indian softshelled turtle (*Lissemys punctata punctata*). Z Mikrosk Anat Forsch 1981;95: 1065–9.

41. Perpinan D, Hernandez-Divers SM, Latimer KS, et al. Hematology of the Pascagoula map turtle (*Graptemys gibbonsi*) and the southeast Asian box turtle (*Cuora amboinensis*). J Zoo Wildl Med 2008;39(3):460–3.

42. Sypek JP, Borysenko M, Findlay SR. Anti-immunoglobulin histamine release from naturally abundant basophils in the snapping turtle, *Chyledra serpentina*. Dev Comp Immunol 1984;8:358.

43. Divers SJ, Redmayne G, Aves EK. Haematological and biochemical values of 10 green iguanas (*Iguana iguana*). Vet Rec 1996;138:203–5.

44. Lamirande EW, Bratthauer AD, Fisher DC, et al. Reference hematologic and plasma chemistry values of brown tree snakes (*Boiga irregularis*). J Zoo Wildl Med 1999;30:516–20.

45. Troiano JC, Vidal JC, Gould J, et al. Haematological and reference intervals of the South American rattlesnake (*Crotalus durissus terrificus*, Laurenti, 1768) in captivity. Comp Haematol Int 1997;1:109–12.
46. Pienaar Ude V. Haematology of some South African reptiles. Johannesburg (South Africa): Witwatersrand University Press; 1962. p. 1–299.
47. Stacy BA, Pessier AP. Host response to infectious agents and identification of pathogens in tissue sections. In: Jacobson ER, editor. Infectious diseases and pathology of reptiles. Boca Raton (FL): CRC Press; 2007. p. 260–1.
48. Gregory CR, Latimer KS, Fontenot DK, et al. Chronic monocytic leukemia in an inland bearded dragon, *Pogona vitticeps*. J Herpetol Med Surg 2004; 14:12–6.
49. George JW, Holmberg TA, Riggs SM, et al. Circulating siderophagocytes and erythrophagocytes in a corn snake (*Elaphe guttata*) after coelomic surgery. Vet Clin Pathol 2008;37(3):308–11.
50. Jacobson ER, Adams HP, Geisbert TW, et al. Pulmonary lesions in experimental ophidian paramyxovirus pneumonia of Aruba island rattlesnakes, *Crotalus unicolor*. Vet Pathol 1997;34:450–9.
51. Dieterlen-Lievre F. Birds. In: Rowley AF, Ratcliffe MA, editors. Vertebrate blood cells. Cambridge (UK): Cambridge University Press; 1988. p. 257–336.
52. Stacy BA, Whitaker N. Hematology and blood chemistry of captive mugger crocodiles (*Crocodylus palustris*). J Zoo Wildl Med 2000;31:339–47.
53. Kakizoe Y, Sakaoka K, Kakizoe F, et al. Successive changes of hematologic characteristics and plasma chemistry values of juvenile loggerhead turtles (*Caretta caretta*). J Zoo Wildl Med 2007;38(1):77–84.
54. Bolten AB, Bjorndal KA. Blood profiles for a wild population of green turtles (*Chelonia mydas*) in the southern Bahamas: size-specific and sex-specific relationships. J Wildl Dis 1992;28(3):407–13.
55. Raphael BL, Klemens MW, Moelman P, et al. Blood values in free-ranging pancake tortoises (*Malacochersus tornieri*). J Zoo Wildl Med 1994;25:63–7.
56. Taylor RW, Jacobson ER. Hematology and serum chemistry of the gopher tortoise *Gopherus polyphemus*. Comp Biochem Physiol 1982;72A:425–8.
57. Zaias J, Norton T, Fickel A, et al. Biochemical and hematologic values for 18 clinically healthy radiated tortoises (*Geochelone radiata*) on St Catherines Island, Georgia. Vet Clin Pathol 2006;35(3):321–5.
58. Chaffin K, Norton TM, Gilardi K, et al. Health assessment of free-ranging alligator snapping turtles (*Macrochelys temminckii*) in Georgia and Florida. J Wildl Dis 2008;44(3):670–86.
59. Wood FE, Ebanks GK. Blood cytology and hematology of the green sea turtle, *Chelonia mydas*. Herpetologica 1984;40:331–6.
60. Cuadadro M, Diaz-Paniagua C, Quevedo MA, et al. Hematology and clinical chemistry in dystocic and healthy post-reproductive female chameleons. J Wildl Dis 2002;38:395–401.
61. Dutton CJ, Taylor P. A comparison between pre- and posthibernation in morphometry, hematology and blood chemistry in viperid snakes. J Zoo Wildl Med 2003;34(1):53–8.
62. Gottdenker NL, Jacobson ER. Effect of venipuncture sites on hematologic and clinical biochemical values in desert tortoises (*Gopherus agassizii*). Am J Vet Res 1995;56:19–21.
63. Crawshaw GJ, Holz P. Comparison of plasma biochemical values in blood and blood-lymph mixtures from red-eared sliders, *Trachemys scripta elegans*. Bull Assoc Rept Amphib Vet 1996;6(2):7–9.

64. Hernandez-Divers SM, Hernandez-Divers SJ, Wyneken J. Angiographic, anatomic, and clinical technique descriptions of a subcarapacial venipuncture site for chelonians. J Herpetol Med Surg 2002;12(2):32–7.

65. Canfield PJ. Comparative cell morphology in the peripheral blood film from exotic and native animals. Aust Vet J 1998;76:793–800.

66. Sykes JM, Klaphake E. Reptile hematology. Vet Clin North Am Exot Anim Pract 2008;11:481–500.

67. Rosskopf WJ Jr, Woerperl RW. Granulocytic leukemia in a Texas tortoise. Mod Vet Pract 1982;9:701–2.

68. Neiffer DL, Lydick D, Burks K, et al. Hematologic and plasma biochemical changes associated with fenbendazole administration in Hermann's tortoises (Testudo hermanni). J Zoo Wildl Med 2005;36:661–72.

69. Tucunduva M, Borelli P, Silva JR. Experimental study of induced inflammation in the Brazilian Boa (Boa constrictor constrictor). J Comp Pathol 2001;125: 174–81.

70. Simpson CF, Jacobson ER, Harvey JW. Electron microscopy of a spiral-shaped bacterium in the blood and bone marrow of a rhinoceros iguana. Can J Comp Med 1981;45:388–91.

71. Jacobson ER, Telford SR. Chlamydial and poxvirus infections of circulating monocytes of the flap-necked chameleon (Chameleo dilepis). J Wildl Dis 1990;26: 572–7.

72. Jacobson ER, Oros J, Tucker SJ, et al. Partial characterization of retroviruses from boid snakes with inclusion body disease. Am J Vet Res 2001;62:217–24.

73. Jacobson ER. Cytologic diagnosis of inclusion body disease of boid snakes. In: Jacobson ER, editor. Proceedings of the North American Veterinary Conference. Orlando (FL); 2001. p. 920.

74. Marquardt WC, Yaeger RG. The structure and taxonomic status of Toddia from the cotton-mouth snake Agkistrodon piscivorus leucostoma. J Protozool 1967; 14:726–31.

75. Allender MC, Fry MM, Irizarry AR, et al. Intracytoplasmic inclusions in circulating leukocytes from an eastern box turtle (Terrapene carolina carolina) with iridoviral infection. J Wildl Dis 2006;42(3):677–84.

76. Telford SR Jr, Jacobson ER. Lizard erythrocytic virus in east African chameleons. J Wildl Dis 1993;29:57–63.

77. Wellehan JFX Jr, Strik NI, Stacy BA, et al. Characterization of an erythrocytic virus in the family Iridoviridae from a peninsula ribbon snake (Thamnophis sauritus sackenii). Vet Microbiol 2008;131:115–22.

78. Daly JJ, Mayhue M, Menna JH, et al. Virus-like particles associated with Pirhemocyton inclusion bodies in the erythrocytes of a water snake, nerodia erythrogaster flavigaster. J Parasitol 1980;66:82–7.

79. Alves de Matos AP, Paperna I, Crespo E. Experimental infection of lacertids with lizard erythrocytic viruses. Intervirology 2002;45:150–9.

80. Johnsrude JD, Raskin RE, Hoge AY, et al. Intraerythrocytic inclusions associated with iridoviral infection in a fer de lance (Bothrops moojeni) snake. Vet Pathol 1997;34:235–8.

81. Jacobson ER. Viruses and viral disease of reptiles. In: Jacobson ER, editor. Infectious diseases and pathology of reptiles. Boca Raton (FL): CRC Press; 2007. p. 395–460.

82. Telford SR. Hemoparasites of the reptilia. Boca Raton (FL): CRC Press; 2008.

83. Wozniak EJ, Telford SR Jr. The fate of Hepatozoon species naturally infecting Florida black racers and watersnakes in potential mosquito and soft tick vectors,

and histological evidence of pathogenicity in unnatural host species. Int J Parasitol 1991;21:511–6.

84. Wozniak EJ, Telford SR, McLaughlin GL. Employment of the polymerase chain reaction in the molecular differentiation of reptilian hemogregarines and its application to preventative zoological medicine. J Zoo Wildl Med 1994;25: 538–49.

85. Lane TJ, Mader DR. Parasitology. In: Mader DR, editor. Reptile medicine and surgery. Philadelphia: WB Saunders Co; 1996. p. 185–203.

86. Keymer IF. Protozoa. In: Cooper JE, Jackson OF, editors. Diseases of reptilia, vol. 1. London: Academic Press; 1981. p. 233–90.

87. Irizarry-Rovira AR, Wolf A, Bolek M, et al. Blood smear from a wild-caught panther cameleon (*Furcifer pardalis*). Vet Clin Pathol 2002;31(3):129–32.

88. Lock B, Heard D, Dumore D, et al. Lymphosarcoma with lymphoid leukemia in an Aruba Island rattlesnake, *Crotalus unicolor.* J Herpetol Med Surg 2001;11:19–23.

89. Georoff TA, Stacy NI, Newton AN. Diagnosis and treatment of chronic T-lymphocytic leukemia in a green tree monitor (*Varanus prasinus*). J Herpe Med Surg 2010;19(4):1–9.

90. Tocidlowski ME, McNamara PL, Wojcieszyn JW. Myelogenous leukemia in a bearded dragon (*Acanthodraco vitticeps*). J Zoo Wildl Med 2001;32:90–5.

91. Garner MM, Hernandez-Divers SM, Raymond JT. Reptile neoplasia: a retrospective study of case submissions to a specialty diagnostic service. Vet Clin North Am Exot Anim Pract 2004;7:653–71.

92. Hernandez-Divers SM, Orcutt CJ, Stahl SJ, et al. Lymphoma in lizards – three case reports. J Herpetol Med Surg 2003;13:14–21.

93. Schultze AE, Mason GL, Clyde VL. Lymphosarcoma with leukemic blood profile in a Savannah monitor lizard (*Varanus exanthematicus*). J Zoo Wildl Med 1999;30: 158–64.

94. Raiti P, Garner MM, Wojcieszyn J. Lymphocytic leukemia and multicentric T-cell lymphoma in a diamond python, *Morelia spilota spilota.* J Herpetol Med Surg 2002;12:26–9.

95. Gyimesi ZS, Garner MM, Burns RB, et al. High incidence of lymphoid neoplasia in a colony of Egyptian spiny-tailed lizards (*Uromastyx aegyptius*). J Zoo Wildl Med 2005;36:103–10.

96. Hruban Z, Vardiman J, Meehan T, et al. Haematopoietic malignancies in zoo animals. J Comp Pathol 1992;106:15–24.

97. Marcus LC. Myeloproliferative disease in a turtle. J Am Vet Med Assoc 1973; 162:4–5.

98. Goldberg SR, Holshuh HJ. A case of leukemia in the desert spiny lizard (*Scelporous magister*). J Wildl Dis 1991;27:521–5.

# The Regenerative Medicine Laboratory: Facilitating Stem Cell Therapy for Equine Disease

Dori L. Borjesson, DVM, PhD[a],*, John F. Peroni, DVM, MS[b]

**KEYWORDS**

- Equine • Stem cell • Mesenchymal stem cell
- Regenerative medicine • Orthopedic disease

Stem cell therapy for tissue regeneration is rapidly gaining momentum as the treatment of choice for many equine orthopedic lesions. Stem cells have significant therapeutic potential because of their ability to regulate inflammation, promote tissue regeneration, and prevent pathologic scar formation. Lameness due to osteoarthritis has long been regarded as a leading cause of reduced or lost performance in horses and a significant reason for economic hardship to the equine industry. With tendon injuries, the damaged tendon is replaced by scar tissue, resulting in a substantial risk for reinjury. The goal of regenerative therapies is to restore normal structural architecture and biomechanical function to an injured tissue.[1] For regeneration to occur, therapy must recapitulate the appropriate spatial and temporal interactions between stem cells, scaffold, and growth factors.[1] The term stem cell encompasses a wide variety of cell types, including hematopoietic stem cells (HSCs), embryonic stem (ES) cells, induced pluripotent stem (iPS) cells, and adult-derived mesenchymal stem cells (MSCs). These cell types differ in their pluripotentiality, tissue of origin, and putative therapeutic uses.

HSCs are pluripotent self-renewing cells, generally derived from umbilical cord blood (CB) or bone marrow (BM) and are capable of reconstituting the hematopoietic environment in primary hematopoietic and nonhematopoietic diseases. Although an active arena for human medical research and laboratory medicine, there are no current

---

The authors have nothing to disclose.

[a] Department of Pathology, Microbiology and Immunology, School of Veterinary Medicine, University of California, One Shields Avenue, Davis, CA 95616, USA

[b] Department of Large Animal Medicine, H-322 College of Veterinary Medicine, University of Georgia, 501 D.W. Brooks Drive, Athens, GA 30602, USA

* Corresponding author.

*E-mail address:* dlborjesson@ucdavis.edu

Clin Lab Med 31 (2011) 109–123

doi:10.1016/j.cll.2010.12.001

therapeutic applications for equine HSCs and these HSCs remain poorly character-ized. Equine ES cell lines have been developed, and a recent review of the state of art for equine ES cell research has been published.[2] Six putative ES cell lines derived from equine embryos have been described. All these cell lines express stem cell–associated markers and exhibit longevity and pluripotency in vitro, but none have been proven to exhibit pluripotency in vivo.[2] As with human medicine, the equine community also struggles with ethical concerns over the use of equine embryos to develop ES cells. In response to these concerns and in alignment with current human medical research, iPS cell line development is an active area of research. Although there are no reports of successful equine iPS cell line development to date, many research groups are working toward this goal, and success in the near future is considered very likely. The research into and development of equine ES and iPS cells is on a fairly typical trajectory for veterinary product development. Research precedes clinical use, and therapy development mirrors and follows human medical advances.

The research and clinical use of equine adult-derived MSCs has followed an entirely different path. MSCs have been in clinical use for equine orthopedic injuries as early as 2003, with only a handful (<5 peer-reviewed articles) of research publications in print at that point. Since that time, the clinical use of MSCs has exploded, with thousands of horses treated all over the world. Basic research has also expanded, but it lags substantially behind rapid product development and clinical experimentation. MSCs are used to treat acute and chronic, primarily orthopedic, lesions, including tendinopa-thies, ligament injuries, fractures, laminitis, and joint diseases, such as subchondral bone cysts, meniscal tears, and cartilage defects. This treatment is in stark contrast to human medicine, whereby MSC therapies are principally focused on immune-medi-ated (eg, steroid refractory acute graft-versus-host disease, and Crohn disease, http://www.osiristx.com/) and ischemic diseases (eg, myocardial infarction and diabetic vasculopathy). Adult-derived MSCs are multipotent (partially lineage committed) and can be obtained and expanded from almost all tissue types; however, the emphasis in horses has been on MSCs derived from BM (BM-MSCs),[3–5] adipose tissue (AT-MSCs),[6–8] and placental tissues (umbilical CB [CB-MSCs][9–13] and umbilical cord tissue [CT-MSCs]) (Fig. 1).[14,15] Equine regenerative medicine is primarily focused on MSCs administered as a single product or in combination with the heterogeneous nonexpanded progenitor cell populations from which they are obtained (BM nucleated cells, adipose-derived stromal vascular fraction, or CB nucleated cells). Similar to human beings, MSCs are being genetically modified in the hopes of augmenting their healing capacity or as a specific way to deliver gene therapy.[16] For example, the oste-ogenic potential of BM-MSCs may be augmented by genes encoding bone morpho-genetic proteins (BMPs). Genetically modified MSCs could be useful for cell-based delivery of BMPs to a site of bone formation.[17,18] Similarly, insulinlike growth factor 1-enhanced BM-MSCs or BMP12-enhanced MSCs may be more specific and beneficial for the treatment of tendonitis with improved tenocyte healing without mineralization.[18,19]

In this article, we focus exclusively on equine MSCs derived from BM, adipose tissues (ATs), and placental tissues. We briefly cover how MSCs are currently defined and what is known about how MSCs work and how tissue source may influence MSC healing properties. Our emphasis is on basic laboratory practices, including the logis-tical aspects of obtaining, processing, and storing equine MSCs. We highlight relevant differences between the human and veterinary MSC arenas in terms of laboratory processes, regulatory issues, and clinical disease applications. Our goal is to make the regenerative medicine laboratory into a state-of-the-art laboratory that adheres to good laboratory practices with oversight by laboratory medicine clinicians and

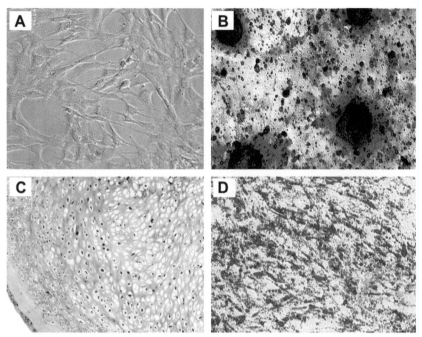

**Fig. 1.** Equine BM-derived MSCs. (*A*) Adherent spindle-shaped MSCs in culture. (*B*) MSCs differentiated toward osteoblasts (alizarin red S stain). (*C*) MSCs differentiated toward chondrocytes (trichome stain). (*D*) MSCs differentiated toward adipocytes (oil red O stain) ([A–D] original magnification ×10).

hematopathologists who work hand in hand with primary care clinicians to facilitate excellent evidence-based medicine and translational research.

## MSC CHARACTERIZATION

MSCs are classically defined as multipotent spindle-shaped stromal cells that adhere to plastic and are capable of differentiation into the mesodermal adipose tissues, cartilage, and bone (see **Fig. 1**A).[3,13,15,20] Techniques used to differentiate MSCs into bone, cartilage, and fat in vitro have been modified for equine tissues, and using these methods, it has been shown that MSCs derived from AT, CB, cord tissue (CT), and BM are all multipotent and capable of trilineage differentiation (see **Fig. 1**B–D).[3,8,11,15,20] Human and rodent MSCs are also defined by a panel of surface protein markers (ie, CD34 and CD45[–] and CD90 and CD105[+]). However, no single defining MSC marker has been recognized in any species.

The ability to fully characterize equine MSCs is hindered by limited antibody availability and variable antibody cross-reactivity. Nonetheless, equine MSC protein expression has been evaluated using flow cytometry and immunocytochemistry, and protein expression, to date, is compatible with findings in rodents and human beings. Established BM-MSCs are negative for the leukocyte antigens CD18 and CD45 and are positive for $\beta_1$ integrins, fibronectin, collagen IV, CD44, CD29, and CD90.[3,21] Equine AT-MSCs similarly express CD90 and CD44.[7] CB and CT-MSCs are negative for CD18, pan cytokeratin (epithelial marker), and von Willebrand factor (factor VIII-related antigen, endothelial marker) and variably positive for smooth muscle actin, osteonectin, and osteocalcin.[13,22] CT-MSCs are vimentin positive; however, early passage, highly proliferative CB-MSCs are mostly negative for vimentin until they undergo senescence.[13,22]

ES cell markers have been reported to be variably expressed by equine MSCs immunocytochemically; however, the absence of antibody validation, including the use of positive control tissue,[23,24] and inappropriate cytochemical antigen localization[24] make interpretation of these data difficult. Recent studies have emphasized other cell characteristics, including long-term proliferation and immunophenotype, to define MSCs because although MSC cell-surface antigens have been extensively explored, there is no conclusive evidence that cell markers confer functional repair outcomes.[25]

## TISSUE SOURCES FOR CELLULAR THERAPIES

Prospective equine clinical trials to determine the optimal regenerative medicine product for treatment of any given lesion have not been completed. Deciding which product or products to be used is at the discretion of the primary clinician after consultation with laboratory personnel and researchers. The availability of multiple tissue sources and cell types for cellular therapy means that decision making for therapeutic use or clinical trials is often based on anecdotal evidence, empirical data, or clinician familiarity with the product rather than solid evidence-based medicine.

Regenerative medicine products can essentially be divided into 2 product categories. The first category includes nonexpanded, patient-side, autologous products, including BM concentrate, CB nucleated cell concentrate, adipose-derived stromal vascular fraction, and platelet-rich plasma. The second category includes culture-expanded, autologous or allogeneic products, including BM-MSCs, CB-MSCs, CT-MSCs, and AT-MSCs. Purported advantages of nonexpanded cell products include the heterogeneity of the cell populations present and the rapid laboratory turn-around time, facilitating treatment of acute lesions (most samples can be concentrated and prepared within a few hours). In addition, as these products are almost exclusively for autologous use, with no additional ancillary materials or additives, they are the least likely to be regulated by the Food and Drug Administration (FDA). CB and BM mononuclear cells and the adipose-derived stromal vascular fraction contain varying numbers of endothelial progenitor cells ($CD34^+$, $CD133^+$), with presumed hematopoietic and angiopoietic properties, monocytes/macrophages ($CD14^+$ cells with antiinflammatory functions such as secretion of interleukin [IL]-10 and IL-1 receptor antagonist, M2 phenotype),[26] MSCs, and HSCs. The heterogeneity of the cell types present in nonexpanded cellular therapies may have some advantages for immunomodulation and angiogenesis-stimulating potential.[26] In contrast, culture-expanded cells are highly enriched in MSCs, which can be delivered to the injured tissue in high number as an autologous or an allogeneic product. Unfortunately, MSC expansion can take 2 to 3 weeks, thus precluding the use of expanded cells for acute injuries. Cultured MSCs may also contain remnant ancillary materials, such as fetal bovine serum (FBS) or other additives, and are likely ultimately regulated as a cell therapy by the Center for Biologics Evaluation and Research, FDA. Regardless of product choice, all cellular therapies should undergo minimal product quality testing, including bacterial culture, to ensure sterility, nucleated cell count, and assessment of cell viability.

MSCs are rare cells, and their number declines with age. These factors strongly influence donor choice for tissue banking (young donors being ideal) and tissue selection. In human beings, there are 1 to 20 MSCs per $1 \times 10^5$ BM cells compared with 0.1 to 5 MSCs per $1 \times 10^5$ BM cells in rodents.[27] In young horses, there are approximately 10 to 100 MSCs (cells with fibroblast colony-forming activity) per $1 \times 10^5$ BM cells.[5] Equine AT has even higher numbers of MSCs[8] with a higher proliferation potential.[7] Human BM-MSCs approximately undergo 23 population doublings, reaching full senescence at 38 population doublings.[28] Equine BM-MSCs are similar (20–30 population doublings) and typically reach senescence by passage 10 or earlier. However, equine CB-MSCs,[13] AT-MSCs, and CT-MSCs are more proliferative, with cell lines reaching more than 70 population doublings (Dori L. Borjesson, unpublished data, 2010). Highly proliferative MSCs are recommended for therapy, regardless of species (for human and equine BM-MSCs, this generally translates to P3-P7 cells). The higher proliferative potential of AT-MSCs, CT-MSCs, and CB-MSCs may make these cell lines more amenable to long-term tissue banking. It is far less expensive to screen a low number of donors and maintain phenotyped and karyotyped proliferative cell lines than to continually screen BM donors and phenotype BM-MSCs. However, this factor is the only one in clinical decision making. Ideally, efficacy would direct product line development.

To date, the efficacy of cell therapy products have been compared in a few in vivo studies, using experimentally induced lesions, and in a few in vitro studies. In the first equine study, autologous BM nucleated cells were compared with autologous culture-expanded BM-MSCs for the treatment of collagen-induced tendonitis. Intralesional injection of either cell type resulted in similar ultrasonographic and histologic improvement in lesion size and tendon fiber pattern.[29,30] These investigators have also reported improvement in 20 horses with spontaneous lesions of the flexor tendons or the suspensory ligament after treatment with BM nucleated cells.[30] In the second model, horses with surgically induced osteoarthritis were treated intra-articularly with either autologous expanded BM-MSCs or the adipose-derived stromal vascular fraction. The clinical, radiographic, biochemical, and histologic effects of stem cell treatment were assessed. Overall, significant improvement was not noted with the use of either therapeutic product.[31]

The intra-articular efficacy of BM-MSCs has also been examined in an osteoarthritis large animal model involving anterior cruciate ligament transection and medial meniscectomy in goats.[32] Autologous BM-MSCs were injected intra-articularly 3 weeks after induction of osteoarthritis. Six weeks postinjection, the degree of cartilage destruction, osteophyte formation, and subchondral sclerosis were all reduced in treated compared with control joints, and the formation of a neomeniscus was also observed that subsequently showed positive results when stained for proteoglycan and type II collagen and had the typical appearance of fibrocartilage. This study highlights the potential for therapeutic intra-articular injection of BM-MSCs in large animals, particularly that have concurrent soft tissue disease.[32]

## HOW MSCs FUNCTION TO HEAL TISSUES

It remains controversial whether MSCs primarily contribute to lesion healing by integrating and differentiating into the injured tissue or by secreting trophic factors. It is likely that MSCs principally contribute to the healing of ischemic, immune-mediated, and acute inflammatory lesions (ie, myocardial infarction, laminitis, graft-versus-host disease, and acute tendonitis) via the secretion of antiinflammatory, vasoactive, and immunomodulatory factors. However, MSCs have also shown efficacy in tissue repair of nonhealing fractures and full-thickness cartilage defects, where they are often administered with a scaffolding material and act more as a tissue graft. For this application, it is still unclear whether ex vivo modification and differentiation of these cells before administration are beneficial for improved healing and tissue repair.

### MSCs as a Tissue Graft, the Cartilage Example

Lameness originating from joint diseases, such as osteoarthritis and osteochondrosis, is a significant source of morbidity and poor performance in equine athletes. Regeneration of articular cartilage presents unique challenges because of its lack of vascularity and innervation, leading to an inefficient and slow intrinsic healing capacity. The tissue produced via normal healing processes typically consists of scar tissue or fibrocartilage that lacks the necessary mechanical properties to withstand physiologic strains. As a result of these challenges, equine articular cartilage restoration using MSCs has been regarded as an attractive option to treat synovial inflammation and articular cartilage degeneration. Research is directed toward defining MSC engraftment within chondral lesions and determining whether chondrogenic differentiation or partial differentiation is best for healing cartilage defects.

In the treatment of joint disease, one concern is the seemingly inefficient engraftment of the cells within the damaged cartilage. Fluorescently labeled MSCs suspended in a gelatin matrix and placed into full-thickness chondral defects in a goat model revealed that MSCs were gradually lost from the implant and that large fragments of the gel could be found in deep marrow spaces.[33] In another study, human MSCs were implanted in utero in sheep and then followed to assess engraftment and survival. MSCs underwent site-specific differentiation into chondrocytes, adipocytes, myocytes, cardiomyocytes, BM stromal cells, and thymic stroma. However, cartilage engraftment was inefficient.[34] Although research indicates that treatment of joint disease with MSCs improves clinical symptoms of osteoarthritis, more work needs to be done to investigate proper engraftment of these cells into the synovial environment.

Researchers have also begun to refine laboratory techniques aimed at promoting chondrogenesis in equine MSCs. Equine MSCs have been chondrogenically differentiated in monolayer culture, micromass pellets, and scaffold matrices. Growth factors, such as transforming growth factor (TGF)-$\beta_1$, TGF-$\beta_3$, and fibroblast growth factor 2 (FGF-2), are added to promote differentiation. In one study, TGF-$\beta_1$ was shown to increase cell density, cell layering, nodule formation, collagen type II messenger RNA (mRNA) expression, and collagen type I mRNA expression in monolayer culture compared with control cells.[35] The effects of culture supplementation with TGF-$\beta_3$ and BMP-6 were also compared in BM-MSCs versus AT-MSCs. BM-MSCs showed hyalinelike cartilage morphology with lacunae formation, rounded chondrocytes, and superior glycosaminoglycan content. In contrast, AT-MSCs produced a mature fibroblastic morphology for the duration of the study.[20] The chondrogenic capacity of BM-MSCs was also superior to AT-MSCs after supplementation with FGF-2, exposure to TGF-$\beta_1$, and encapsulation in a hydrogel matrix.[25] Equine BM-MSCs and CB-derived MSCs have also been compared in their capacity for chondrogenic differentiation. CB-derived cells produced larger pellets with hyalinelike cartilage morphology, higher concentrations of cartilage-derived proteins, and higher gene expression of collagen 21 and aggrecan. This study concluded that CB-MSCs may possess a higher capacity for chondrogenic differentiation than BM-MSCs.[36] Although the details of these studies are vastly different, for example, culture conditions and markers used to determine regenerative potential, these types of studies are critical first steps to help define the most appropriate cell source for orthopedic lesions.

## MSCs as Modulators of the Immune System

The therapeutic value of MSCs may be based not only on their contribution to the restoration of the architecture of damaged tissues but also on their proven ability to modulate the inflammatory response. MSCs exhibit potent antiinflammatory and immunomodulatory effects through cell-cell interactions and/or release of soluble factors into the local environment. MSCs have a distinct immunophenotype or profile of bioactive trophic factors, inflammatory mediators, and adhesion molecules that work to inhibit scar formation, inhibit apoptosis, increase angiogenesis, and stimulate intrinsic progenitor cells to regenerate function. MSCs influence host immune responses in vivo and in vitro by interacting with immune cells such as T and B lymphocytes, natural killer cells, and dendritic cells.[37,38] These immunomodulatory properties have formed the basis for their use in the treatment of autoimmune diseases and graft-versus-host disease.[39-43]

MSCs downregulate inflammation and are also considered immune privileged. Because of these properties, the use of non–tissue matched, nonself (allogeneic) MSCs is being pursued. Typically, MSCs are obtained from ex vivo culture of the patient's own tissues (autologous). However, the use of cryogenically preserved MSCs obtained from unrelated donor horses (allogeneic treatment) offers the advantage of more rapid treatment and the use of a more homogenous selected cell population with proven regenerative and differentiation capacity. Pilot studies have evaluated the injection of allogeneic BM-MSCs in surgically induced lesions of the equine superficial digital flexor tendon and the intra-articular injection of allogeneic placentally derived MSCs into equine joints.[22,44] In the tendon study, BM-MSCs, transduced with green fluorescent protein, were placed into superficial digital flexor tendon core lesions 7 days after surgery. Histopathologic examination of the tendons revealed similar numbers of BM-MSCs within the uninjured tendon and within the lesion itself regardless of whether MSCs were allogeneic or autologous. There was no difference in infiltrating leukocyte density between allogeneic and autologous treatments.[44] In the joint study, the injection of MSCs induced joint inflammation (increased leukocyte and total protein concentrations in synovial fluid); however, the inflammation was self-limiting, and there was no difference in the type or severity of the inflammatory response elicited by autologous versus allogeneic MSCs.[22] These studies may help alleviate concerns about the potential negative effects of an immune-mediated response, such as engrafted MSC destruction or induction of a hypersensitivity reaction, after administration of allogeneic MSCs.

Allogeneic MSCs do not induce a significant immune response in part because of differential expression of major histocompatibility complexes (MHCs) on the cell surface.[45] Equine MSCs, similar to murine and human MSCs, express MHC class I but not MHC class II molecules.[22,45,46] Equine MSCs also do not express T-cell costimulatory molecules.[22] This is important because MHC class II molecules, typically found on the cell surface of specialized cells, such as macrophages, dendritic cells, and B cells, stimulate T cells to differentiate into either cytotoxic or helper cells. Although cell membrane expression of MHC class II is lacking in MSCs, there is a substantial intracellular accumulation of this molecule.[38,47] This accumulation may be especially relevant in the context of MSC interaction with cells associated with tissue inflammation. Understanding the environment into which MSCs are introduced during therapeutic use is critical, and research aimed at elucidating the inflammatory niche and MSC function is lacking. For example, MSCs treated with interferon γ (IFN-γ) increase expression of MHC class I and class II molecules.[48] These effects may be dose dependent. Exposure to low levels of IFN-γ leads MSCs to express MHC class

II and acquire phagocytic functions, whereas exposure to high levels of IFN-$\gamma$ decreases MHC class II expression and allows MSCs to acquire an immunomodulatory function.[49]

## ANIMALS AS MODELS

Work to date highlights the need to establish appropriate models for studying the efficacy of MSCs in tissue regeneration. These studies could be paired with well-designed clinical trials. Compared with human medicine, veterinary medicine has a strong advantage because research can be translated directly into clinical (animal) patients. There is far less stringent study regulation compared with similar studies conducted in humans. Animal models are also needed to demonstrate benefits associated with new therapies or products, which are sufficiently different from human standard of care treatment. In addition, preclinical testing of new treatments or devices is required to prove efficacy and safety. In a typical example, the FDA recommends that agents used to enhance bone repair or address treatment of osteoporosis be evaluated in 2 different animal species, rats and a second nonrodent large animal that has a bone structure and remodeling pattern similar to that of humans.[50,51] These animal models of human disease also directly benefit veterinary patients. What remains clear about cellular therapy in both veterinary and human medicine is the large number of unanswered questions regarding MSC dose, MSC tissue source, timing of MSC administration, and cellular augmentation (growth factors and so forth), which may refine and improve clinical outcome. Animal models, in addition to studies performed in large animal species to directly test novel cell therapies for animal use, are critical to answer these questions.

## LABORATORY TECHNIQUES AND PROTOCOLS

There are a few public and private human stem cell companies that have developed veterinary medicine subsidiaries. Most of these companies offer cell storage and/or cell processing for immediate autologous use. Laboratories that offer MSC isolation and expansion from primary tissues for equine patients are limited to a few veterinary companies, academic institutions (eg, the University of California Davis Veterinary Regenerative Medicine Laboratory and the University of Georgia), and a few large equine veterinary referral hospitals (eg, Alamo Pintado Equine Medical Center, Los Olivos, CA, USA and Rood and Riddle Equine Hospital, Lexington, KY, USA). At present, MSC laboratories operate essentially without regulation or oversight; however, ongoing clinical use of these products increases the pressure to maintain high quality standards for cellular therapy products. Our goal is to place the regenerative medicine laboratory and its oversight under the umbrella of good practices followed by Veterinary Clinical Laboratories.

### Tissue Collection

There are several important considerations regarding tissue collection. The first is that the amount of sample tissue harvested (AT, BM, and CB) generally does not predict MSC recovery.[6,13,52] The second is that there is a tremendous amount of intrinsic donor-to-donor variation that influences the success of MSC isolation. The most reliable predictor for successful MSC isolation seems to be donor age (for BM and AT), with young horses (up to 7 years of age) ideal for MSC isolation.[6,52] Some investigators believe that MSCs are blood vessel pericytes and thus that tissue vessel density, generally higher in younger patients, dictates MSC recovery.[37,52] For CB, postprocessing nucleated cell count best predicts the chance of successful MSC isolation.[13]

The isolation technique used (or digestion technique in the case of AT and CT) also contributes to the number of cells isolated. For example, a new method of CB and BM processing markedly improves cellular recovery compared with Ficoll and auto-mated methods for concentrating nucleated cells (Dori L. Borjesson, unpublished data, 2010).[12]

MSCs can be isolated from several tissues. CB and CT are of fetal origin and can only be obtained during foaling. These tissues are easy to collect and, when collected together, provide autologous sources of several different stem cell types. Ideally, CB is processed and frozen for later use as a source of mixed cells with pluripotent potential. High numbers of MSCs can be expanded from CT. Together, these 2 tissues provide a wide range of autologous therapeutic potential for a valuable animal. If placental tissues are not obtained, BM and AT are the most readily available tissues for MSC isolation. Collection is moderately invasive for both techniques.

BM can be successfully harvested from either the sternum or tuber coxae, depend-ing on horse age, temperament, and clinician preference. No differences between sites have been noted for MSC isolation.[5,15] Up to 120 mL of BM can be collected into heparinized syringes, although MSCs have been isolated from as little as 10 mL of BM. The collection of equine CB is safe, and the procedure is well documented.[9] At least 60 mL of CB should be collected; with experience, more than 200 mL of CB can be obtained. CB should be collected into citrate phosphate dextrose adenine 1 anticoagulant to promote cell viability, especially when CB needs to be shipped to a laboratory.[9] Umbilical CT can be readily collected after foaling (videos for equine CB, BM and CT collection can be found at http://www.vetmed.ucdavis.edu/ceh/events_vets.cfm). Because of the inherent environmental contamination of samples collected in a barn, thorough washing of CT samples is recommended as described.[9,15] AT (5–50 g) is generally harvested from the region above the dorsal gluteal muscle, at the base of the tail, because of easy access and the absence of large veins.[6,7,52,53] Fat can be collected into phosphate-buffered saline or media before processing. Collected tissues need to be delivered overnight to an MSC labo-ratory for processing and collection. Many equine patients are presented to an equine referral center or academic institution where processing and MSC expansion occur on-site. However, many regenerative medicine laboratories also receive samples from outside, referring veterinarians.

### Tissue Processing

After collection, BM and CB volumes should be reduced, red blood cells removed, and, if possible, mononuclear cells concentrated. In a laboratory that receives very few samples, this processing can be accomplished manually through ammonium chloride lysis of red blood cells[31,54] or through density gradient centrifugation (Ficoll).[3] Sample processing using these methods may result in bacterial contamination of the sample. Closed systems, such as PrepaCyte (BioE, St Paul, MN, USA)[12] or MXP AutoXpress (Thermogenesis, Rancho Cordova, CA, USA),[13] facilitate sterile, rapid, and standardized volume and red blood cell depletion with maximal nucleated cell recovery. The absence of cross-reactive monoclonal antibodies to deplete lineage committed cells from BM or CB prevents further enrichment or purification of stem cell populations from equine tissues.

The processing of AT and CT both involve tissue mincing and enzymatic digestion of connective tissue before cell isolation and culture. Protocols for the isolation of adipose-derived progenitor cells (or the stromal vascular fraction) vary but all generally include mincing with a scalpel blade or scissors followed by tissue digestion at 37°C with enzymes (generally including collagenase type I) in media for 1 to 12 hours, with or without agitation.[6–8,31,53,54] Nucleated cells are pelleted, washed, enumerated, and seeded at a concentration of $3.5 \times 10^3$ nucleated cells/$cm^2$.[7,8,53,54] CT needs to be thoroughly washed, disinfected, and incubated with high concentrations of antibiotics before mincing and tissue digestion.[9,15] The umbilical vessels should be stripped from the cord to avoid culture contamination with endothelial cells. Commercially available tissue homogenizers are recommended for CT mincing because equine CT is very fibrous and manual mincing is difficult. After homogenization, the tissue is incubated with an enzyme cocktail that includes collagenases, elastase, and hyaluronidase[15] or trypsin[10] for 1 to 3 hours at 37°C. After multiple washings and filtration steps, the recovered nucleated cells are ready for culture.[9,15]

### MSC Culture

Ideal culture conditions maintain MSCs with phenotypic and functional characteristics similar to those exhibited in their original niche, with indefinite proliferation and the capacity to differentiate into multiple lineages.[27] Long-term culture and high cell density are determinants of loss of differentiation potential for human and equine MSCs. Similar to human and rodent MSCs, equine MSCs grow readily in minimal essential media (usually low glucose, Dulbecco modified essential medium or $\alpha$ minimal essential medium) with glutamine and 1% penicillin/streptomycin. This media facilitates MSC expansion while limiting growth of other hemic cells (including hematopoietic cells and macrophages).[3,14,24,27,54] Media must be supplemented with serum (10%–20% FBS) or other supplements that mimic serum (serum-free media). To date, there are no reports of the growth and expansion of equine MSCs in commercially available serum-free media, and the expense of serum-free media may preclude their use until mandated by regulatory agencies. High protein platelet lysate has also been shown to support MSC proliferation in the absence of FBS[53]; however, the variability and complication induced by the addition of autologous or allogeneic cells and proteins to MSC culture are not acceptable for commercial laboratories.

Culture conditions can be modified to enhance MSC isolation and proliferation from different tissue sources or to promote differentiation toward a specific cell lineage. For example, the frequency of MSCs in CB is low; as such, methods to optimize their initial isolation and growth include the addition of dexamethasone ($10^{-7}$ M) to the media[11,12,36] and the use of fibronectin-coated culture plates.[13] CT-MSCs increased their population doublings with the addition of epidermal growth factor supplement to the media while not altering in vitro differentiation ability.[14] Although increased cell proliferation is perceived as useful to decrease culture time, decrease turnaround time for product administration, and potentially increase cell dose, it is unknown whether MSCs are best administered in a fully naive state or whether initiating MSC differentiation toward a selected committed lineage is preferential.

Although there is much debate about initial cell plating density for optimal MSC recovery,[55] it is clear from the literature that plating density is highly variable both between labs and between tissue types (ranges from $2 \times 10^3$ to $5 \times 10^6$ cells/$cm^2$).[3,29] Nonetheless, reported MSC expansion kinetics are remarkably similar between labs, and no data are available that compare initial plating density and success of MSC culture for MSCs derived from the different equine tissue sources. As such, initial and expansion cell plating density remains an uncontrolled variable in the shift toward standardization of MSC culture. Equine MSCs can be plated in standard tissue culture flasks and cultured in standard incubator conditions (37°C with 5% $CO_2$ and 21% $O_2$). Early incubation in a relatively hypoxic environment (5% $O_2$) improved MSC recovery from CB-MSCs[13]; however, the maintenance of a hypoxic incubator (obtained through high nitrogen concentration) may be cost and time prohibitive in most clinical laboratories. Similar to other species, MSC proliferation occurs after an initial lag phase of 5 to 10 days followed by rapid expansion with an average population doubling time of 12 to 36 hours.[28] During the rapid growth stage, MSCs are typically passed every 2 to 3 days using enzymatic dissociation, frequently with 0.05% trypsin EDTA. Inherent limitations of trypsin include cleavage of surface proteins and the need for a serum deactivation step. Gentler, commercially available, proprietary, nonenzymatic dissociation solutions[56] (ie, HyQTase [Hyclone, Logan, UT, USA]) work very well with equine MSCs and result in increased long-term cell viability (Dori L. Borjesson, unpublished data, 2010). Nonenzymatic dissociation solutions can be readily combined with protocols using commercially available serum-free media for clinical trial protocols or for patients receiving multiple MSC doses to minimize exposure to bovine proteins.

After initial outgrowth, MSC media can be altered to include growth factors that facilitate cell expansion. The most common additive is FGF-2.[31,54] Similar to human and rodent MSC culture, the addition of FGF induces a morphologic change (increased spindle shape, associated with increased cell proliferation) with a concurrent increase in growth rate and population doublings, regardless of MSC tissue origin.[6,54,57] FGF treatment may also enhance osteogenic and chondrogenic differentiation of MSC in vitro and bone synthesis in in vivo models by stimulating osteoprogenitor cells.[6,57,58]

### MSC Cryopreservation

Equine MSCs have been safely cryopreserved (up to years) with no significant adverse effects. Cryopreservation has been well described for BM-MSCs,[3] CT-MSCs,[15] CB-MSCs,[10,13] AT-MSCs, and peripheral blood–derived MSCs.[59] Cryopreservation does not alter proliferation, multipotentiality, or morphology. Work with equine peripheral blood–derived MSCs also confirmed that these MSCs retained telomerase activity, karyotype profile, cluster of differentiation expression pattern and in vitro differentiation potential.[59] Cryopreservation permits standardization of cell lines for research use and storage of expanded MSCs in multiple "doses" for autologous or allogeneic clinical use. Cryopreservation media (containing media, FBS, and dimethyl sulfoxide), cell concentrations, and freezing/thawing techniques are compatible with those described for human tissue and cell banks.[60] Controlled rate freezers are recommended; however, overnight storage at $-80^\circ$C in an isopropanol freezing canister followed by a liquid nitrogen plunge also works for long-term storage at smaller facilities.[11]

## LABORATORY REGULATORY ISSUES

The FDA currently does not regulate veterinary use of MSCs because most clinical use to date uses an autologous product. At the FDA, stem cells largely fall under the purview of the Center for Biologics Evaluation and Research and the Office of Cellular, Tissue and Gene Therapies. The FDA regulates tissues on the basis of section 361 of the Public Health Safety Act, which has the intent of preventing the introduction, transmission, and spread of communicable diseases (http://www.fda.gov/cber/summaries/). In this light, because private or public enterprises seek to license allogeneic MSC products, it is likely that the regulatory capacity of the FDA will come into effect. For this reason, veterinary laboratories that are involved in clinical application of allogeneic cell-based products should implement quality laboratory practices, such as donor screening for infectious diseases, standards for cell manufacturing and preservation, and record keeping. Especially important may be the regulations that are needed to ensure that appropriate laboratory practices are met, if and when pharmacologic manipulation for alteration of the biologic characteristics of MSCs is pursued.

## SUMMARY

The clinical use of autologous and allogeneic MSCs derived from fat, BM, and placental tissues in equine regenerative medicine has far outpaced basic research to delineate how MSCs function to restore tissue architecture and modulate the immune system. Although equine success stories can be found throughout the popular press and significant adverse reactions have not been reported, careful laboratory oversight and more in-depth research are mandatory to fully realize the potential of cellular therapy for equine and human patients. Although equine MSCs have been primarily used to treat a wide variety of orthopedic lesions, their clinical use has also expanded into the treatment of neurologic, inflammatory, and ischemic disorders. This tremendous experimentation is exciting but also worthy of critical review, well-designed prospective clinical trials, and thoughtful oversight.

## REFERENCES

1. Fortier LA, Smith RK. Regenerative medicine for tendinous and ligamentous injuries of sport horses. Vet Clin North Am Equine Pract 2008;24(1):191–201.
2. Paris DB, Stout TA. Equine embryos and embryonic stem cells: defining reliable markers of pluripotency. Theriogenology 2010;74(4):516–24.
3. Arnhold SJ, Goletz I, Klein H, et al. Isolation and characterization of bone marrow-derived equine mesenchymal stem cells. Am J Vet Res 2007;68(10):1095–105.
4. Fortier LA, Nixon AJ, Williams J, et al. Isolation and chondrocytic differentiation of equine bone marrow-derived mesenchymal stem cells. Am J Vet Res 1998;59(9):1182–7.
5. Vidal MA, Kilroy GE, Johnson JR, et al. Cell growth characteristics and differentiation frequency of adherent equine bone marrow-derived mesenchymal stromal cells: adipogenic and osteogenic capacity. Vet Surg 2006;35(7):601–10.
6. Colleoni S, Bottani E, Tessaro I, et al. Isolation, growth and differentiation of equine mesenchymal stem cells: effect of donor, source, amount of tissue and supplementation with basic fibroblast growth factor. Vet Res Commun 2009;33:811–21.
7. de Mattos Carvalho A, Alves AL, Golim MA, et al. Isolation and immunophenotypic characterization of mesenchymal stem cells derived from equine species adipose tissue. Vet Immunol Immunopathol 2009;132(2–4):303–6.
8. Vidal MA, Kilroy GE, Lopez MJ, et al. Characterization of equine adipose tissue-derived stromal cells: adipogenic and osteogenic capacity and comparison with bone marrow-derived mesenchymal stromal cells. Vet Surg 2007;36(7):613–22.
9. Bartholomew S, Owens SD, Ferraro GL, et al. Collection of equine cord blood and placental tissues in 40 thoroughbred mares. Equine Vet J 2009;41(8):724–8.
10. Cremonesi F, Violini S, Lange Consiglio A, et al. Isolation, in vitro culture and characterization of foal umbilical cord stem cells at birth. Vet Res Commun 2008;32(Suppl 1):S139–42.
11. Koch TG, Heerkens T, Thomsen PD, et al. Isolation of mesenchymal stem cells from equine umbilical cord blood. BMC Biotechnol 2007;7:26.
12. Koch TG, Thomsen PD, Betts DH. Improved isolation protocol for equine cord blood-derived mesenchymal stromal cells. Cytotherapy 2009;11(4):443–7.

13. Schuh EM, Friedman MS, Carrade DD, et al. Identification of variables that optimize isolation and culture of multipotent mesenchymal stem cells from equine umbilical-cord blood. Am J Vet Res 2009;70(12):1526–35.
14. Passeri S, Nocchi F, Lamanna R, et al. Isolation and expansion of equine umbilical cord-derived matrix cells (EUCMCs). Cell Biol Int 2009;33(1):100–5.
15. Toupadakis CA, Wong A, Genetos DC, et al. Comparison of the osteogenic potential of equine mesenchymal stem cells from bone marrow, adipose tissue, umbilical cord blood, and umbilical cord tissue. Am J Vet Res 2010;71(10):1237–45.
16. Ishihara A, Zachos TA, Bartlett JS, et al. Evaluation of permissiveness and cytotoxic effects in equine chondrocytes, synovial cells, and stem cells in response to infection with adenovirus 5 vectors for gene delivery. Am J Vet Res 2006;67(7):1145–55.
17. Carpenter RS, Goodrich LR, Frisbie DD, et al. Osteoblastic differentiation of human and equine adult bone marrow-derived mesenchymal stem cells when BMP-2 or BMP-7 homodimer genetic modification is compared to BMP-2/7 heterodimer genetic modification in the presence and absence of dexamethasone. J Orthop Res 2010;28(10):1330–7.
18. Murray SJ, Santangelo KS, Bertone AL. Evaluation of early cellular influences of bone morphogenetic proteins 12 and 2 on equine superficial digital flexor tenocytes and bone marrow-derived mesenchymal stem cells in vitro. Am J Vet Res 2010;71(1):103–14.
19. Schnabel LV, Lynch ME, van der Meulen MC, et al. Mesenchymal stem cells and insulin-like growth factor-I gene-enhanced mesenchymal stem cells improve structural aspects of healing in equine flexor digitorum superficialis tendons. J Orthop Res 2009;27(10):1392–8.
20. Vidal MA, Robinson SO, Lopez MJ, et al. Comparison of chondrogenic potential in equine mesenchymal stromal cells derived from adipose tissue and bone marrow. Vet Surg 2008;37(8):713–24.
21. Radcliffe CH, Flaminio MJ, Fortier LA. Temporal analysis of equine bone marrow aspirate during establishment of putative mesenchymal progenitor cell populations. Stem Cells Dev 2010;19(2):269–82.
22. Carrade DD, Owens SD, Galuppo LD, et al. Clinicopathologic findings following intra-articular injection of autologous and allogeneic placentally derived equine mesenchymal stem cells in horses. Cytotherapy 2010. [Epub ahead of print].
23. Reed SA, Johnson SE. Equine umbilical cord blood contains a population of stem cells that express Oct4 and differentiate into mesodermal and endodermal cell types. J Cell Physiol 2008;215(2):329–36.
24. Violini S, Ramelli P, Pisani LF, et al. Horse bone marrow mesenchymal stem cells express embryo stem cell markers and show the ability for tenogenic differentiation by in vitro exposure to BMP-12. BMC Cell Biol 2009;10:29.
25. Riekstina U, Cakstina I, Parfejevs V, et al. Embryonic stem cell marker expression pattern in human mesenchymal stem cells derived from bone marrow, adipose tissue, heart and dermis. Stem Cell Rev 2009;5(4):378–86.
26. Riordan NH, Ichim TE, Min WP, et al. Non-expanded adipose stromal vascular fraction cell therapy for multiple sclerosis. J Transl Med 2009;7:29.
27. Alison M, Wobus AM, Boheler KR. Stem cells. Berlin: Springer; 2006.
28. Marion N, Mao J. Mesenchymal stem cells and tissue engineering. Methods in enzymology, vol. 420. New York: Elsevier Inc; 2006. p. 339–44.
29. Crovace A, Lacitignola L, De Siena R, et al. Cell therapy for tendon repair in horses: an experimental study. Vet Res Commun 2007;31(Suppl 1):281–3.
30. Lacitignola L, Crovace A, Rossi G, et al. Cell therapy for tendinitis, experimental and clinical report. Vet Res Commun 2008;32(Suppl 1):S33–8.

31. Frisbie DD, Kisiday JD, Kawcak CE, et al. Evaluation of adipose-derived stromal vascular fraction or bone marrow-derived mesenchymal stem cells for treatment of osteoarthritis. J Orthop Res 2009;27(12):1675–80.
32. Murphy JM, Fink DJ, Hunziker EB, et al. Stem cell therapy in a caprine model of osteoarthritis. Arthritis Rheum 2003;48(12):3464–74.
33. Quintavalla J, Uziel-Fusi S, Yin J, et al. Fluorescently labeled mesenchymal stem cells (MSCs) maintain multilineage potential and can be detected following implantation into articular cartilage defects. Biomaterials 2002;23(1):109–19.
34. Liechty KW, MacKenzie TC, Shaaban AF, et al. Human mesenchymal stem cells engraft and demonstrate site-specific differentiation after in utero transplantation in sheep. Nat Med 2000;6(11):1282–6.
35. Worster AA, Nixon AJ, Brower-Toland BD, et al. Effect of transforming growth factor beta1 on chondrogenic differentiation of cultured equine mesenchymal stem cells. Am J Vet Res 2000;61(9):1003–10.
36. Berg L, Koch T, Heerkens T, et al. Chondrogenic potential of mesenchymal stromal cells derived from equine bone marrow and umbilical cord blood. Vet Comp Orthop Traumatol 2009;22(5):363–70.
37. Caplan AI. Why are MSCs therapeutic? New data: new insight. J Pathol 2009; 217(2):318–24.
38. Noel D, Djouad F, Bouffi C, et al. Multipotent mesenchymal stromal cells and immune tolerance. Leuk Lymphoma 2007;48(7):1283–9.
39. Kode JA, Mukherjee S, Joglekar MV, et al. Mesenchymal stem cells: immunobiology and role in immunomodulation and tissue regeneration. Cytotherapy 2009; 11(4):377–91.
40. Wang L, Zhao RC. Mesenchymal stem cells targeting the GVHD. Sci China C Life Sci 2009;52(7):603–9.
41. Weng JY, Du X, Geng SX, et al. Mesenchymal stem cell as salvage treatment for refractory chronic GVHD. Bone Marrow Transplant 2010;45(12):1732–40.
42. Zhang X, Jiao C, Zhao S. Role of mesenchymal stem cells in immunological rejection of organ transplantation. Stem Cell Rev 2009;5(4):402–9.
43. Zhao S, Wehner R, Bornhauser M, et al. Immunomodulatory properties of mesenchymal stromal cells and their therapeutic consequences for immune-mediated disorders. Stem Cells Dev 2010;19(5):607–14.
44. Guest DJ, Smith MR, Allen WR. Monitoring the fate of autologous and allogeneic mesenchymal progenitor cells injected into the superficial digital flexor tendon of horses: preliminary study. Equine Vet J 2008;40(2):178–81.
45. Krampera M, Pasini A, Pizzolo G, et al. Regenerative and immunomodulatory potential of mesenchymal stem cells. Curr Opin Pharmacol 2006;6(4):435–41.
46. Krampera M, Franchini M, Pizzolo G, et al. Mesenchymal stem cells: from biology to clinical use. Blood Transfus 2007;5(3):120–9.
47. Le Blanc K. Immunomodulatory effects of fetal and adult mesenchymal stem cells. Cytotherapy 2003;5(6):485–9.
48. Krampera M, Cosmi L, Angeli R, et al. Role for interferon-gamma in the immunomodulatory activity of human bone marrow mesenchymal stem cells. Stem Cells 2006;24(2):386–98.
49. Stagg J, Galipeau J. Immune plasticity of bone marrow-derived mesenchymal stromal cells. Handb Exp Pharmacol 2007;180:45–66.
50. Egermann M, Goldhahn J, Schneider E. Animal models for fracture treatment in osteoporosis. Osteoporos Int 2005;16(Suppl 2):S129–38.
51. Food and Drug Administration. Guidelines for preclinical and clinical evaluation of agents used in the prevention or treatment of postmenopausal osteoporosis.

Washington, DC: FDA, Division of Metabolism and Endocrine Drug Products; 1994.

52. da Silva Meirelles L, Sand TT, Harman RJ, et al. MSC frequency correlates with blood vessel density in equine adipose tissue. Tissue Eng Part A 2009;15(2): 221–9.

53. Del Bue M, Ricco S, Ramoni R, et al. Equine adipose-tissue derived mesenchymal stem cells and platelet concentrates: their association in vitro and in vivo. Vet Res Commun 2008;32(Suppl 1):S51–5.

54. Kisiday JD, Kopesky PW, Evans CH, et al. Evaluation of adult equine bone marrow- and adipose-derived progenitor cell chondrogenesis in hydrogel cultures. J Orthop Res 2008;26(3):322–31.

55. Neuhuber B, Swanger SA, Howard L, et al. Effects of plating density and culture time on bone marrow stromal cell characteristics. Exp Hematol 2008;36(9): 1176–85.

56. Loring J, Wesselschmidt R, Schwartz P. Human stem cell manual, a laboratory guide. New York: Academic Press, Elsevier Inc; 2007.

57. Stewart AA, Byron CR, Pondenis H, et al. Effect of fibroblast growth factor-2 on equine mesenchymal stem cell monolayer expansion and chondrogenesis. Am J Vet Res 2007;68(9):941–5.

58. Stewart AA, Byron CR, Pondenis HC, et al. Effect of dexamethasone supplementation on chondrogenesis of equine mesenchymal stem cells. Am J Vet Res 2008; 69(8):1013–21.

59. Martinello T, Bronzini I, Maccatrozzo L, et al. Cryopreservation does not affect the stem characteristics of multipotent cells isolated from equine peripheral blood. Tissue Eng Part C Methods 2010;16(4):771–81.

60. Rubinstein P, Dobrila L, Rosenfield RE, et al. Processing and cryopreservation of placental/umbilical cord blood for unrelated bone marrow reconstitution. Proc Natl Acad Sci U S A 1995;92(22):10119–22.

# The Equine Neonatal Intensive Care Laboratory: Point-of-Care Testing

Pamela A. Wilkins, DVM, MS, PhD

**KEYWORDS**

- Hematologic • Blood gas • Point-of-care testing devices
- Neonate

Critically ill equine neonates are increasingly being treated by trained specialists at equine neonatal intensive care units (eNICUs) throughout the world. Treatment at these units is costly but sought after for equine neonates of high economic or personal value. Knowledge regarding the care, treatment, and prognosis of these small patients is increasing, and awareness of the differences between, and needs of, these patients and the adult horse is important to obtain a good outcome, meaning not just survival but preserving the athletic potential. Delivery of intensive care to critically ill neonates of veterinary species requires both age-specific and species/breed-specific knowledge for appropriate interpretation of results of clinical laboratory tests. In addition, because close and frequent monitoring of several clinical laboratory parameters is needed to deliver appropriate intensive care to critically ill neonates, additional specific knowledge relating to the performance capabilities of various point-of-care (POC) clinical laboratory monitors is also required. This article provides an overview of the age-specific differences expected in clinical laboratory testing for critically ill equine neonates and also discusses the potential confounders that may exist when POC devices developed for use in one species are used in another. Horse is the veterinary species in which most work has been done, specifically to evaluate some of these issues. Techniques used in different laboratories on different normal reference populations frequently result in different reference values. Therefore, rather than focusing on specific laboratory values the author focuses on the differences between

Financial disclosure: The author has no financial interest in any device or system discussed within this article to disclose.

Equine Medicine and Surgery, Department of Veterinary Clinical Medicine, College of Veterinary Medicine, University of Illinois at Champaign-Urbana, 1008 West Hazelwood Drive, Urbana, IL 61802, USA

E-mail address: pawilkin@ad.uiuc.edu

age and maturity groups and on the effects of important disorders in foals in the eNICU in this article.

## HEMATOLOGIC DIFFERENCES IN THE NEONATE

Normal hematologic values in children, and foals, differ significantly from those in adults, and even among children there are substantial variations in different age groups.[1–3] These differences are more pronounced at birth and during the neonatal period. Although neonatal samples in laboratories generally constitute a small proportion of the overall laboratory load, they bring considerable preanalytic, analytic, and postanalytic challenges that should be known and understood for proper testing and result interpretation.

The unique characteristics of fetal hematopoiesis and the changes that occur at and around birth are important for understanding the differences between neonatal and adult blood. Experimental animal studies support a model in which 3 waves of erythroid progenitors emerge in the mammalian embryo.[4] The first wave consists of primitive erythroid progenitors that originate in the yolk sac and generate erythroid precursors that mature in the bloodstream. The second wave is transient and consists of definitive erythroid precursors that originate in the yolk sac and seed the liver. The final wave consists of a continuous stream of definitive erythroid progenitors in the liver during late gestation and bone marrow during the postnatal period, which generate adult-repopulating hematopoietic stem cells. There is considerable overlap and gradual transition between the stages.

The hematologic values of 19 equine fetuses between 202 and 238 days' gestation were compared with those of their dams in one study.[5] The red blood cell (RBC) count, hemoglobin (Hb) concentration, hematocrit (HCT), and mean corpuscular Hb concentration were significantly lower in the fetal blood, whereas the mean corpuscular volume, mean corpuscular Hb, and RBC distribution width were significantly higher. Mares had a significantly higher nucleated blood cell count than fetuses, and in mares, all nucleated cells were leukocytes (white blood cells [WBCs]). The majority of WBCs in mare blood were segmented neutrophils and lymphocytes. In contrast, more than half of the nucleated cells in fetal blood were nucleated RBCs and the majority of WBCs in fetal blood were lymphocytes. Mares also had significantly higher plasma protein and fibrinogen concentrations than their fetuses. Mild macrocytosis and mild polychromasia were observed in most fetal blood samples but not in blood samples from mares. All fetal blood samples contained reticulocytes, and most samples contained Heinz bodies and Howell-Jolly bodies.

Specific values reported for equine neonates for components of the hemogram appeared in a recent review.[6] In general, the RBC count, Hb concentration, and HCT are maximal at birth, whereas the erythrocyte size and volume is variable because of different sites of production during the second half of gestation.[3,7] The premature foal will, as a consequence, have a lower RBC count and Hb concentration and a larger erythrocyte size.

There is no fetal Hb in the horse fetus, and the Hb structure of the fetus is identical to that of the adult.[8,9] Instead, oxygen diffusion across the placenta is facilitated by the lower fetal erythrocyte concentration of 2,3-diphosphoglycerate, shifting the oxyhemoglobin dissociation curve to the left,[9,10] and a counterplacental circulatory pattern.[11] While the HCT and Hb concentration increase transiently at birth, possibly because of placental blood transfusion during parturition, it is not unusual to see the packed cell volume (PCV) decrease by up to 10% in normal foals over the first day of life. A progressive slower decrease follows until foal PCV is in the lower range of adult values.

The WBC count gradually increases after birth, primarily associated with an increase in neutrophils. In normal foals, the neutrophil:lymphocyte ratio is greater than 2.5:1.0. The neutrophil count then decreases slightly, reaching a nadir at about 6 months of age. Band (immature) neutrophils are very low in number to absent in normal foals. Although neutrophils are functionally mature at birth, phagocytic ability is limited until about 3 weeks of age because of limitation of the serum of the foal to induce opsonization.[12] Neutropenia is a relatively common finding in septic and premature foals. In premature foals in particular, failure of increase neutrophil numbers after birth may indicate a decreased chance of survival, thought to be associated with relative nonresponsiveness to endogenous or exogenous corticotropin.[13] Neutrophilia is primarily associated with infection, prepartum or postpartum, the presence of the systemic inflammatory response syndrome, and stress, whereas the presence of toxic neutrophils (Döhle bodies, basophilia, toxic granulation) inform endotoxemia or bacterial infection as the more probable causes of alterations in the neutrophil count outside of the reference range.

Lymphocyte numbers are initially increased at birth but decrease thereafter. Lymphocyte numbers then approximate adult values at about 3 months of age. Persistent lymphopenia is commonly seen in critically ill foals and should not be overinterpreted in breeds not at risk for primary immunodeficiency. T and B lymphocytes found in the circulation of foal are functional. Eosinophils are generally not found in the circulation of neonatal foals but increase to adult values at around 4 months of age. Both basophils and monocytes are rare to absent in the equine neonate but reach adult values after the first year of life. Platelet numbers in newborn foals are the same or are greater than that of the adult horse but are less responsive to collagen or ADP aggregation in the first week, possibly contributing to the slightly longer bleeding time reported in neonatal foals.[14,15]

## CLINICAL CHEMISTRY DIFFERENCES IN THE NEONATE

There is an excellent recent review of clinical chemistry finding in healthy and abnormal neonatal foals in the veterinary literature.[6] Biochemistry values for the neonatal foal change over the first month of life and should be evaluated with these changes in mind. Before parturition, the placenta performs many functions for the fetus and is responsible for fluid and electrolyte homeostasis, in addition to excretion of waste, and gas and nutrient exchange. It is incumbent on the clinician to be fully aware of what the normal values are for these parameters at differing ages for their laboratoriesin order to properly assess and treat critically ill neonatal foals.

### Concentrations of Fibrinogen and Proteins

The total protein concentration in foals is generally lower than that of adults for a variety of reasons but should increase after birth following acquisition of maternal immunoglobulins. Foals with inadequate maternal transfer of immunoglobulin, primarily of the IgG class, are classified as having failure of passive transfer (FPT) of immunity. The albumin concentration approximates that of the adult from the time of birth and remains constant. Agammaglobulinemia has been reported in male foals and is associated with a lack of B lymphocytes.[16]

The fibrinogen concentration is lower in the foal than in the adult at birth, gradually reaches a maximal value at about 5 months of age, and then reaches the adult values between 7 to 9 months of age. Hyperfibrinogenemia in the neonatal foal indicates infection and, if present when the foal is younger than 2 days, is highly suggestive of an in utero infection. Resolving hyperfibrinogenemia is understood to be an indication of appropriate response to therapy. Hypofibrinogenemia, as estimated by heat precipitation or measured by quantitative methods, is not an indication of disseminated intravascular coagulation as suggested in other species but may be recognized with significant blood loss.

The serum amyloid A (SAA) protein concentration is being evaluated more commonly in critically ill foals. Physiologically, SAA levels transiently increase approximately 2 days after birth in normal foals. Increased SAA values (more than physiologic levels) are associated with infection and, similar to fibrinogen levels, its decreasing values are associated with disease resolution.[17]

## Activity of Enzymes

Alkaline phosphatase (ALP) activity is greatly increased in the first week of life, with a gradual decrease to adult values by 4 weeks of age. As such, ALP activity is not useful in assessing liver function in the equine neonate.[18] γ-Glutamyl transferase activity transiently increases during the second week of life in the normal equine neonate, being in the normal adult range thereafter.[19,20] Sorbitol dehydrogenase activity appears to not be affected by age.[19] The creatinine kinase level is within the adult range in foals, whereas aspartate aminotransferase activity increases slightly above adult values in the first week of life, probably associated with increased muscle activity.

## Levels of Electrolytes

Electrolyte levels are maintained within a relatively narrow range during the first 6 months of life, and abnormal values at birth reflect an altered placental function and an abnormal uterine environment. Exception are the total and ionized calcium concentrations, which may be more than 25% increased over adult values at birth and then decrease to approximately 20% less than adult values within a few hours. The inorganic phosphorus concentration is generally the same as that in adults but then slowly increases over the next 8 weeks, likely associated with bone metabolism.

## Creatinine and Urea Concentrations

Creatinine concentrations may be mildly increased at birth physiologically but should return to the adult range, or lower, within 24 hours after birth. Significant increases in the creatinine concentration may be seen in newborn foals, associated with adverse peripartum conditions, including placental dysfunction and in utero stress, but should also rapidly return to lower normal values. This condition has been termed spurious hypercreatininemia and is not associated with renal dysfunction in the neonate.[21] Increases in creatinine concentrations at birth that do not resolve should prompt investigation of other causes of azotemia including renal and postrenal causes. The urea concentration is initially in the adult range at birth because of placental function but decreases to less than the adult values between 3 days and 8 weeks of age.[22]

## Levels of Bilirubin and Bile Acids

Neonatal hyperbilirubinemia is normal and is associated with an increase in the level of unconjugated (indirect reacting) bilirubin, which is thought to be caused by a high rate of turnover of fetal RBCs. Bilirubin concentrations should approximate the adult range by the end of the first week of life. The bile acid concentration is higher than that of the adult range for the first 6 weeks of life.

### Glucose Levels

At birth, glucose concentrations should be approximately 50% that of the dam. The glucose concentration reaches a nadir at about 2 hours after birth, before ingestion of the first meal.[23] The blood glucose concentration then increases over the next 48 hours and remains greater than the adult values until 2 to 3 months of age. Abnormalities in blood glucose concentrations, too high or too low, should prompt investigation of caloric intake and disease states that can alter glucose homeostasis.

### Lactate Concentration

Lactate concentration is normally increased at birth and subsequently decreases to adult values over the following 24 to 72 hours. Hyperlactatemia, acute or persistent, of any neonatal foal should prompt investigation for occult infection and/or abnormalities in tissue perfusion, gas exchange, muscle activity, glucose metabolism, liver function, increased metabolic demands, catecholamine surges, or protein catabolism. Lactate concentration has been, and continues to be, investigated as an indicator of disease severity and prognosis for survival in critically ill neonatal foals.[24–28]

### Levels of Cholesterol and Triglycerides

Cholesterol and triglyceride concentrations are greater in the neonate than in the adult for the first 2 weeks of life. Transient postprandial hyperlipemia can give serum or plasma an opaque appearance, but true hyperlipemia/hyperlipidemia is associated with several disease states in foals from sepsis to deranged lipid metabolism.

## MEASURES OF HEMOSTASIS IN THE NEONATE

Hemostatic indices in foals differ from those in adults and also vary with age. Foals, in general, have lower liver-derived clotting factors and vitamin K–dependent factors, which contribute to higher prothrombin time and activated partial thromboplastin time compared with adults.[14,15,29–31] Assays of clotting such as Sonoclot (Sienco Inc, Arvada, CO, USA), thromboelastography, and thromboelastometry demonstrate differences from results in adults in those studies reported to date.[32–34]

## POC TESTING IN THE ENICU

POC testing can be defined in laboratory medicine as "the analysis of clinical specimens as close as possible to the patient, including bedside, ward–unit, or 'stat' regional response labs that service specified areas–eg, the ER (emergency room) or ICU (intensive care unit)" or as "testing that is performed near or at the site of a patient with the result leading to possible change in the care of the patient." These definitions also hold true in veterinary laboratory medicine. Veterinarians have measured blood glucose and IgG levels and performed urinalysis using POC tests for many years. Testing of blood gases, L-lactate concentration, blood coagulation, troponin I concentration, and infectious disease markers at the POC are more recent developments in veterinary POC laboratories. The key objective of POC testing is to generate a result quickly so that appropriate treatment can be implemented, leading to an improved clinical or economic outcome. POC testing should be based not on what tests can be done at the POC but on what tests should be done to expedite the patient care process.

POC devices have the following 3 main advantages over central laboratory devices (CLDs): first, they are considerably less expensive; second, they give almost immediate results compared with the time taken to label, package, and send a sample to the laboratory and await the result to be reported; and third, the sample volume needed is minimal. The main disadvantages of POC devices are their lack of accuracy compared with CLDs and the differences in reference intervals.

### Glucose Levels

POC or stall-side glucometry has become a standard approach to measure blood glucose concentrations in the eNICU worldwide. However, glucometry has not been fully evaluated in critically ill foals in a systematic manner, and aberrations in glucose homeostasis are not unusual in these patients, ranging from hypoglycemia to hyperglycemia. The routine monitoring of blood glucose concentration and the use of drugs affecting glucose homeostasis, such as corticosteroids and insulin, in addition to dextrose infusions and parenteral nutrition, has become more common in neonatal intensive care units (NICUs), and, with the recent discussions of tight glucose control affecting outcome in critically ill human patients, the need for accuracy in POC glucometry has increased.[35–39]

Inaccuracies in measuring glucose levels using POCs can originate from several different sources.[40] Glucose measurement techniques use enzymatic indirect approaches that can be affected by environmental (oxygen tension, electrochemical currents) and patient factors (azotemia, interfering drugs, presence of other measured sugars, severe polycythemia).

Because the glucose concentration is reported by CLDs as the concentration in plasma or serum, rather than in whole blood, most POC monitors use conversion algorithms to report the result as a plasma value, despite the glucose concentration being measured in whole blood. These algorithms are based on the ratio of glucose concentrations in plasma to that in erythrocytes, which varies with species and age.[41,42] In devices aimed at human use, the correction multiplier used to convert the whole blood measurement to the reported plasma value is 1.11 based on the higher water content of plasma (93%) when compared with erythrocytes (73%).[43] In the neonatal foal, however, glucose is largely present in plasma (approximately 82 mg/dL), with little measurable glucose (approximately 15 mg/dL) in erythrocytes, quite different from other species, and this difference seems to persist into adulthood.[42] Fructose, apparently, is the primary sugar present in equine erythrocytes, and it seems that equine erythrocytes are differentially permeable to glucose and fructose.

Anemia decreases and polycythemia increases the difference between whole blood and plasma glucose concentrations not only by altering the ratio of plasma to erythrocytes but also by altering the impedance of plasma diffusion into the test strip by viscosity changes associated with abnormal HCT.[44–46] To date, no peer-reviewed study of the critically ill or normal equine neonate or adult has been done to demonstrate whether or not there is a potential important effect of HCT on POC glucose monitoring. The lack of differences found in studies that casually examined this effect may be because of the previously discussed low concentration of glucose present in the equine erythrocyte, although other factors may also play a role.

Arterial blood glucose concentrations have been shown to be significantly higher than both capillary and venous blood glucose concentrations in humans.[47,48] The difference between capillary and venous glucose levels is typically not significant in nonhypotensive fasting subjects. Circulatory shock results in an increased tissue glucose extraction and a lower glucose value in capillary as opposed to venous blood. Arterial and central venous blood glucose levels are more likely to be underestimated when measuring capillary blood glucose specimens from severely hypotensive patients, resulting in an incorrect diagnosis of systemic hypoglycemia compared with normotensive patients.[49] In general, it is recommended that venous blood be used for determination of glucose concentration using POC glucometry, and this recommendation holds for most eNICUs.

Several POC devices using glucose oxidase reactions in their testing media are susceptible to errors caused by high or low oxygen concentrations. Tang and colleagues[50] showed that errors of more than 15% could occur in patients with a $Pao_2$ greater than 100 mm Hg. Conversely, these devices have been shown to underestimate blood glucose levels at altitude by 1% to 2% per 300 m of elevation,[51,52] and errors of more than 15% have been shown when analyzing hypoxic blood ($Po_2$ approximately 44 mm Hg).[53] The severity of the errors at low $Pao_2$ is highly dependent on the type of test strip (electrochemical vs photometric) and the particular enzyme used.

In 1 foal study, using a target range of 60 to 180 mg/dL of glucose, several patients' glucose tests (3 of 38, 8%) would have been differently classified if glucometry values rather than the standard laboratory chemistry values were used for classification: 2 as hypoglycemic (<60 mg/dL) and 1 as within the reference interval (60–180 mg/dL). In each case, glucometry underestimated the CLD value.[54] Two recent studies have evaluated glucometers in adult horses,[55,56] with one[56] also evaluating the glucometer in foals. Results were accurate only for the glucometer that had been specifically designed for veterinary use.[56]

POC glucometry as practiced in many NICU's is practical, rapid, and affordable. However, glucometry frequently had a less-than-ideal agreement with both laboratory plasma chemistry standard and another POC blood gas analyzer in one study.[54] Because there are many glucometers currently marketed, and each may react differently to confounding effects, resulting in its own characteristic signature, method-specific target values are needed and should be developed for each technique used in any patient setting.[44,57,58] Each NICU needs to evaluate its glucometry method by periodically comparing results to its laboratory standard and recognizing that the very competitive glucometry market drives constant modifications by the manufacturers, necessitating repeated evaluation. In human medicine, many glucometers have performed quite poorly in the hypoglycemic range, with inaccuracies leading to treatment errors that could result in death of the patient.[40] Given this, the investigators of one recent review stated "it is our opinion that they should not be used in conjunction with perioperative insulin therapy, and we appeal to investigators not to use them as diagnostic tools during investigator-initiated clinical trials."[40] Differences may be clinically important, and decisions regarding management of glucose concentrations in critically ill foals should be made with these concerns in mind.

### IgG Levels

Sepsis is the leading cause of disease and death in newborn foals, and the results of multiple studies indicate a positive correlation between FPT and bacterial sepsis.[59–64] Radial immunodiffusion (RID) is recognized as the gold standard for determination of IgG concentrations in equine serum, and assays are commercially available from various manufacturers.[65] The major disadvantage of RID, beyond a requirement for trained personnel, is that it takes 18 to 24 hours to obtain test results, even if the testing is done in-house, potentially resulting in a serious delay in the treatment of foals with FPT. It is generally recommended that foals at risk for developing sepsis with IgG concentrations between 400 and 800 mg/dL at 18 to 24 hours after birth be administered intravenous plasma.

Estimation of the total protein concentration in serum or plasma by refractometry represents a rapid, inexpensive, and accurate test for the diagnosis of FPT in calves.[66]

However, refractometry is an unreliable indicator of FPT in foals because of the wide range of normal protein concentrations in newborn foals. Several other rapid POC screening tests have been used to estimate the concentration of IgG in neonatal foals, including those based on zinc sulfate turbidity, glutaraldehyde coagulation, latex agglutination, turbidimetric immunoassays, and enzyme immunoassays.[59,67–71] Many of these assays are commercially available as kits and are commonly used by horse owners and veterinarians. The diagnostic performance of several of these kits was evaluated in 2005,[72] such as zinc sulfate turbidity (Equi Z Equine FPT Test Kit, VMRD Inc, Pullman, WA, USA), glutaraldehyde coagulation (Gamma-Check-E, Plasvacc USA Inc, Templeton, CA, USA), 3 semiquantitative enzyme immunoassays [Plasma Foal IgG Midland Quick Test Kit (400 mg/dL), Midland BioProducts Corporation, Boone, IA, USA; Plasma Foal IgG Midland Quick Test Kit (800 mg/dL), Midland BioProducts Corp, Boone, IA, USA; SNAP Foal IgG, IDEXX Laboratories, Westbrook, ME, USA], and a handheld quantitative colorimetric immunoassay (DVM Stat, VDx Inc, Belgium, WI, USA).

When used for screening, a test with a high sensitivity should be used to ensure a high predictive value of a negative test and accurate identification of most foals with FPT. Ideally, to confirm FPT, foals with positive results in the screening test should be tested with a different confirmatory test. In a second test, high specificity and positive predictive values are required. In the 2005 study, at a cutoff value of 400 mg/dL, sensitivity was similar for each assay evaluated, resulting in negative predictive values greater than 95%. As a result, all assays evaluated were thought to be suitable screening tests. One assay (DVM Stat) outperformed the others but because of variable agreement with the RID standard in the range of 600 to 800 mg/dL IgG would have resulted in unnecessary treatment of some foals. The cost of unnecessary treatment, primarily economic, should be weighed against the cost of failure to treat, potential sepsis and death, when making choices regarding which POC IgG test to use. In this study, interestingly, the 2 RID tests evaluated did not have good agreement with each other in the 400 to 800 mg/dL range, previously unreported, although there was excellent agreement in the samples when IgG concentration was less than 400 mg/dL. Refractometry was not recommended as a screening test for FPT based on the results of this study.

### Levels of Blood Gases

There are several reported studies evaluating POC blood gas analyzers and their use in horses.[73–77] In these studies, POC analyzers were compared with CLD blood gas analyzers and were found to be sufficient for diagnostic purposes. None of the studies specifically evaluated the use of these POC devices in the foal, however, and these studies should be performed.

### Lactate Levels

POC monitoring of lactate concentrations in critically ill foals is performed almost as commonly as determination of blood glucose levels in eNICUs. Several studies have been published evaluating the utility of POC lactate concentration monitoring in terms of determining both disease severity and prognosis in critically ill foals,[24–26,78] although to date only one study has been performed prospectively.[27,28]

In POC lactate monitors in general, the lactate concentration is measured by placing a drop of sample fluid on a reagent pad, similar to many POC glucometers. Plasma is separated from erythrocytes within a glass-fiber layer, which lies beneath a covering mesh on a test strip. Below the separation layer is the actual reaction layer in which the lactate concentration is determined by reflectance photometry using an enzyme-mediated colorimetric reaction. The total test time for the POC lactate monitors range from 30 seconds to a little more than 60 seconds. The monitor's light source generally lies below the strip and shines up through the sample. Lactate is oxidized to pyruvate by the action of lactate oxidase. A mediator transfers electrons from lactate to phosphomolybdic acid, which then forms a dye whose reflectance can be measured. The reactions are specific for L-lactate and do not measure D-lactate. The monitors measure the plasma lactate concentration, the but whole blood concentration can be calculated using a proprietary algorithm.

Based on the results of one study,[79] it is clear that for the adult horse, plasma and whole blood samples are not equivalent when measured on POC monitors, although similar studies have yet to be performed in foals. This finding was similar to the findings of some earlier reports examining the accuracy and reliability of the same POC monitor in exercising Thoroughbred horses.[80–82] The reasons for the poorer performance, and an effect of HCT on the accuracy of the POC monitor when using equine but not human whole blood samples, are not clear but may be related to differences in erythrocytes between species. Other possible limitations of accuracy and consistency include the proprietary algorithms used by the lactate analyzers and the movement of lactate between blood compartments. Because the POC monitors measure plasma lactate, whole blood lactate concentration is expected to decrease with an increase in HCT because of dilution by the increased erythrocyte portion, leading to an underestimation of the whole blood lactate concentration, depending on the algorithms used to calculate the whole blood lactate concentration.

Despite these limitations, POC monitoring of lactate concentrations seems to be useful clinically. As with glucometry, POC monitors should be chosen with care and their performance against a CLD determined before being put into clinical use. In the hospital situation, the use of POC lactate analysis will decrease analytical time, making an important diagnostic parameter immediately available in the critical care setting. Furthermore, the monitor and test strips are inexpensive, making frequent lactate measurements possible and economical.

## SUMMARY

Differences between the neonate and the adult, differences associated with maturity at the time of birth, and changes over time from birth all need to be considered when evaluating laboratory results relating to the care of a critically ill foal. The increasing availability and use of POC laboratory devices are allowing for improved care of these patients and more rapid intervention, but care must be taken to ensure that these devices are properly evaluated before their use in patient populations for which they were not originally intended. Given this caution, most eNICUs should be able to provide, at minimum, POC evaluation of blood gas, glucose, IgG, and lactate concentrations.

## REFERENCES

1. Proytcheva MA. Issues in neonatal cellular analysis. Am J Clin Pathol 2009; 131(4):560–73.
2. Lumsden JH, Rowe R, Mullen K. Hematology and biochemistry reference values for the light horse. Can J Comp Med 1980;44(1):32–42.
3. Harvey JW, Asquith RL, McNulty PK, et al. Haematology of foals up to one year old. Equine Vet J 1984;16(4):347–53.
4. Palis J. Ontogeny of erythropoiesis. Curr Opin Hematol 2008;15(3):155–61.

5. Allen AL, Myers SL, Searcy GP, et al. Hematology of equine fetuses with comparisons to their dams. Vet Clin Pathol 1998;27(3):93–100.

6. Axon JE, Palmer JE. Clinical pathology of the foal. Vet Clin North Am Equine Pract 2008;24(2):357–85.

7. Jeffcott LB, Rossdale PD, Leadon DP. Haematological changes in the neonatal period of normal and induced premature foals. J Reprod Fertil Suppl 1982;32: 537–44.

8. Stockell A, Perutz MF, Muirhead H, et al. A comparison of adult and fetal horse hemoglobin. J Mol Biol 1961;3:112–6.

9. Kitchen H, Bunn HF. Ontogeny of equine haemoglobins. J Reprod Fertil Suppl 1975;23:595–8.

10. Bunn HF, Kitchen H. Hemoglobin function in the horse: the role of 2,3-diphosphoglycerate in modifying the oxygen affinity of maternal and fetal blood. Blood 1973; 42(3):471–9.

11. Silver M, Comline RS. Transfer of gases and metabolites in the equine placenta: a comparison with other species. J Reprod Fertil Suppl 1975;23:589–94.

12. Gröndahl G, Johannisson A, Demmers S, et al. Influence of age and plasma treatment on neutrophil phagocytosis and CD18 expression in foals. Vet Microbiol 1999;65(3):241–54.

13. Silver M, Ousey JC, Dudan FE, et al. Studies on equine prematurity 2: post natal adrenocortical activity in relation to plasma adrenocorticotrophic hormone and catecholamine levels in term and premature foals. Equine Vet J 1984;16(4):278–86.

14. Darien BJ, Feldman BF. Hemostasis in the newborn foal. In: Robinson N, editor. Current therapy in equine medicine. 3rd edition. Philadelphia: WB Saunders Co; 1992. p. 427–31.

15. Clemmons RM, Dorsey-Lee MR, Gorman NT, et al. Haemostatic mechanisms of the newborn foal: reduced platelet responsiveness. Equine Vet J 1984;16(4): 353–6.

16. Davis JL, Jones SL. Equine primary immunodeficiencies. Compend Contin Educ Vet 2003;25(7):548–55.

17. Stoneham SJ, Palmer L, Cash R, et al. Measurement of serum amyloid A in the neonatal foal using a latex agglutination immunoturbidimetric assay: determination of the normal range, variation with age and response to disease. Equine Vet J 2001;33(6):599–603.

18. Rose RJ, Backhouse W, Chan W. Plasma biochemistry changes in thoroughbred foals during the first 4 weeks of life. J Reprod Fertil Suppl 1979;27:601–5.

19. Barton MH, LeRoy BE. Serum bile acids concentrations in healthy and clinically ill neonatal foals. J Vet Intern Med 2007;21(3):508–13.

20. Patterson WH, Brown CM. Increase of serum gamma-glutamyltransferase in neonatal Standardbred foals. Am J Vet Res 1986;47(11):2461–3.

21. Chaney KP, Holcombe SJ, Schott HC 2nd, et al. Spurious hypercreatininemia: 28 neonatal foals (2000–2008). J Vet Emerg Crit Care (San Antonio) 2010;20(2): 244–9.

22. Bauer JE, Harvey JW, Asquith RL, et al. Clinical chemistry reference values of foals during the first year of life. Equine Vet J 1984;16(4):361–3.

23. Palmer JE. Recognition and resuscitation of the critically ill foal. In: Paradis MR, editor. Equine neonatal medicine: a case-based approach. Philadelphia: Elsevier Saunders; 2006. p. 135–48.

24. Corley KT, Donaldson LL, Furr MO. Arterial lactate concentration, hospital survival, sepsis and SIRS in critically ill neonatal foals. Equine Vet J 2005;37(1): 53–9.

25. Wotman K, Wilkins PA, Boston RC, et al. Association of blood lactate concentration and outcome in foals. J Vet Intern Med 2009;23(3):598–605.
26. Henderson ISF, Franklin RP, Boston RC, et al. Association of hyperlactataemia with age, diagnosis and survival in equine neonates. J Vet Emerg Crit Care 2008;18(5):496–502.
27. Borchers A, Wilkins PA, Marsh PS, et al. Preliminary results from a prospective multi-center study of the association of lactate concentration with survival in sick neonatal foals. J Vet Intern Med 2010;24(3):711–2, 787.
28. Borchers A, Wilkins PA, Marsh PM, et al. Survival and major diagnosis of sick neonatal foals are associated with L-Lactate concentration: preliminary results of a prospective multicenter study [abstract]. In: Proceedings of International Veterinary Emergency and Critical Care Society Annual Meeting. San Antonio (TX), September, 2010.
29. Barton MH, Morris DD, Crowe N, et al. Hemostatic indices in healthy foals from birth to one month of age. J Vet Diagn Invest 1995;7(3):380–5.
30. Barton MH, Morris DD, Norton N, et al. Hemostatic and fibrinolytic indices in neonatal foals with presumed septicemia. J Vet Intern Med 1998;12(1):26–35.
31. Bentz AI, Palmer JE, Dallap BL, et al. Prospective evaluation of coagulation in critically ill neonatal foals. J Vet Intern Med 2009;23(1):161–7.
32. Dallap Schaer BL, Bentz AI, Boston RC, et al. Comparison of viscoelastic coagulation analysis and standard coagulation profiles in critically ill neonatal foals to outcome. J Vet Emerg Crit Care (San Antonio) 2009;19(1):88–95.
33. Dallap Schaer BL, Wilkins PA, Boston R, et al. Preliminary evaluation of hemostasis in neonatal foals using a viscoelastic coagulation and platelet function analyzer. J Vet Emerg Crit Care (San Antonio) 2009;19(1):81–7.
34. Dallap Schaer BL, Epstein K. Coagulopathy of the critically ill equine patient. J Vet Emerg Crit Care (San Antonio) 2009;19(1):53–65.
35. Van den Berghe G, Wouters P, Weekers P, et al. Intensive insulin therapy in critically ill patients. N Engl J Med 2001;345:1539–67.
36. Chrousos G, Kaltsas G. How accurate are currently used methods of determining glycemia in critically ill patients, and do they affect their clinical course? Crit Care Med 2005;33(12):2849–50.
37. Kanji S, Buffie J, Hutton B, et al. Reliability of point-of-care testing for glucose measurement in critically ill adults. Crit Care Med 2005;33(12):2778–85.
38. Kulkarni A, Saxena M, Price G, et al. Analysis of blood glucose measurements using capillary and arterial blood samples in intensive care patients. Intensive Care Med 2005;31(1):142–5.
39. Finkielman JD, Oyen LJ, Afressa B, et al. Agreement between bedside blood and plasma glucose measurement in the ICU setting. Chest 2005;127(5):1749–51.
40. Rice MJ, Pitkin AD, Coursin DB. Review article: glucose measurement in the operating room: more complicated than it seems. Anesth Analg 2010;110(4):1056–65.
41. Jacquez JA. Red blood cell as glucose carrier: significance for placental and cerebral glucose transfer. Am J Physiol 1984;246(3 Pt 2):R289–98.
42. Goodwin RFW. The distribution of sugar between red cells and plasma: variations associated with age and species. J Physiol 1956;134:88–101.
43. D'Orazio P, Burnett RW, Fogh-Andersen N, et al. Approved IFCC recommendation on reporting results for blood glucose: International Federation of Clinical Chemistry and Laboratory Medicine Scientific Division, Working group on Selective Electrodes and Point-of-Care Testing (IFCC-SD-WG-SEPOCT). Clin Chem Lab Med 2006;44:1486–90.

44. Dungan K, Chapman J, Braithwaite SS, et al. Glucose measurement: confounding issues in setting targets for inpatient management. Diabetes Care 2007;30:403–9.
45. Tang Z, Lee JH, Louie RF, et al. Effects of different hematocrit levels on glucose measurements with handheld meters for point-of-care testing. Arch Pathol Lab Med 2000;124:1135–40.
46. Dacombe CM, Dalton RG, Goldie DJ, et al. Effect of packed cell volume on blood glucose estimations. Arch Dis Child 1981;56:789–91.
47. Karon BS, Gandhi GY, Nuttall GA, et al. Accuracy of Roche Accu-Chek Inform whole blood capillary, arterial, and venous glucose values in patients receiving intensive intravenous insulin therapy after cardiac surgery. Am J Clin Pathol 2007;127:919–26.
48. Maser RE, Butler MA, DeCherney GS. Use of arterial blood with bedside glucose reflectance meters in an intensive care unit: are they accurate? Crit Care Med 1994;22:595–9.
49. Atkin SH, Dasmahapatra A, Jaker MA, et al. Fingerstick glucose determination in shock. Ann Intern Med 1991;114:1020–4.
50. Tang Z, Louie RF, Payes M, et al. Oxygen effects on glucose measurements with a reference analyzer and three handheld meters. Diabetes Technol Ther 2000;2: 349–62.
51. Giordano BP, Thrash W, Hollenbaugh L, et al. Performance of seven blood glucose testing systems at high altitude. Diabetes Educ 1989;15:444–8.
52. Fink KS, Christensen DB, Ellsworth A. Effect of high altitude on blood glucose meter performance. Diabetes Technol Ther 2002;4:627–35.
53. Kilpatrick ES, Rumley AG, Smith EA. Variations in sample pH and pO2 affect ExacTech meter glucose measurements. Diabet Med 1994;11:506–9.
54. Russell C, Palmer JE, Boston RC, et al. Agreement between point-of-care glucometry, blood gas and laboratory based measurement of glucose in an equine neonatal intensive care unit. J Vet Emerg Crit Care 2007;17(3):236–42.
55. Hollis AR, Dallap Schaer BL, Boston RC, et al. Comparison of the Accu-Chek Aviva point-of-care glucometer with blood gas and laboratory methods of analysis of glucose measurement in equine emergency patients. J Vet Intern Med 2008;22(5):1189–95.
56. Hackett ES, McCue PM. Evaluation of a veterinary glucometer for use in horses. J Vet Intern Med 2010;24(3):617–21.
57. Flore KM, Delanghe JR. Analytical interferences in point-of care testing glucometers by icodextrin and its metabolites: an overview. Perit Dial Int 2009;29: 377–83.
58. Bhatia A, Cadman B, Mackenzie I. Hypoglycemia and cardiac arrest in a critically ill patient on strict glycemic control. Anesth Analg 2006;102:549–51.
59. Clabough DL, Levine JF, Grant GL, et al. Factors associated with failure of passive transfer of colostral antibodies in Standardbred foals. J Vet Intern Med 1991;5:335–40.
60. Haas SD, Bristol F, Card CE. Risk factors associated with the incidence of foal mortality in an extensively managed mare herd. Can Vet J 1996;37:91–5.
61. McGuire TC, Crawford TB, Hallowell AL, et al. Failure of colostral immunoglobulin transfer as an explanation for most infections and deaths of neonatal foals. J Am Vet Med Assoc 1977;170:1302–4.
62. Raidal SL. The incidence and consequences of failure of passive transfer of immunity on a Thoroughbred breeding farm. Aust Vet J 1996;73:201–6.
63. Perryman LE, McGuire TC. Evaluation for immune system failures in horses and ponies. J Am Vet Med Assoc 1980;176:1374–7.

64. Cohen ND. Causes of and farm management factors associated with disease and death in foals. J Am Vet Med Assoc 1994;204:1644–51.
65. Young KM, Lunn DP. Immunodiagnostic testing in horses. Vet Clin North Am Equine Pract 2000;16:79–103.
66. Tyler JW, Hancock DD, Parish SM, et al. Evaluation of 3 assays for failure of passive transfer in calves. J Vet Intern Med 1996;10:304–7.
67. Bauer JE, Brooks TP. Immunoturbidimetric quantification of serum immunoglobulin G concentration in foals. Am J Vet Res 1990;51:1211–4.
68. Beetson SA, Hilbert BJ, Mills JN. The use of the glutaraldehyde coagulation test for detection of hypogammaglobulinaemia in neonatal foals. Aust Vet J 1985;62:279–81.
69. Bertone JJ, Jones RL, Curtis CR. Evaluation of a test kit for determination of serum immunoglobulin G concentration in foals. J Vet Intern Med 1988;2:181–3.
70. Pusterla N, Pusterla JB, Spier SJ, et al. Evaluation of the SNAP foal IgG test for the semiquantitative measurement of immunoglobulin G in foals. Vet Rec 2002;151:258–60.
71. Davis DG, Schaefer DM, Hinchcliff KW, et al. Measurement of serum IgG in foals by radial immunodiffusion and automated turbidimetric immunoassay. J Vet Intern Med 2005;19:93–6.
72. Davis R, Giguère S. Evaluation of five commercially available assays and measurement of serum total protein concentration via refractometry for the diagnosis of failure of passive transfer of immunity in foals. J Am Vet Med Assoc 2005;227(10):1640–5.
73. Mitten LA, Hinchcliff KW, Sams R. A portable blood gas analyzer for equine venous blood. J Vet Intern Med 1995;9(5):353–6.
74. Looney AL, Ludders J, Erb HN, et al. Use of a handheld device for analysis of blood electrolyte concentrations and blood gas partial pressures in dogs and horses. J Am Vet Med Assoc 1998;213(4):526–30.
75. Grosenbaugh DA, Gadawski JE, Muir WW. Evaluation of a portable clinical analyzer in a veterinary hospital setting. J Am Vet Med Assoc 1998;213(5):691–4.
76. Klein LV, Soma LR, Nann LE. Accuracy and precision of the portable StatPal II and the laboratory-based NOVA stat profile 1 for measurement of pH, P(CO2), and P(O2) in equine blood. Vet Surg 1999;28(1):67–76.
77. Peiró JR, Borges AS, Gonçalves RC, et al. Evaluation of a portable clinical analyzer for the determination of blood gas partial pressures, electrolyte concentrations, and hematocrit in venous blood samples collected from cattle, horses, and sheep. Am J Vet Res 2010;71(5):515–21.
78. Castagnetti C, Pirrone A, Mariella J, et al. Venous blood lactate evaluation in equine neonatal intensive care. Theriogenology 2010;73(3):343–57.
79. Tennent-Brown BS, Wilkins PA, Lindborg S, et al. Assessment of a point-of-care lactate monitor in adult equine emergency admissions to a referral hospital. J Vet Intern Med 2007;21:1090–8.
80. Evans DL, Golland LC. Accuracy of Accusport for measurement of lactate concentrations in equine blood and plasma. Equine Vet J 1996;28:398–402.
81. Lindner A. Measurement of plasma lactate concentration with Accusport. Equine Vet J 1996;28:403–5.
82. Williamson CC, James EA, James MP, et al. Horse plasma lactate determinations: comparison of wet and dry chemistry methods and the effect of storage. Equine Vet J 1996;28:406–8.

# Comparative Hemostasis: Animal Models and New Hemostasis Tests

Marjory B. Brooks, DVM[a], Tracy Stokol, BVSc, PhD[b],*,
James L. Catalfamo, PhD[a]

**KEYWORDS**

- Hemostasis • Animal model • Thromboelastography
- Flow cytometry

Hemostasis is vital for the restoration of endothelial integrity after vascular injury. Effective hemostasis requires complex interactions among enzymes, enzymatic cofactors, protease and nonprotease inhibitors, matrix proteins, and cells. These fluid phase, membrane-bound, and subendothelial components cooperate to create a finely tuned system that deftly balances activation and inhibition of coagulation and fibrinolysis in a temporal and spatial-specific manner. Engineered and naturally occurring animal models have provided a remarkable insight into the mechanisms of physiologic and pathologic hemostasis and thrombosis (**Tables 1** and **2**).[1–3] The goal of this review is to provide an overview of animal model systems and their strengths and limitations in the study of hemostasis. Examples of animal models are described in the context of cell-based hemostasis, and new assay techniques applicable to comparative hemostatic studies are summarized.

## OVERVIEW OF ANIMAL MODELS

Laboratory animal models serve as surrogate systems that recapitulate, and ideally describe with high fidelity, common biologic processes such as the molecular and cellular events of hemostasis and thrombosis.[4] The significance and validity of data obtained using an animal model and its extrapolation coefficient to human and/or veterinary medicine depend on the selection of a suitable model. This selection

---

The authors declare no conflicts of interest.

[a] Department of Population Medicine and Diagnostic Sciences, College of Veterinary Medicine, Cornell University, S1-084 Schurman Hall, Upper Tower Road, Ithaca, NY 14853, USA

[b] Department of Population Medicine and Diagnostic Sciences, College of Veterinary Medicine, Cornell University, S1-058 Schurman Hall, Upper Tower Road, Ithaca, NY 14853, USA

* Corresponding author.

*E-mail address:* ts23@cornell.edu

Clin Lab Med 31 (2011) 139–159
doi:10.1016/j.cll.2010.10.009
**labmed.theclinics.com**

**Table 1**
Spontaneous and genetically engineered animal models of hemostasis

| Hemostatic Component | Species | Defect |
|---|---|---|
| **Platelets** | | |
| *Adhesion* | | |
| Gp1b | M | Bernard-Soulier syndrome: macroplatelets, bleeding phenotype. No thrombus formation (M) |
| GpVI | M | Defective thrombus formation on collagen |
| vWF | M, C, E, F, P | Bleeding phenotype, severity depends on type and inheritance of vWD. There are species differences in platelet-vWF expression. Spontaneous vWD in RIIIS/J mouse due to glycosyltransferase defect, which promotes vWF clearance. Defective thrombus formation (M) |
| *Aggregation* | | |
| GpIIb-IIIa | M, C, E | Bleeding phenotype, reduced aggregation |
| Rap1b | M | Neonatal mortality, reduced aggregation, resistant to thrombosis |
| CalDAG-GEF1 | M, C, B | Bleeding phenotype, reduced aggregation (agonist is species dependent) |
| Kindlin-3 | M, C | Bleeding phenotype, neonatal mortality (hemorrhage, M) |
| *Procoagulant activity* | | |
| Phosphatidylserine exposure | C | Scott syndrome: bleeding phenotype, unable to exteriorize PS or shed microparticles in response to agonists |
| *Granule secretion* | | |
| δ-Storage pool disease | M, C, F, B | Dense granule deficiency, bleeding phenotype due to decreased ADP and serotonin content or secretion |
| | | Chédiak-Higashi syndrome (F, B) |
| **Coagulation Cascade** | | |
| *Initiation of fibrin formation* | | |
| TF | M | Embryonically lethal due to defective yolk sac development (vasculogenesis), rescued with human tissue factor transgene or gene insertion (knock in). Adult mice with low expression of human TF bleed in specific vascular beds |
| Factor VII | M, C | Perinatally lethal due to vascular bed–specific bleeding (M). Mild to moderate bleeding phenotype in dogs (exon 5 mutation) |

*Amplification of fibrin formation*

| | | |
|---|---|---|
| Factor XI | M, C, B | No thrombus formation (M). Injury-induced hemorrhage (C, F), mild to minimal hemorrhage (B) |
| Factors IX and VIII | Factor IX: M, C, F; Factor VIII: M, C, F, B, O, E | Mild to moderate hemorrhage, particularly into joints and soft tissue; usually injury-induced. Spontaneous rodent hemophilia: hemophilia A in WAG-F8 rats; hemophilia B in PLJ mice |
| Factors X and V | M, C, F (factor X) | Neonatal mortality (M), bleeding phenotype (C, F) |
| Prothrombin | M, C | Neonatal lethality due to hemorrhage (M) |
| Factor XIII | M | Bleeding tendency into body cavities and subcutaneous tissue |
| *Coagulation factor binding to PS* | | |
| Defective carboxylation of glutamic acid | F, B | Severe bleeding tendency, partially vitamin K responsive. Carboxylation of glutamic acid residues in the amino-terminal domain of coagulation factors II, VII, IX, and X is required for calcium-dependent binding to PS |
| *Contact pathway factors* | | |
| Factor XII, prekallikrein, high-molecular-weight kininogen | Factor XII: birds, whales, C, F, M; Prekallikrein: E, C | No bleeding tendency (factor XII), reported bleeding tendency (prekallikrein, E). Reduced arterial thrombosis (M) |
| **Fibrinolysis** | | |
| tPA, uPA | M | No overt phenotype unless combined deficiency (spontaneous fibrin deposition) |
| Plasminogen | M, C | Severe thrombosis, rescued by fibrinogen deficiency. Ligneous conjunctivitis (C) |
| **Inhibitors** | | |
| TFPI, thrombomodulin, antithrombin, protein C, endothelial protein C receptor | M, E (protein C) | Neonatal lethality. TFPI, thrombomodulin-, and endothelial protein C receptor–knockout mice rescued by transgenic mice expressing low amounts of human tissue factor (low-tissue factor mice). TFPI-knockout mice are also rescued by factor VII deficiency. Thrombotic tendency associated with reduced protein C level (E) |
| Protein S | — | Cofactor for protein C, no murine model |
| TAFI | M | No overt phenotype |

Unless otherwise indicated, all murine models are genetically engineered.

A complete list of all available animal models is beyond the scope of this review. For a more extensive list, please refer Refs.[1,3,9,10]

*Abbreviations:* B, bovine; CalDAG-GEF1, calcium and diacylglycerol guanine-exchange factor 1; C, canine; E, equine; F, feline; Gp, glycoprotein; M, mouse; O, ovine; P, porcine; TAFI, thrombin-activatable fibrinolytic inhibitor; TFPI, TF pathway inhibitor; tPA, tissue plasminogen activator; uPA, urokinase plasminogen activator; vWD, von Willebrand disease; vWF, von Willebrand factor.

**Table 2**
**Murine models of induced pathologic thrombosis**

| Model | Description |
|-------|-------------|
| Ferric Chloride | Induces severe endothelial injury with exposure of subendothelial collagen and thrombus formation in arterioles. Platelet activation is mediated by collagen binding (GpVI and vWF dependent) |
| Laser | Can induce superficial or deep injury. Platelet activation is thrombin dependent (tissue factor exposure) |
| Rose Bengal | Photoreactive dye that induces oxidant injury |
| Systemic Collagen/Epinephrine | Induces pulmonary thromboembolism |
| Mechanical Trauma | Denudation with a guide wire, compression, or ligation |

For additional information, please see Refs.[2,3]
*Abbreviations:* Gp, glycoprotein; vWF, von Willebrand factor.

requires knowledge of the comparative anatomy, cell and molecular biology, physiology, and biochemistry of the animal model relative to the target species. More highly conserved mechanisms or pathways are easier to extrapolate from an animal model to a distant target species. However, modeling species far removed phylogenetically can provide a substantial insight into fundamental processes; one obvious example is the use of the fruit fly to model human and animal genetics.

Animal studies are used to model biologic structure or function. They can be designed to describe mechanisms in healthy individuals or an aberrant pathway causing dysfunction. Moreover, animal models can be tailored to mimic specific human disease phenotypes within a broad category of disease.[5] The combination of animal studies and physical or mathematical modeling has proven invaluable for elucidating complex multistep pathways. Animal models have also been developed to predict clinical outcomes. Animal models are often used to discover and measure the effect of a drug or surgical intervention, assess treatment complications, and detect toxicity. Predictive animal models, however, must share relevant biologic systems and mirror reactions in the target species.

## CLASSIFICATION OF ANIMAL MODELS OF HEMOSTASIS
### Induced Models

Historically, animal model studies involved the experimental induction of hemostatic disease in healthy animals, for example, the intravenous administration of endotoxin to rats to produce disseminated intravascular coagulation.[6] Since the early 1990s, there has been a tremendous increase in the use of genetically altered mice to develop in vivo systems to study intravascular thrombus formation. In 2007, a comprehensive review of murine thrombosis models was published.[3] This review highlighted more than 150 reports that used ferric chloride, direct laser, and photochemical or mechanical wire injury to study thrombosis in genetically engineered mice or specific strains. In addition to chemical or mechanical injury, intravenous injection of systemic collagen or epinephrine has been used to induce pulmonary thromboembolism to test the in vivo antithrombotic effects of pharmacologic compounds. The onset and progression of thrombotic disease has been extensively studied using mice engineered to underexpress or overexpress virtually all genes known to be involved in hemostasis. Those studies dissected pathways to identify which gene products exerted relative prothrombotic and antithrombotic influences.[3] However, it is difficult to develop experimental vascular injury techniques that demonstrate consistent occlusion time end points. It may take weeks to months before reliable and reproducible end point results can be obtained. Nonspecific variables that influence in vivo thrombus formation include depth of anesthesia, levels of oxygen administration, and maintenance of physiologic body temperature. Transgenic mice can display phenotypic variability in thrombosis susceptibility and vascular endothelial response depending on the strain background.[7] Appropriate strain controls for murine thrombosis models include the use of paired experiments with engineered and wild-type littermates and age- and sex-matched study populations.

### Spontaneous Models

Spontaneous mutations may produce genetic variants whose phenotypes manifest as hemorrhagic or thrombotic disorders. Hundreds of disease strains of mice have been characterized and conserved, including those that model hereditary coagulation factor deficiencies, platelet function defects, and thrombotic disorders.[8] In addition to spontaneous rodent models, a wide range of naturally occurring genetic variants have been identified in other species including dogs.[9–11] Spontaneous hemophilia A has been recently characterized in WAG-F8 rats[12]; this animal model has the potential to overcome limitations currently associated with murine models of hemophilia. The canine models of hemophilia A, hemophilia B, Glanzmann thrombasthenia, and von Willebrand disease (vWD) display a very high phenotypic similarity with the corresponding human disease. This phenotypic similarity often extends to response to treatment in the model animal and the human patient. These models have been critical for the development of effective treatment modalities for corresponding human disease.[13–15] The severity of disease expression may vary according to the mutation type and residual factor activity. In general, mild bleeding phenotypes result from mild factor deficiencies; however, a fatal hemorrhagic diathesis was associated with experimental manipulation and instrumentation of PL/J mice with mild factor IX (FIX) deficiency.[16]

### Genetically Engineered Models

The rapid advances and refinements in molecular and cell biology technologies have led to genetically modified mice becoming the predominant model system in terms of animal numbers and research dollars. The popularity of mouse models is because of their relatively low cost and the ease and flexibility in targeted disease expression. Recent breakthroughs in rat stem cell biology and new techniques for targeted and random mutation insertion in this species hold promise that rats may someday rival mice as the rodent model of choice.[17] In addition, other mammalian species and fish are being developed specifically for hemostasis modeling.[18,19]

The insertion of DNA into the genome of animals or the deletion of specific genes can result in unpredictable outcomes; in part due to the polygenic nature of many physiologic reactions. Transgenic lines need to be selected and bred or cloned for a specific phenotype. The development of genetic maps of the mouse, dog, and other animals facilitates research in comparative genomics and proteomics. These maps provide the tools to assess the importance of genetic background and modifier genes on disease phenotypes. The use of genetically modified animals now extends beyond the identification of disease genes to the study of genetic pathways, gene-gene interactions, and gene-environment effects.

### Negative Models

In contrast to animal models that display a disease phenotype, negative models refer to animals with disease resistance. This category comprises naturally occurring and genetically modified species, strains, and breeds, in which selected diseases fail to develop. These models have been used effectively in studies to characterize the physiologic basis of the observed resistance and to relate resistance to normal or pathologic pathways.

### Orphan Models

Orphan models include functional disorders that occur naturally in a nonhuman species but have not yet been recognized in humans. Spontaneous mutations in calcium and diacylglycerol guanine-exchange factor 1 (CalDAG-GEF1) in dogs[20] and cattle[21] with platelet dysfunction are examples of orphan models. A murine knockout of the CalDAG-GEF1 gene has been generated[22] and it has a platelet phenotype similar to, but not identical to, that of spontaneous models.

## EXTRAPOLATION FROM ANIMAL MODELS

Most animal studies do not yield data for direct extrapolation in the mathematical sense. The predictive value of animal model studies may seem high when designed with scientific rigor; however, uncritical reliance on animal test results can be dangerously misleading. For example, the unanticipated prothrombotic effects of the 3 widely prescribed cyclooxygenase-2 inhibitors rofecoxib (Vioxx), valdecoxib (Bextra), and celecoxib (Celebrex) led to the withdrawal of Vioxx and Bextra from the market. Celebrex has not been withdrawn; however, in the United States, Celebrex can be prescribed only with a prominent warning of possible cardiovascular risks, including an increased risk of heart attack. Genetically defined and uniform rodent strains may not be appropriate models for human target populations that are genetically diverse and influenced by many cultural, dietary, and environmental conditions.

Pharmacologic studies to detect hemostatic side effects have proven particularly difficult to model in rodents. The general assumption that conservation of biologic systems among animal species allows for direct comparisons has not proven true. One striking difference is the relative size difference between mouse and man. This size difference translates into significantly higher metabolic rates for small animal models, affecting comparative respiration rate, blood pressure, and drug metabolism. Murine models pose special challenges for evaluating coagulation, platelet function, and thrombosis. It is often difficult to obtain adequate blood sample volumes for analysis. In animals smaller than rabbits, capillary density increases dramatically with decreasing body weight,[5] a difference that may influence hemostasis and thrombotic reactions. As the importance of species differences has become obvious, federally regulated toxicology studies now require testing in at least 2 species and in at least 1 nonrodent species. The choice of any laboratory animal model must factor in costs, availability of reagents, similarities between target and model disease phenotype, relevance of the animal model for prediction of adverse reactions, and drug or treatment efficacy. The dominance of mouse models will likely continue; however, new genetic tools and assay systems hold promise for expanding the repertoire of animal systems to study hemostasis.

## ANIMAL MODELS AND CELL-BASED HEMOSTASIS

The cell-based model of hemostasis takes into account the role of circulating blood platelets, vessel wall, endothelial cells, and tissue factor (TF)-bearing cells.[23] Hemostasis is conceptually separated into 3 stages: platelet plug formation (primary hemostasis), fibrin clot formation (secondary hemostasis), and clot dissolution (fibrinolysis). In vivo, these stages overlap rather than proceeding sequentially.

Thrombin generation is the crucial determinant of fibrin formation and occurs in 3 phases: initiation, amplification, and propagation. All the phases take place on cell membranes, predominately on those that express the negatively charged phospholipid phosphatidylserine (PS). Activated platelets are considered the major source of cell membrane–associated PS for amplification and propagation of hemostasis. In resting platelets, PS is sequestered on the inner leaflet of the cell membrane; however, PS is translocated to the outer leaflet on cell activation. PS-enriched membranes provide physical scaffolding and binding sites for coagulation factor complexes, protect against inhibitors, and function as a cofactor that amplifies coagulation factor complex activity. Exteriorization of PS is accompanied by the shedding of tiny (<1 μm) membrane-derived vesicles or microparticles (MPs). MPs are enriched with PS and coagulation factors and vastly expand the surface area for hemostasis. Localization of hemostasis to PS-bearing membranes, now termed the cell-based model of hemostasis, restricts fibrin formation to the injured site. The importance of PS-containing surfaces is exemplified by Scott syndrome, a rare bleeding diathesis in humans[24] and German shepherd dogs.[25] Platelets of affected patients are unable to exteriorize PS or shed MPs. Intravital microscopy in mice with laser-induced vascular injury has demonstrated MPs being actively incorporated into the developing fibrin thrombus.[26]

Primary and secondary hemostases begin simultaneously on vessel injury (**Fig. 1**). Injury activates endothelial cells and exposes thrombogenic subendothelial matrix

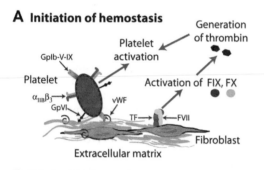

**Fig. 1.** Overview of primary and secondary hemostasis. (*A*) Initiation of hemostasis culminates in the activation of platelets and the generation of trace amounts of thrombin mediated via the action of the TF-FVII complex on FIX and FX. (*B*) Fibrin clot formation results from a burst of thrombin generated by the assembly of highly active coagulation complexes on the surface of procoagulant platelets and platelet-derived MPs. TF-bearing monocyte-derived MPs likely contribute to localized generation of thrombin. FVII, factor VII; FX, factor X; Gp, glycoprotein; vWF, von Willebrand factor.

components (eg, collagen and von Willebrand factor [vWF]) and TF-expressing perivascular cells. Circulating platelets adhere by surface receptors that bind to the exposed matrix proteins. Key receptors involved in adhesion, signaling and anchoring include the glycoprotein (Gp) complex GpIb-V-IX, which binds vWF, and GpVI and the integrin $\alpha_2\beta_1$, which bind collagen. Adherent platelets undergo activation through intracellular calcium signaling and phospholipid metabolism and secrete preformed and synthesized agonists, coagulation factors, and growth factors from storage granules. Animal models of platelet secretion defects have been described in mice, dogs, cats, and cattle.[27,28] The release of bioactive proteins recruits new platelets to the injured site and contributes to endothelial activation. Agonist- or adhesion receptor–induced intracellular signaling alters the conformation of the fibrinogen receptor $\alpha_{IIb}\beta_3$ (GpIIb-IIIa). Fibrinogen binding to $\alpha_{IIb}\beta_3$ on adjacent platelets mediates platelet aggregation, formation of the primary platelet plug, and stabilization of the plug to the vessel wall. Agonist-stimulated adherent platelets undergo a series of signaling events that activate the small GTPase, Rap1b, and protein kinase C. These proteins in turn sustain the conformational change in $\alpha_{IIb}\beta_3$ and bound fibrinogen required to support platelet aggregation.[29]

The importance of Rap1b-mediated platelet signaling was illustrated by spontaneous and induced mutations of its activator, CalDAG-GEF1. CalDAG-GEF1 null knockout mice demonstrate severe platelet aggregation defects to various agonists.[22] Similarly, clinically severe platelet function defects have been described in Simmental cattle and 3 dog breeds, including basset hounds, because of mutations in CalDAG-GEF1.[20,21] Additional signaling partners necessary for platelet aggregation continue to be discovered. Kindlin-3, a protein that links the actin cytoskeleton to the cytoplasmic tail of integrin receptors, has a recently identified role in platelet aggregation. Mutations in Kindlin-3 have been associated with a combined bleeding disorder and immune dysfunction in humans[30] and a dog.[31] Defective or deficient receptors for fibrinogen ($\alpha_{IIb}\beta_3$) or vWF (Gp1b) and functional or quantitative defects in vWF result in the bleeding disorders Glanzmann thrombasthenia, Bernard-Soulier syndrome, and vWD, respectively. Spontaneous models of human Glanzmann thrombasthenia[15] and quantitative and functional vWD variants have been well characterized in several breeds of dogs and horses; however, murine knockouts remain the only model of Bernard-Soulier syndrome to date (see **Table 1**).

Exposure of extravascular TF, which is constitutively expressed on perivascular cells, initiates fibrin formation through activation of the coagulation cascade. Coagulation reactions occur concurrently and with extensive integration with platelet activation (see **Fig. 1**). Plasma factor VII (FVII) adheres to exposed TF, forming a membrane-bound enzymatic complex that activates factor X (FX) and FIX. TF is crucial for hemostasis and vascular development. There are no reports of spontaneous TF deficiency in humans or animals, and a complete deficiency of TF is lethal at day 9.5 postconception in knockout mice embryos.[32] FVII-knockout mice die perinatally of severe abdominal and cranial hemorrhage from apparently normal vessels.[33] In contrast, FVII deficiency in humans and dogs does not seem to be lethal and causes variable bleeding (from none to moderate), presumably due to residual FVII activity.[34,35]

The TF-FVIIa-FXa complex on cell surfaces activates small amounts of prothrombin but is rapidly inhibited by TF pathway inhibitor (TFPI), which is released from activated endothelial cells. The trace amounts of thrombin generated through this pathway are insufficient to produce fibrin or to inhibit fibrinolysis through thrombin-activatable fibrinolytic inhibitor (TAFI). The generated thrombin, however, does provide positive feedback to amplify its own production by activating intrinsic pathway cofactors (factor VIII [FVIII] and factor V [FV]), factor XI (FXI), and platelets (by binding to protease-activated receptors). This amplification phase (1) produces a sudden localized increase in the level of thrombin, which then cleaves fibrinogen to soluble fibrin, (2) activates factor XIII (FXIII), which then cross-links the soluble fibrin, and (3) activates TAFI, which inhibits fibrinolysis. Simultaneously, thrombin-activated platelets externalize PS and shed PS-expressing MPs to serve as binding sites for enzymatic coagulation complex assembly. Platelet degranulation also releases key coagulation factors, including FV, FXIII, and fibrinogen, from alpha granule stores, thereby producing high local factor concentrations. Together, these platelet responses facilitate thrombin generation and fibrin production, with the fibrin becoming incorporated into the growing platelet plug. Thus, the intimate physical and costimulatory relationships among platelets and coagulation factors are essential for stable fibrin clot formation. When coagulation factors are unable to bind or assemble on activated platelets, a hemorrhagic diathesis ensues. This diathesis occurs with Scott syndrome in German shepherd dogs and glutamic acid carboxylation defects in Devon rex cats[36] and Rambouillet sheep[37] (see **Table 1**).

Leukocytes and erythrocytes are frequently incorporated into the developing fibrin clot. Like activated platelets, these cells release MPs that express markers specific for the cell of origin. These surface antigens can be identified and quantified using flow cytometric techniques. In particular, monocyte-derived MPs express TF and PS[38] and are incorporated into the fibrin thrombus as it forms.[26] TF-enriched MPs likely facilitate continued local activation of the coagulation cascade and are thought to contribute to dissemination of coagulation in inflammatory or septic states. Their pathologic role in various diseases, including cancer, is an area of intense investigation.[39]

The contact pathway factors of the coagulation cascade factor XII (FXII), high-molecular-weight kininogen (HMWK), and prekallikrein have no demonstrated role in physiologic thrombin generation. Indeed, reptiles, birds, marsupials, and all cetaceans lack the FXII gene.[40] A hereditary FXII deficiency syndrome is common in domestic cats, with no associated signs of a bleeding diathesis.[41] However, FXII does seem to be involved in arterial thrombosis as demonstrated by attenuation of thrombus formation in studies of severe mechanically induced or chemically induced arteriolar injury in FXII-knockout mice.[42]

As fibrin formation proceeds, fibrinolysis is activated through the release of tissue plasminogen activator from injured endothelium and concomitant activation of prekallikrein and HMWK. Just as fibrin formation is localized to cell surfaces, fibrinolysis is restricted primarily to the fibrin clot. There are few reports of naturally occurring fibrinolytic defects in animals. Most experimental information has been obtained from genetically engineered mice and in vitro studies.

Numerous checks and balances limit hemostasis to prevent dissemination beyond the primary site of injury. These checks include platelet adhesion directly to vascular injury sites, spatial restriction of fibrin formation to PS-bearing cell surfaces, and action of specific coagulation factor inhibitors that downregulate each phase of hemostasis. The extrinsic (TF-FVII-FX) pathway is inhibited by soluble and endothelium-bound TFPI. The anticoagulant effect of antithrombin, the main inhibitor of serine protease coagulation factors, is enhanced in vivo by heparin-sulfated glycosaminoglycans on endothelial surfaces. Thrombin not only amplifies its own production but also triggers its own inhibition, by binding to thrombomodulin on endothelial cells. The thrombin-thrombomodulin complex, in concert with the endothelial protein C receptor, activates protein C, which inhibits the activated coagulation cofactors FVIIIa and FVa. Decreased cofactor activity slows thrombin generation and the thrombin-mediated inhibition of fibrinolysis, thereby allowing clot dissolution. Complete deficiencies of TFPI, antithrombin, or any component of the protein C pathway results in neonatal mortality in mice, demonstrating the importance of these inhibitors.[1] Thus, a delicate balance exists between procoagulant, anticoagulant, and profibrinolytic forces. Procoagulants are favored initially as a fibrin clot forms, and then, as the endothelium heals, the impetus for fibrin production decreases. Thrombin generation slows, and fibrinolysis then dominates to restore vessel patency. Alterations in this finely tuned system can result in excessive hemorrhage or thrombosis. For example, a mutation in FV (FV Leiden) renders this activated factor resistant to protein C inhibition. This defect is a common risk factor for deep vein thrombosis in humans,[43] for which there is no natural animal counterpart.

Recent studies emphasize the influence of the microvascular environment on the mechanisms that activate and inhibit hemostasis. Local shear rates dictate whether platelets bind to extracellular matrix via vWF-Gp1b-V-IX or collagen-GpVI interactions, with vWF adhesive contacts dominating at high shear rates.[2] Studies in genetically modified mice have shown vascular bed–specific expression of coagulation factors, receptors, and inhibitors. This differential expression of hemostatic components dictates which procoagulant and anticoagulant pathways are operative in specific vascular beds or tissues.[1] These concepts of cell-based and tissue-specific regulation of hemostasis provide novel approaches and targets for pharmacologic modification of hemostasis.

## ASSAY SYSTEMS FOR CELL-BASED HEMOSTASIS

The model of cell-based hemostasis has led to the development of new instrumentation and assay techniques to assess cellular reactions and membrane dependent-reactions, thrombin generation, and qualitative characteristics of a nascent fibrin clot. Thromboelastography, thrombin generation assays, and cytometric detection of platelet reactivity are among the tests that are now used for characterizing physiologic hemostasis, pathologic thrombosis, and refractory hemorrhage. Application of these assays to animal model systems requires consideration of blood collection site, sample volume, and the availability of cross-reactive or species-specific reagents. As previously outlined, comparative studies provide valuable mechanistic insights into the signaling and regulatory pathways that modulate thrombus formation. Knowledge of species differences, however, should influence the choice of animal models to maximize their predictive value for human disease and drug studies.

### Thromboelastography

Thromboelastography refers to the graphic display of the viscoelastic properties of fibrin clots generated in whole blood samples under conditions of low shear.[44,45] The TEG system (Haemonetics Corp, Braintree, MA, USA. www.haemoscope.com/index.html) uses a tabletop coagulation device and associated software to detect the motion of a pin suspended in a small volume (approximately 350 µL) of whole blood. The sample cup rotates through a defined angle, with torque on the immersed pin detected after a fibrin-platelet thrombus has linked the cup and pin together. The rate and strength of fibrin formation affects pin motion, which is transduced to an electric signal and ultimately displayed as the TEG output tracing (**Fig. 2**). In addition to this qualitative tracing, the TEG software performs direct measurements and derived calculations that describe various parameters of clot formation and subsequent clot lysis. Among the routinely reported parameters are reaction time (R), clotting time (K), angle (α), maximal amplitude (MA), and lysis index (LY30 or LY60). The parameter R is the interval from the assay start till the first deviations of the tracing from baseline denoting initial fibrin formation; K is arbitrarily assigned as the time for deflection from 2 to 20 mm from

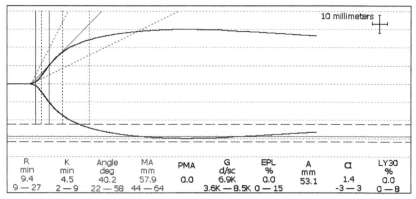

| R min | K min | Angle deg | MA mm | PMA | G d/sc | EPL % | A mm | α | LY30 % |
|---|---|---|---|---|---|---|---|---|---|
| 9.4 | 4.5 | 40.2 | 57.9 | 0.0 | 6.9K | 0.0 | 53.1 | 1.4 | 0.0 |
| 9 — 27 | 2 — 9 | 22 — 58 | 44 — 64 | | 3.6K — 8.5K | 0 — 15 | | -3 — 3 | 0 — 8 |

**Fig. 2.** Canine thromboelastograph tracing (TEG). TEG tracing generated by recalcification of citrated whole blood from a healthy control dog displays instrument-derived parameters: A, amplitude; α, angle; CI, coagulation index; EPL, estimated percent lysis; G, clot firmness; K, clotting time; LY30, lysis index at 30 minutes; MA, maximal amplitude; PMA, projected MA; R, reaction time.

baseline; α is the slope of a line drawn from R to K; MA is the widest vertical amplitude of the TEG tracing, reflecting maximum clot strength; and LY60 is the TEG amplitude at 60 minutes after the time of MA, denoting the extent of fibrinolysis. A derived parameter summarizing overall clot firmness (G) is expressed in dyne/second and calculated from the formula $G = (5000 \times MA)/(100-MA)$. The TEG software can perform more complex data analyses, including first derivative measures of the standard TEG waveform.[46] This transformation yields a thrombus generation velocity curve and derived parameters that are thought to provide indirect information on thrombin generation in the assay mixture.

Thromboelastography is typically performed on whole blood samples. Native blood drawn with no anticoagulant must be assayed within 5 minutes, thereby limiting this sample type to point-of-care testing. Sodium citrate is the most common anticoagulant used for laboratory TEG. In this method, coagulation is initiated in citrate samples by the addition of calcium. Citrated blood, however, demonstrates variable changes in TEG parameters during storage[47]; initiation of the assay after a fixed time point improves standardization of results within and among laboratories. The addition of different "trigger" reagents to activate coagulation shortens the assay time, removes some of the variability of sample storage, and limits the influence of sample contact with the reaction cup for initial serine protease activation.[48,49] Recombinant human TF (Innovin) is often chosen as a trigger reagent to mimic the physiologic initiation of coagulation by tissue injury and TF expression in the vascular space. The TEG manufacturer-supplied kaolin and phospholipid solution (Kaolin) is also frequently used as an initiator of coagulation by activation of the contact pathway factors. In addition to these reagents, the TEG manufacturer supplies modified reaction cups containing heparinase to monitor coagulation independent of therapeutic heparin levels. Specialized trigger reagents containing reptilase and FXIII (Activator F) are used with either ADP or arachidonic acid platelet activators to monitor antiplatelet therapy in heparinized blood samples (Platelet Mapping assay, Haemoscope, Niles, IL, USA).

Numerous other assay modifications can be performed, such as using corn trypsin inhibitor collection tubes to inhibit contact activation during sample storage, varying the concentration or composition of the trigger reagent (eg, dilute TF reagents, celite contact activators), and adding drugs or blood products ex vivo to the reaction mixture.[50–52] Ultimately, this flexibility in TEG assay configuration requires careful consideration of the study population and clinical question or hypothesis under investigation to ensure optimal assay conditions. The choice of trigger reagent affects assay sensitivity to coagulation factor deficiencies in the same manner as traditional clotting time tests. For example, thromboplastin reagents used in both the prothrombin time screening test and TF-activated TEG generate thrombin by FVII-mediated activation of FX, thereby reducing the sensitivity of both assays to deficiencies of the intrinsic pathway factors (**Fig. 3**).

Thromboelastography has wide use in basic, translational, and comparative hemostatic studies as a kinetic monitor of fibrin and platelet plug formation under defined reaction conditions. Interpretation of TEG tracings in any setting requires concomitant evaluation of standard hematology and hemostatic tests, for example, platelet count, fibrinogen and coagulation screening, and/or individual factor assays. The TEG reaction proceeds under low shear conditions and is insensitive to vWF deficiency or dysfunction or primary platelet adhesion defects. Thromboelastography is considered a cost-effective diagnostic aid to guide transfusion therapy for people undergoing complex surgical procedures including orthotopic liver transplant and cardiac bypass.[53] The TEG system is also used to characterize hypercoagulable syndromes and monitor some anticoagulant and antiplatelet drugs; however, the diagnostic utility of these applications is not yet well defined.

The use of TEG in clinical veterinary settings has been recently described, primarily in dogs having diseases associated with thrombosis.[54,55] The assay methodology is broadly applicable to many species, with sample volume being the major limitation precluding its use in small rodents. The standard TEG sample volume of 340 μL of whole blood is feasible for serial determinations in rabbits and larger animal models. Trigger reagent and reaction conditions must be optimized to account for species differences in contact activation, relative sensitivity to human TF, and variable reactivity to platelet agonists. A recent comparative study revealed that among sheep, rats, pigs, and rabbits, the viscoelastic properties of fibrin formed in recalcified citrated blood from sheep most closely matched that of humans.[56]

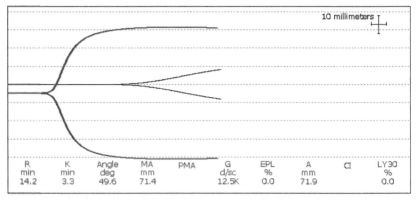

| R<br>min<br>14.2 | K<br>min<br>3.3 | Angle<br>deg<br>49.6 | MA<br>mm<br>71.4 | PMA | G<br>d/sc<br>12.5K | EPL<br>%<br>0.0 | A<br>mm<br>71.9 | CI | LY30<br>%<br>0.0 |
|---|---|---|---|---|---|---|---|---|---|

**Fig. 3.** Thromboelastograph tracing from a hemophiliac dog depicting effects of a TF-activating reagent. Citrated whole blood from a dog with severe hemophilia A (FVIII <1%) was recalcified without an activator or activated by the addition of recombinant human TF (Innovin, 1:50,000 final concentration). The tracing from nonactivated blood (*black tracing*) depicts aberrant fibrin formation, with no coupling of the TEG pin and cup. In contrast, TF activation generates thrombin through the extrinsic pathway, producing a qualitatively normal tracing (*green tracing*). A, amplitude, CI, coagulation index; EPL, estimated percent lysis; G, clot firmness; PMA, projected MA.

### Thrombin Generation Assays

The in vitro capacity of plasma to generate thrombin over time is referred to as the endogenous thrombin potential (ETP).[57,58] Newly developed automated assay systems allow kinetic measurements of thrombin's cleavage of a fluorogenic substrate, with calculation and display of a thrombin generation curve or thrombogram (**Fig. 4**). The 4 main parameters derived from the thrombogram include lag time, peak thrombin, time to peak thrombin, and ETP. Lag time (minutes) is defined as the interval from assay start till the tracing moves beyond 2 SDs from baseline, indicating early thrombin formation. The peak thrombin and time to peak thrombin refer to the maximal thrombin value (nM thrombin) and the time interval (minutes), respectively, required from the start of the assay to reach this value. ETP is the area under the thrombogram (minutes × nM) and is a summary of the overall capacity for thrombin production. ETP provides a global measure of net forces that promote thrombin formation (displayed as the upward deflection of the thrombogram) and the subsequent activity of endogenous thrombin inhibitors (displayed as the downward deflection toward baseline).

Commercially available thrombin generation assays (Calibrated Automated Thrombogram [CAT], Thrombinoscope, Maastricht, The Netherlands; Technothrombin TGA, Technoclone, Dorking, Surrey, UK) are generally performed on either platelet-rich plasma (PRP) or platelet-poor plasma (PPP) collected with citrate-based anticoagulants. Reactions require approximately 40 to 50 μL of plasma, thereby allowing replicates and serial determinations from small-volume blood draws. The assays are configured with trigger reagents that contain calcium, phospholipid, and TF. Preanalytic variables, particularly blood collection and processing techniques, greatly influence thrombogram results and assay interpretation.[59] Storage and centrifugation conditions determine the cellular and cell-derived MP concentration and activation status in the test sample. Centrifugation conditions to prepare PPP (eg, 1500 g × 10 minutes) may produce wide interindividual variation in residual platelet and MP concentration.[60] Sequential high-speed

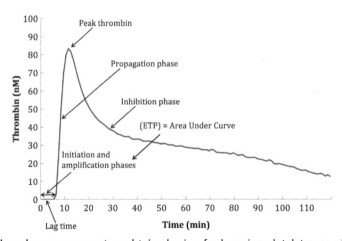

**Fig. 4.** Thrombogram parameters obtained using fresh canine platelet-poor plasma (PPP). PPP was isolated from citrated (3.8%) whole blood by centrifugation at 2500 g for 15 minutes at 4° to 8°C and analyzed within 2 hours. Thrombin generation was triggered by the simultaneous addition of excess calcium chloride and PS-enriched synthetic phospholipid vesicles containing 2 pM of recombinant human TF. Thrombin calibrator and data analysis software used to generate thrombograms were purchased from Technoclone GmbH, Vienna, Austria. ETP, endogenous thrombin potential.

centrifugation (eg, 15,000 g × 30 minutes) and/or microfiltration are required to produce MP-free supernatants. The use of frozen-thawed PRP or PPP samples results in cold-induced platelet activation, membrane damage, and procoagulant phospholipid exposure[61]; these samples accelerate thrombin generation and yield increased amounts of thrombin compared with corresponding fresh sample types. Ultimately, reliable and interpretable thrombin generation data require rigorously defined preanalytic conditions.

As in TEG and traditional clotting time tests, varying the trigger reagent and other components of the assay mixture influences the sensitivity and specificity of thrombin generation assays.[57,62] A low TF concentration (eg, <1 pmol/L) in trigger reagents increases the assay sensitivity to activities of the intrinsic pathway factors (FVIII, FIX, FXI), contact activation (FXII, prekallikrein, HMWK), and protein S inhibitory activity. Trigger reagents containing higher TF concentrations (eg, >5 pmol/L) reduce the influence of contact activation and residual MP content of the test samples. Corn trypsin inhibitor added to the reaction mixture directly blocks the contribution of contact activation and is used often to increase assay specificity in FVIII-deficient samples.[63] Phospholipid concentrations less than 3 to 5 μM/L become rate limiting in cell- and MP-free samples. Assays configured with a low amount of or no phospholipid-containing reagents are therefore used to study the effects of endogenous MP content on thrombin generation.[60] Numerous other assay variables can be manipulated, including the addition of activated serine protease factors (eg, FIXa, FXa) to bypass the TF trigger and the addition of thrombomodulin to increase assay sensitivity to the protein C pathway.

Thrombin generation assays, in numerous configurations, have become important research tools to explore the procoagulant and anticoagulant forces contributing to net thrombin production. The clinical utility of these assays is currently under investigation for a variety of hemorrhagic and thrombotic disorders in humans. Among these applications, studies of hemophilia A aim to better differentiate bleeding severity among patients with similar residual FVIII activities and to assess the efficacy of inhibitor bypass therapy for patients with anti-FVIII antibodies. Thrombin generation assays are also under investigation as predictors of incipient thrombosis among at-risk patient populations. As a measure of cumulative pro- and antithrombin generating forces, thrombin generation assays may provide unique information that complements other clinical and laboratory parameters of venous and arterial thrombosis.[62]

Thrombin generation assays have many desirable features for comparative studies, including the use of relatively small sample volumes, standardized assay end points, and comprehensive assessment of net hemostatic forces. The amino acid sequence of prothrombin is approximately 75% similar among vertebrates.[64] The most highly conserved regions include the active site and primary substrate-binding residues, whereas the least conserved regions include inhibitor (thrombomodulin and hirudin)-binding sites. Thrombin's action on the peptide substrate in thrombin generation assays is likely to be similar among species; however, the composition of the trigger reagent, sample preparation, residual cell membrane content, and contact activation are potential sources of wide variation in thrombogram results among species.[40] The appropriate configuration of thrombin generation assays for animal model studies must consider the species-specific variables in addition to the underlying pathophysiology or drug targets under investigation.

## FLOW CYTOMETRIC CHARACTERIZATION OF PLATELET FUNCTION

In contrast to global hemostatic tests that aim to characterize net thrombin and fibrin formation, flow cytometric assays examine platelet function on a single-cell basis. The advantages of cytometric assays include small sample volumes, simultaneous multi-parameter analyses, characterization of variable response among platelet subpopula-tions, and detection of platelet-leukocyte interactions and platelet-derived MPs.[65,66] The inherent challenges of platelet flow cytometry include the small cell size and size heterogeneity of platelets. The presence of any bacterial contaminants, immune complexes, or protein precipitates can interfere with discrimination of platelets and derived MPs. Platelet variations in size, volume, and activation status influence its light scattering properties, which in turn correlate with other measured parameters of forward scatter and fluorescence.

Evaluating the complex repertoire of platelet activation requires a combination of tests and the ability to assess different response parameters. Cytometric assays can be configured to detect platelet activation based on alterations in the density of expressed or bound surface Gps and ligands, the expression of granule proteins and neoepitopes, changes in ion flux, protein phosphorylation status, the permeability of cell and mitochondrial membranes, the outer membrane lipid composition, and membrane vesiculation.[67–69]

The aspects of platelet function to be studied dictate assay configuration and choice of activation markers (**Table 3**). In addition, tests may be performed to deter-mine basal in vivo platelet activation status or the in vitro reactivity of platelets to a variety of agonist stimuli. Detection of membrane expression of the alpha granule protein P-selectin (CD62P) is among the most commonly used marker of platelet reac-tivity in clinical and comparative studies (**Fig. 5**).

Preanalytic variables greatly influence flow cytometric assays, regardless of which activation parameters are evaluated. These variables include the choice of cytometer, fluorescent probe combinations, and gating strategies used for data collection and anal-ysis. In particular, methods for characterization and quantification of platelet-derived MPs have yet to be standardized among laboratories.[70,71] Blood collection and process-ing techniques are critical determinants of platelet activation status and therefore influ-ence the validity of all subsequent tests. Platelet reactivity differs for samples collected in EDTA, citrate, and heparin, which is in part due to the availability of extracellular calcium. Anticoagulant mixtures, such as CTAD (citrate, theophylline, adenosine, dipyr-idamole), provide greater sample stability during short-term (hours) storage.[72] The use of fixatives for long-term storage precludes in vitro activation studies and has been shown to differentially affect platelet activation parameters, including CD62P expression levels.[73] Whole blood assays using directly conjugated fluorescent probes and quench-dilute termination are generally preferred to avoid platelet activation resulting from cell separation and washing.[74] Constitutively expressed high-density antigens, such as CD42 (Gplb) and CD61 (GpIIIa), used in combination with specific activation markers then allow flow cytometric isolation of platelets in whole blood.

Flow cytometric tests provide rapid clinical diagnosis of hereditary platelet defects affecting constitutive receptors, such as Glanzmann thrombasthenia (GpIIb/IIIa defects), and have been used in animal model and clinical veterinary settings.[27] Assay techniques to monitor the effects of antiplatelet drug therapy are widely used in research laboratories. Selection of activation markers is based on a specific targeted receptor (eg, Abciximab binding to GpIIb/IIIa) or a targeted signaling pathway (eg, clopidogrel [Plavix] blocking of ADP-mediated vasodilator-stimulated phosphoprotein phosphorylation). Cytometric assays are also ideal in blood banking studies to monitor the activation status of platelets under various storage conditions.[67] The detection of "hyperfunctional" platelets in patients with thrombotic disorders is another common application, with numerous clinical studies examining patient populations with cardiac syndromes and other diseases associated with arterial or venous thrombosis. These

**Table 3**
Cytometric detection of platelet activation

| Activation Response | Markers | Molecule or Process Detected |
|---|---|---|
| Adhesion | CD42 (a, b, c, d) | vWF receptor complex (GpIb-V-IX) |
| | CD49b/CD29 | Collagen receptor (GpIa/GpIIa) |
| | CD49e/CD29 | Fibronectin receptor (GpIc/GpIIa) |
| | CD41/CD61 | Fibrinogen receptor (GpIIb/GpIIIa) |
| Aggregation | CD41/CD61 | Fibrinogen receptor (GpIIb/GpIIIa) |
| | PAC-1 (human) | Ligand-induced binding site neoepitope denoting occupied fibrinogen receptor |
| | JON/A (mouse) | |
| | Fibrinogen | Fibrinogen bound to platelet membrane |
| Degranulation | CD62P | P-selectin (alpha granule membrane protein) |
| | CD63 | Lysosomal integral membrane protein |
| | Mepacrine | Concentrated in dense granules, lost on release |
| Signaling | Fluo-3 | Cytosolic free calcium |
| | Vasodilator-stimulated phosphoprotein | ADP (P2Y12) receptor activation and target phosphorylation |
| | JC-1 | Mitochondrial membrane potential |
| | Tetramethylrhodamine ethyl ester | Mitochondrial membrane potential |
| Procoagulant activity | Annexin V | PS exposure |
| | Lactadherin | PS exposure |
| | FV | FV bound to platelet outer membrane |
| | Calcein | Lost through outer membrane pore on MP release |
| | Fibrinogen | Derivatized fibrinogen bound to outer membrane |
| MP release | CD42b, CD41/CD61 | Constitutive high-density membrane proteins to define platelet-origin membrane fragments |
| Platelet-leukocyte aggregates | CD42b, CD41/CD61 | Constitutive high-density membrane proteins to identify platelets bound to leukocytes; detected in combination with a leukocyte marker (eg, CD18, CD45) |

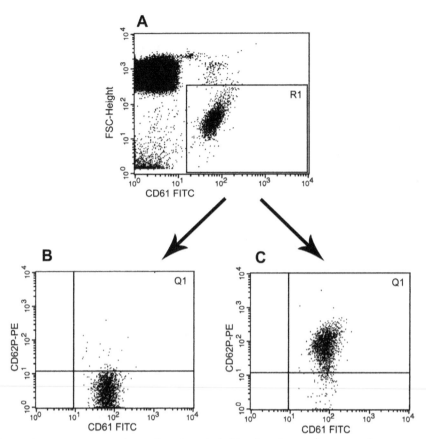

**Fig. 5.** Flow cytometric analyses of canine whole blood to detect platelet P-selectin expression. Whole blood from a healthy dog was treated with thrombin (1 U/mL) or vehicle control and then double-labeled with cross-reactive fluorescent antibodies to CD61 (GpIIIa) and CD62P (P-selectin). (*A*) Dot plot depicting gating strategy to identify platelets (R1) based on forward and side scatter properties and labeling with a cross-reactive CD61 antibody. (*B*) Dot plots of the gated region (R1) from unstimulated platelets, demonstrating a lack of P-selectin expression (Q2). (*C*) Dot plots of the gated region (R1) from thrombin-stimulated platelets depicting more than 90% platelets expressing P-selectin (Q1).

populations are now being studied to determine whether characterization of MPs originating from platelets and other cells will provide useful diagnostic or prognostic information.

Adaptation of functional flow cytometric assays for comparative studies may be challenging because of the lack of reagents and the difficulty (in any species) in obtaining and processing quality samples. Suboptimal phlebotomy techniques and lag times between blood collection and analysis often result in ex vivo platelet activation, precluding meaningful test results. Sample collection artifacts are important considerations for animal model studies. Practices such as cardiac puncture in small rodents generally activate platelets and yield blood samples that are not representative of the peripheral circulation. Lack of availability of species-specific or cross-reactive platelet antibodies presents another difficulty in configuring activation assays for many species. Finally, species differ in relative reactivity to various physiologic platelet agonists such as ADP, and the platelets of some species fail to respond to venom-derived and peptide agonists that trigger human platelet activation.[75,76] Comparative and animal model studies invariably require initial optimization to define appropriate agonists, agonist concentration, and the relevant parameters of activation response among those demonstrating cross-species reactivity.

## SUMMARY

Spontaneous and engineered hemostatic defects in animals have provided a wealth of information to model physiologic and pathologic hemostasis and thrombosis. Laboratory and domestic animals have also proven to be invaluable tools for testing efficacy and safety of new pharmacologic and genetic therapies. However, due to species-dependent differences in the hemostatic system, findings made in such animal models may not be directly applicable to human diseases.

## REFERENCES

1. Mackman N. Tissue-specific hemostasis in mice. Arterioscler Thromb Vasc Biol 2005;25(11):2273–81.
2. Furie B, Furie BC. In vivo thrombus formation. J Thromb Haemost 2007;5(Suppl 1): 12–7.
3. Westrick RJ, Winn ME, Eitzman DT. Murine models of vascular thrombosis. Arterioscler Thromb Vasc Biol 2007;27:2079–93.
4. Wessler S. Animals models of thrombosis and hemorrhagic diseases. DHEW Pub. No. NIH 76982. Washington, DC: U.S. Department of Health, Education and Welfare; 1976.
5. Hau J. Animal models for human diseases. In: Conn PM, editor. Source book of models for biomedical research. Totowa (NJ): Humana Press Inc; 2008. p. 3–8.
6. Aoshima K, Asakura H, Yamazaki M, et al. Treatment of disseminated intravascular coagulation (DIC) with all trans retinoic acid in an endotoxin-induced rat model. Semin Thromb Hemost 1998;24(3):227–31.
7. Bodary PF, Westrick RJ, Wickenheiser KJ, et al. Effect of leptin on arterial thrombosis following vascular injury in mice. JAMA 2002;287:1706–9.
8. The Jackson Laboratory. Available at: http://www.jax.org. Accessed September 20, 2010.
9. Hamosh A. John Hopkins University School of Medicine, On-line Mendelian Inheritance in Man, OMIM. Available at: http://www.ncbi.nlm.nih.gov/omim/. Accessed September 20, 2010.
10. Nicholas F. University of Sydney, On-line Mendelian Inheritance in Animals (OMIA). Available at: http://www.ncbi.nlm.nih.gov/sites/omia. Accessed September 20, 2010.
11. Brooks M. A review of canine inherited bleeding disorders: biochemical and molecular strategies for disease characterization and carrier detection. J Hered 1999;90(1):112–8.
12. Booth CJ, Brooks MB, Rockwell S, et al. WAG-F8 rats harboring a factor VIII gene mutation provide a new animal model for hemophilia A. J Thromb Haemost 2010; 8:2472–7.
13. Wolfe JH. Gene therapy in large animal models of human genetic diseases. ILAR J 2009;50(2):107–11.
14. Nichols TC, Dillow AM, Franck HW, et al. Protein replacement therapy and gene transfer in canine models of hemophilia A, hemophilia B, von Willebrand disease, and factor VII deficiency. ILAR J 2009;50(2):144–67.

15. Boudreaux MK, Lipscomb DL. Clinical, biochemical, and molecular aspects of Glanzmann thrombasthenia in humans and dogs. Vet Pathol 2001;38: 249–60.
16. Trammell RA, Brooks M, Cox L, et al. Fatal hemorrhagic diathesis associated with mild factor IX deficiency in pl/J mice. Comp Med 2006;56(5):426–34.
17. Tong C, Li P, Wu NL, et al. Production of p53 knockout rats by homologous recombination of embryonic stem cells. Nature 2010;467(7312):211–3.
18. Yang X, Tian XC, Dai Y, et al. Transgenic farm animals: applications in agriculture and biomedicine. Biotechnol Annu Rev 2000;5:269–92.
19. Lang MR, Gihr G, Gawaz MP, et al. Hemostasis in *Danio rerio*: is the zebra fish a useful model for platelet research? J Thromb Haemost 2010;8:1159–69.
20. Boudreaux MK, Schmutz SM, French PS. Calcium diacylglycerol guanine nucleotide exchange factor I (CalDAG-GEFI) gene mutations in a thrombopathic Simmental calf. Vet Pathol 2007;44(6):932–5.
21. Boudreaux MK, Catalfamo JL, Klok M. Calcium-diacylglycerol guanine nucleotide exchange factor I gene mutations associated with loss of function in canine platelets. Transl Res 2007;150(2):81–92.
22. Crittenden JR, Bergmeier W, Zhang Y, et al. CalDAG-GEFI integrates signaling for platelet aggregation and thrombus formation. Nat Med 2004;10(9):982–6.
23. Hoffman M, Monroe D. A cell-based model of hemostasis. Thromb Haemost 2001;85(6):958–65.
24. Satta N, Toti F, Fressinaud E, et al. Scott syndrome: an inherited defect of the procoagulant activity of platelets. Platelets 1997;8(2–3):117–24.
25. Brooks MB, Catalfamo JL, Brown HA, et al. A hereditary bleeding disorder of dogs caused by a lack of platelet procoagulant activity. Blood 2002;99(7):2434–41.
26. Falati S, Liu Q, Gross P, et al. Accumulation of tissue factor into developing thrombi in vivo is dependent upon microparticle P-selectin glycoprotein ligand 1 and platelet P-selectin. J Exp Med 2003;197(11):1585–98.
27. Boudreaux MK. Characteristics, diagnosis, and treatment of inherited platelet disorders in mammals. JAMA 2008;233(8):1251–9.
28. Shiraishi M, Ogawa H, Ikeda M, et al. Platelet dysfunction in Chediak-Higashi syndrome-affected cattle. J Vet Med Sci 2002;64(9):751–60.
29. Cifuni SM, Wagner DD, Bergmeier W. CalDAG-GEFI and protein kinase C represent alternative pathways leading to activation of integrin alphaIIbbeta3 in platelets. Blood 2008;112(5):1696–703.
30. Malinin NL, Zhang L, Choi J, et al. A point mutation in KINDLIN3 ablates activation of three integrin subfamilies in humans. Nat Med 2009;15(3):313–8.
31. Boudreaux MK, Wardrop KJ, Kiklevich V, et al. A mutation in the canine Kindlin-3 gene associated with increased bleeding risk and susceptibility to infections. Thromb Haemost 2010;103(2):475–7.
32. Toomey JR, Kratzer KE, Lasky NM, et al. Targeted disruption of the murine tissue factor gene results in embryonic lethality. Blood 1996;88(5):1583–7.
33. Rosen ED, Chan JC, Idusogie E, et al. Mice lacking factor VII develop normally but suffer fatal perinatal bleeding. Nature 1997;390(6657):290–4.
34. Perry DJ. Factor VII deficiency. Br J Haematol 2002;118(3):689–700.
35. Callan MB, Aljamali MN, Margaritis P, et al. A novel missense mutation responsible for factor VII deficiency in research Beagle colonies. J Thromb Haemost 2006;4(12):2616–22.
36. Soute BA, Ulrich MM, Watson AD, et al. Congenital deficiency of all vitamin K-dependent blood coagulation factors due to a defective vitamin K-dependent carboxylase in Devon rex cats. Thromb Haemost 1992;68(5):521–5.

37. Johnson JS, Soute BA, Olver CS, et al. Defective gamma-glutamyl carboxylase activity and bleeding in Rambouillet sheep. Vet Pathol 2006;43(5):726–32.
38. Satta N, Toti F, Feugeas O, et al. Monocyte vesiculation is a possible mechanism for dissemination of membrane-associated procoagulant activities and adhesion molecules after stimulation by lipopolysaccharide. J Immunol 1994;153(7):3245–55.
39. Piccin A, Murphy WG, Smith OP. Circulating microparticles: pathophysiology and clinical implications. Blood Rev 2006;21:157–71.
40. Ponczek MB, Gailani D, Doolittle RF. Evolution of the contact phase of vertebrate blood coagulation. J Thromb Haemost 2008;6(11):1876–83.
41. Kier AB, Bresnahan FJ, White FJ, et al. The inheritance pattern of factor XII (Hageman) deficiency in domestic cats. Can J Comp Med 1980;44:309–14.
42. Renne T, Pozgajova M, Gruner S, et al. Defective thrombus formation in mice lacking coagulation factor XII. J Exp Med 2005;202(2):271–81.
43. Segers O, Castoldi E. Factor V Leiden and activated protein C resistance. Adv Clin Chem 2009;49:121–57.
44. Ganter MT, Hofer CK. Coagulation monitoring: current techniques and clinical use of viscoelastic point-of-care coagulation devices. Anesth Analg 2008;106(5): 1366–75.
45. Luddington RJ. Thrombelastography/thromboelastometry. Clin Lab Haematol 2005;27(2):81–90.
46. Rivard GE, Brummel-Ziedins KE, Mann KG, et al. Evaluation of the profile of thrombin generation during the process of whole blood clotting as assessed by thrombelastography. J Thromb Haemost 2005;3(9):2039–43.
47. Camenzind V, Bombeli T, Seifert B, et al. Citrate storage affects Thrombelastograph analysis. Anesthesiology 2000;92(5):1242–9.
48. Johansson PI, Bochsen L, Andersen S, et al. Investigation of the effect of kaolin and tissue factor-activated citrated whole blood, on clot forming variables, as evaluated by thromboelastography. Transfusion 2008;48(11):2377–83.
49. Thalheimer U, Triantos CK, Samonakis DN, et al. A comparison of kaolin-activated versus nonkaolin-activated thromboelastography in native and citrated blood. Blood Coagul Fibrinolysis 2008;19(6):495–501.
50. Nielsen VG, Steenwyk BL, Gurley WQ, et al. Argatroban, bivalirudin, and lepirudin do not decrease clot propagation and strength as effectively as heparin-activated antithrombin in vitro. J Heart Lung Transplant 2006;25(6):653–63.
51. Sorensen B, Ingerslev J. Whole blood clot formation phenotypes in hemophilia A and rare coagulation disorders. Patterns of response to recombinant factor VIIa. J Thromb Haemost 2004;2(1):102–10.
52. Nielsen VG. Corn trypsin inhibitor decreases tissue-type plasminogen activator-mediated fibrinolysis of human plasma. Blood Coagul Fibrinolysis 2009;20(3):191–6.
53. Hobson AR, Agarwala RA, Swallow RA, et al. Thrombelastography: current clinical applications and its potential role in interventional cardiology. Platelets 2006; 17(8):509–18.
54. Otto CM, Rieser TM, Brooks MB, et al. Evidence of hypercoagulability in dogs with parvoviral enteritis. J Am Vet Med Assoc 2000;217(10):1500–4.
55. Wiinberg B, Jensen AL, Johansson PI, et al. Thromboelastographic evaluation of hemostatic function in dogs with disseminated intravascular coagulation. J Vet Intern Med 2008;22(2):357–65.
56. Siller-Matula JM, Plasenzotti R, Spiel A, et al. Interspecies differences in coagulation profile. Thromb Haemost 2008;100(3):397–404.
57. Baglin T. The measurement and application of thrombin generation. Br J Haematol 2005;130(5):653–61.

58. Hemker HC, Al Dieri R, De Smedt E, et al. Thrombin generation, a function test of the haemostatic-thrombotic system. Thromb Haemost 2006;96(5):553–61.
59. Chantarangkul V, Clerici M, Bressi C, et al. Standardization of the endogenous thrombin potential measurement: how to minimize the effect of residual platelets in stored plasma. Br J Haematol 2004;124(3):355–7.
60. Berckmans RJ, Neiuwland R, Boing AN, et al. Cell-derived microparticles circulate in healthy humans and support low grade thrombin generation. Thromb Haemost 2001;85(4):639–46.
61. Lippi G, Salvagno GL, Montagnana M, et al. Reliability of the thrombin-generation assay in frozen-thawed platelet-rich plasma. Clin Chem 2006;52(9):1827–8.
62. van Veen JJ, Gatt A, Makris M. Thrombin generation testing in routine clinical practice: are we there yet? Br J Haematol 2008;142(6):889–903.
63. Chantarangkul V, Clerici M, Bressi C, et al. Thrombin generation assessed as endogenous thrombin potential in patients with hyper- or hypo-coagulability. Haematologica 2003;88(5):547–54.
64. Kimura A, Ikeo K, Nonaka M. Evolutionary origin of the vertebrate blood complement and coagulation systems inferred from liver EST analysis of lamprey. Dev Comp Immunol 2009;33(1):77–87.
65. Ault KA. The clinical utility of flow cytometry in the study of platelets. Semin Hematol 2001;38(2):160–8.
66. Schmitz G, Rothe G, Ruf A, et al. European Working Group on clinical cell analysis: consensus protocol for the flow cytometric characterisation of platelet function. Thromb Haemost 1998;79:885–96.
67. Cardigan R, Turner C, Harrison P. Current methods of assessing platelet function: relevance to transfusion medicine. Vox Sang 2005;88(3):153–63.
68. Favaloro EJ, Lippi G, Franchini M. Contemporary platelet function testing. Clin Chem Lab Med 2010;48(5):579–98.
69. Michelson AD, Barnard MR, Krueger LA, et al. Evaluation of platelet function by flow cytometry. Methods 2000;21(3):259–70.
70. Bode AP, Hickerson DH. Characterization and quantitation by flow cytometry of membranous microparticles formed during activation of platelet suspensions with ionophore or thrombin. Platelets 2000;11(5):259–71.
71. Kim HK, Song KS, Lee ES, et al. Optimized flow cytometric assay for the measurement of platelet microparticles in plasma: pre-analytic and analytic considerations. Blood Coagul Fibrinolysis 2002;13(5):393–7.
72. Macey M, McCarthy D, Azam U, et al. Ethylenediaminetetraacetic acid plus citrate-theophylline-adenosine-dipyridamole (EDTA-CTAD): a novel anticoagulant for the flow cytometric assessment of platelet and neutrophil activation ex vivo in whole blood. Cytometry B Clin Cytom 2003;51(1):30–40.
73. Hu H, Daleskog M, Li N. Influences of fixatives on flow cytometric measurements of platelet P-selectin expression and fibrinogen binding. Thromb Res 2000; 100(3):161–6.
74. Ritchie JL, Alexander HD, Rea IM. Flow cytometry analysis of platelet P-selectin expression in whole blood–methodological considerations. Clin Lab Haematol 2000;22(6):359–63.
75. Derian CK, Santulli RJ, Tomko KA, et al. Species differences in platelet responses to thrombin and SFLLRN. Receptor-mediated calcium mobilization and aggregation, and regulation by protein kinases. Thromb Res 1995;78(6):505–19.
76. Nylander S, Mattsson C, Lindahl TL. Characterisation of species differences in the platelet ADP and thrombin response. Thromb Res 2006;117(5):543–9.

# Preclinical Safety Assessment: Current Gaps, Challenges, and Approaches in Identifying Translatable Biomarkers of Drug-Induced Liver Injury

Shashi K. Ramaiah, DVM, PhD

KEYWORDS

- Biomarkers • Liver • Preclinical • Translatable
- Laboratory animal

Before new chemical or biopharmaceutical entities enter human clinical trials, they need to be tested preclinically in animal species, such as rats and nonrodents (dogs or nonhuman primates), to establish a robust therapeutic index, so that only the safest compounds progress to the clinic. During preclinical safety evaluation, efforts are directed at characterizing the toxic effects of a therapeutic agent with respect to underlying mechanisms of toxicity, target organs, dose dependence, exposure relationships, and when appropriate, reversibility. In addition to toxicologists, veterinary clinical pathologists are involved in discovery, optimization, and drug candidate evaluation. During these stages of drug development, veterinary clinical pathologists engage in biomarker development and evaluation of new technologies in addition to providing clinical pathology services and laboratory management to effectively build assays to address critical biomarker gaps.

---

Disclosures: There are no conflicts of interest, although the author is an employee of Pfizer.
Disclaimer: The views expressed in this article by the author may not be understood or quoted as being made on behalf of or reflecting the position of Pfizer, the US Food and Drug Administration, European Medicines Agency, the Predictive Safety Testing Consortium, and the Innovative Medicine Initiative and its membership companies.
Pfizer-Biotherapeutics Research Division, Drug Safety Research and Development, 35 Cambridge Park Drive, Cambridge, MA 02140, USA
*E-mail address:* shashi.ramaiah@pfizer.com

Clin Lab Med 31 (2011) 161–172
doi:10.1016/j.cll.2010.10.004
0272-2712/11/$ – see front matter © 2011 Elsevier Inc. All rights reserved.

During preclinical assessment, the liver is one of the more common target organs for toxicity, which can manifest as acute liver injury and is often noted at moderate to high doses of the therapeutic agent. Toxicity is often the result of off-target or chemical class (chemotype)-driven mechanisms. Such toxicities are usually predictable and exhibit a dose-response relationship, manifest in a shorter period, and are referred to as predictive drug-induced liver injury (DILI). Compounds that have a robust therapeutic index or wide safety margin for predictive DILI usually progress in drug development to eventual human dosing.

In contrast to predictive DILI, some compounds cause hepatic injury that cannot be detected or that is missed preclinically. The toxic effects typically lack clear dose-response relationships (although not always) and manifest clinically in only a small number of patients at readily achievable doses. This type of injury is commonly referred to as idiosyncratic DILI.[1,2] There are many examples of compounds that initially failed to elicit clear preclinical signals of hepatic toxicity but subsequently failed clinical trials or raised concerns postmarketing.[3,4] Idiosyncratic DILI can lead to program termination, to regulatory action with postmarket warnings, to withdrawal of the drug from the market (eg, troglitazone, benoxaprofen, bromfenac, ticrynafen), or can require a black-box designation be added to the label (eg, tolcapone, trovafloxacin, felbamate, isoniazid, telithromycin). The mechanisms underlying DILI are largely unknown but are thought to be multifactorial and include genetics, cytochrome P450 polymorphisms, lack of adaptation, age, gender, nutrition, drug-drug interactions, and immune-mediated responses.[3,5–8] Of all these mechanisms, compelling evidence exists for an immune-mediated/hapten hypothesis for idiosyncratic DILI, although definitive evidence is still lacking.[5–8]

The goal of this review is to summarize the available hepatic biomarkers and identify the important gaps related to detection of both predictive and idiosyncratic DILI in laboratory animals with translational relevance to human toxicity. In addition, ongoing research within the field of hepatic biomarkers to identify novel hepatic signals is discussed. Because the focus is on translatable biomarkers, available preclinical models or mechanisms related to DILI are not discussed; however, readers are encouraged to refer to other review articles in this area.[5–11]

## ATTRIBUTES OF A PERFECT HEPATIC BIOMARKER

The definition of an ideal hepatic biomarker may differ somewhat between the preclinical context of predictive liver injury and the clinical context of idiosyncratic liver injury. It is particularly challenging and almost impossible to define an idiosyncratic hepatic biomarker preclinically because the precise mechanisms for idiosyncratic DILI are not completely understood. With this caveat, it is important to have a biomarker that can accurately predict liver injury, even though the mechanisms for liver injury may be different between humans and preclinical species. It is equally important for hepatic biomarkers to track the underlying mechanisms of liver injury. Because an immune-mediated mechanism of liver injury seems to be the widely accepted hypothesis for causation of idiosyncratic DILI, a biomarker that can detect hapten-mediated adverse events before the occurrence of liver injury would be valuable. The ideal clinical biomarker would also differentiate between DILI and other causes of liver disease, such as alcoholism, herbal supplements, drug-drug interactions. For example, it is not clear whether the increase in alanine aminotransferase (ALT) activity noted clinically is caused by DILI or nonhepatic causes. The ideal biomarker should track the degree or severity of hepatic injury and also the restoration of normal liver function. In addition, the ideal hepatic biomarker would predict the ultimate outcome of injury; whether the patient will adapt and recover or progressively worsen, leading to hepatic failure.

## CURRENT STATUS OF SERUM BIOMARKERS TO ASSESS LIVER DAMAGE

Traditional serum biochemical parameters of hepatic injury, such as leakage enzymes that spill from damaged hepatocytes, are routinely assayed in preclinical and clinical situations to signal or monitor DILI.[12–17] The serum leakage enzymes that are widely used in both preclinical and clinical situations include ALT and aspartate aminotransferase (AST).[12,15,16] Other leakage enzymes that are variably used include sorbitol dehydrogenase and glutamate dehydrogenase (GLDH).[16,17] Generally, the degree of increase in serum enzyme activity depends on the severity and extent of hepatic injury. In contrast, alkaline phosphatase and γ-glutamyltransferase (γ-glutamyl peptidase) are parameters of cholestatic induction, and serum activities increase with biliary or hepatobiliary changes. 5′-Nucleotidase is another cholestatic-induction enzyme, the level of which is occasionally measured preclinically.[16,17] Cholestatic enzymes are not discussed further in this review because cholestasis does not usually contribute to the occurrence of DILI.[1,2,13]

Preclinically, ALT is well accepted as a highly sensitive biomarker for the detection of liver injury. In routine preclinical safety studies, ALT in combination with AST and GLDH are used to confirm hepatocellular injury, and serum activities often correlate with the severity of histopathologic findings.[12,14–17] Neither serum ALT activity nor bilirubin concentration accurately reflect hepatic function in animals; in fact, serum bilirubin level is usually only evaluated in the context of cholestasis.[16] Despite this, serum ALT level elevations in combination with total bilirubin level elevations are well-accepted specific predictors of severe DILI in human clinical medicine.[2,3] Although increases in serum ALT activity correlate with hepatic injury in most cases, serum total bilirubin concentration represents the functional capacity of the human liver. This important finding is based on the original work of Hy Zimmerman,[2] who initially noted that patients with concurrent marked elevations in serum ALT and total bilirubin levels had at least a 10% chance of mortality from liver failure. In clinical trials, "Hy's Law cases" are defined as subjects who have serum ALT concentration more than 3 times the upper limit of normal and serum total bilirubin concentration more than 2 times the upper limit of normal, with mostly hepatocellular alterations, who lack a concurrent disease such as viral hepatitis, and who are not on medications.[1–3] It should be noted that Hy's Law is not applicable to preclinical species because there is no validated sensitive marker of hepatic function. A schematic outlining the current state of hepatic biomarkers and the advantage of bringing forward newer biomarkers is depicted in **Fig. 1**.

## CURRENT GAPS IN THE ABILITY OF ALT TO ACCURATELY DETECT HEPATIC INJURY

Although there is consensus on the pitfalls of ALT and other serum transaminases for identifying hepatic injury, ALT remains the most commonly used biomarker of DILI by default. Although ALT is a highly sensitive biomarker of liver injury, limitations and gaps exist regarding its ability to accurately predict acute liver injury (see **Fig. 1**). First, there are concerns about specificity. It is known that serum ALT activity can increase in the absence of hepatocyte necrosis, such as in metabolic disorders (eg, type 1 diabetes) and nonalcoholic fatty liver disease, or as a result of skeletal muscle disorders.[13,15] Furthermore, in some instances, serum ALT levels are not elevated despite the presence of liver injury because of inhibitory factors (eg, vitamin B12 cofactor deficiency) that can affect the measurement of serum ALT activity.[16] Second, ALT is most useful for signaling predictable types of hepatic injury and is not known to forecast the occurrence of or determine the susceptibility to idiosyncratic DILI. Serum ALT level is usually elevated after an injury or after the pathogenesis of injury is initiated and thus is not seen as a predictor of DILI. Third, ALT alone does not detect hepatic function, although

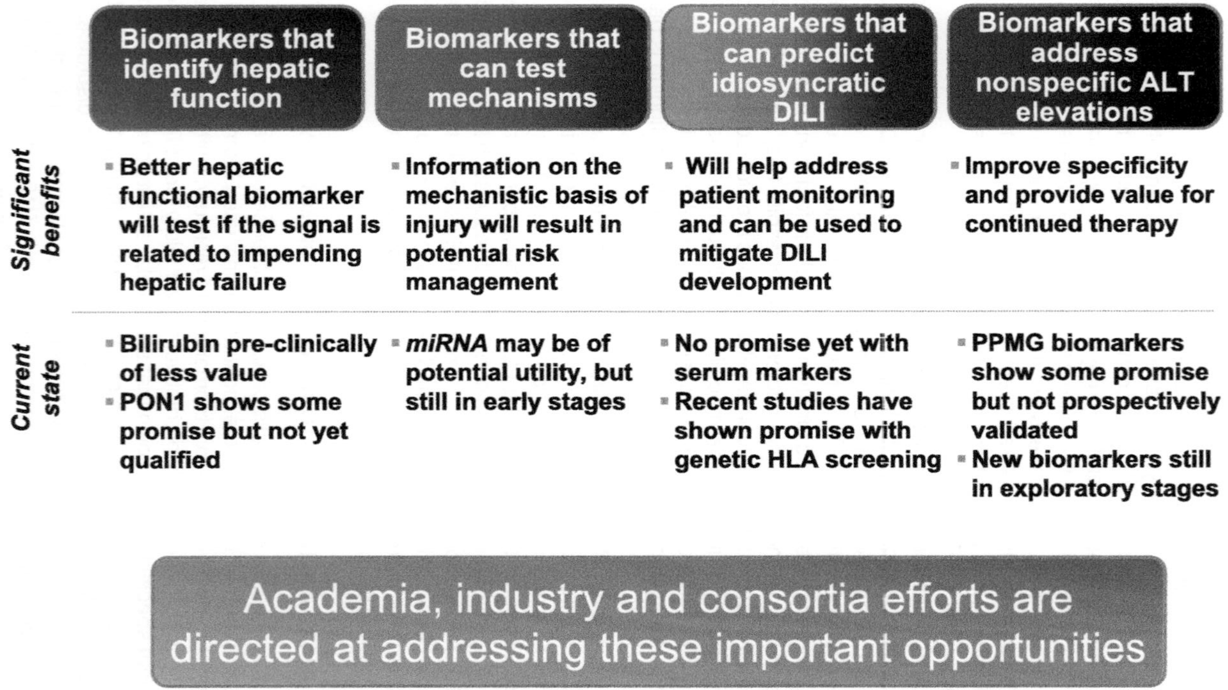

**Fig. 1.** The current status of biomarkers and the benefits of new biomarkers in addressing the limitations and gaps in ALT, a conventional biomarker used to identify DILI. The ultimate goal is the generation of biomarkers superior to those used currently, which can be applied to both preclinical and clinical samples. miRNA, microRNA; PON1, paraoxonase 1; PPMG, paraoxonase 1, purine-nucleoside phosphorylase, malate dehydrogenase, and glutamate dehydrogenase.

it is used in combination with serum total bilirubin concentration to assess hepatic function clinically. In spite of these issues, ALT is routinely used by regulatory agencies to assess patient safety in clinical trials. Thus, it is clear that additional biomarkers are needed to address these important gaps (see **Fig. 1**).

## ONGOING RESEARCH ON HEPATIC BIOMARKERS TO ADDRESS GAPS IN ALT

Serum biomarker candidates to fill gaps in the utility of ALT are tested within the Predictive Safety Testing Consortium (PSTC), Severe Adverse Event Consortium, Drug-Induced Liver Injury Network, and Innovative Medicine Initiative. These efforts focus on different platform approaches, use varying experimental designs, and are being tested in both preclinical and clinical situations. For example, serum enzyme markers such as purine-nucleoside phosphorylase (PNP), paraoxonase (PON) 1, and malate dehydrogenase (MDH) are being tested preclinically through the PSTC.[14,18] In addition, other novel biomarkers (see later discussion) continue to be explored and have been reported in the literature. In spite of these efforts, none of the emerging novel biomarkers have been thoroughly validated in prospective studies. A major challenge to validating novel biomarkers that could potentially address the issue of ALT specificity involves their testing in preclinical and clinical settings. In addition, there is a clear lack of annotation of clinical samples available to test the validity of these biomarkers. Finally, assay technology, reagents, and platform capability may be the limiting factors for high throughput testing of novel hepatic biomarkers.

PNP, PON1, and MDH were initially discovered during exploratory work to identify serum biomarkers whose signals were altered following the administration of mechanistically dissimilar and chemically diverse hepatotoxicants such as acetaminophen, α-naphthylisocyanate, phenobarbital, and WY-14632.[19] Alterations in differential protein expression signatures in both liver and serum were identified by proteomic analysis. From this study, approximately 19 proteins were found to be significantly altered and strongly associated with hepatotoxicity, including PON1, PNP, and MDH. To prioritize the list of hepatic biomarkers, the investigators defined criteria such as alterations in these proteins should occur at the earliest time point before hepatic injury and the origin of the biomarker comes mainly from the liver. To ensure clinical translatability, the investigators also confirmed expression of these biomarkers in both rat and human liver samples.[19]

Similar to ALT, PNP and MDH are leakage enzymes whose serum activities increase during hepatic injury, whereas PON1 is considered to be indicative of liver function because its levels decrease considerably after liver injury.[12] PON1 is a high-density lipoprotein-1-esterase secreted by the liver and involved in organophosphate detoxification; it protects low-density lipoproteins from oxidative modification. All the 3 enzymes are found mostly within hepatocytes, although small quantities are present in the cytoplasm of endothelial cells and Kupffer cells.[12] There also are differences in the regiospecific location of these enzymes within the liver. For example, MDH is a periportal enzyme located within the cytoplasm and mitochondria and released into the serum following tissue injury.[14,17,19]

Since their discovery, 2 clinical studies have shown alterations in the serum activities of these enzymes following treatment with hepatotoxicants.[20,21] These studies have shown that PNP may also be a biomarker of nonparenchymal hepatic injury. Clearly, this new set of biomarkers has the potential to increase confidence in the detection of true hepatic injury caused by drugs. Whether these analytes improve specificity concerns related to ALT and can detect decreased hepatic function still need to be addressed, as does their ability to assess DILI. Comprehensive analysis of data and prospective use of these analytes should shed more light on their potential to help fill existing gaps in hepatic biomarkers.

## CAN ALT ISOZYMES IMPROVE ALT SPECIFICITY?
### ALT Isozymes in Normal Liver

Liver is the primary source of increased serum ALT levels during hepatic injury because hepatic tissue contains greater amounts of the enzyme compared with other tissues, on a per gram basis. Other tissues that also contain substantial amounts of ALT in rats, dogs, and humans include skeletal muscle and those of heart, fat, and intestines.[17,22,23] Because ALT plays a critical role in carbohydrate and amino acid metabolism and is distributed in multiple tissues, significant but mild elevations of serum ALT levels resulting from enzyme induction can be detected in the absence of liver injury in rats during gluconeogenesis, with diabetes, or after administration of corticosteroids.[15,17,23] Such mild elevations in ALT levels in the absence of hepatic injury have historically been noted and are usually associated with nonnecrotic events or background hepatocyte turnover; however, prodromal hepatic injury or ALT originating from nonhepatic tissues remains a possibility.

To evaluate subtle increases in ALT levels in the absence of hepatic injury, investigations have focused on ALT isozymes (ALT1 and ALT2) in rats in which hepatocytes contain soluble cytosolic and mitochondrial forms of the enzyme.[23] The investigators reported differential expression of ALT isozymes within tissues and subcellular compartments, with ALT2 likely localized to mitochondria and ALT1 to the cytosolic fraction of hepatocytes.[23] Therefore, the measurement of ALT isozymes could potentially differentiate between hepatic injury and hepatic induction/adaptation events such as mitochondrial gluconeogenesis. Because ALT2 is present within mitochondria and is known to play a role in gluconeogenesis, mild elevations in serum ALT2 (and thus total ALT) activity due to mitochondrial gluconeogenesis would be expected. Much like total serum ALT, both isozymes seem to catalyze similar processes and function similarly in amino acid metabolism and gluconeogenesis. To confirm this finding, the biochemical activities of ALT1 and ALT2 in rat samples were measured using D-cycloserine, which differentially inhibits the 2 isozymes. By using recombinant rat ALT1 and ALT2 proteins as standards, serum isozyme activities could be calculated. The results suggested there was higher ALT1 than ALT2 activity in rat liver.[17,23] Human hepatocytes similarly contain both ALT1 and ALT2, although investigators detected only a weak ALT2 signal by immunohistochemical staining.[22] In this study, more ALT2 protein, as measured by immunohistochemistry and Western blot analysis, was detected within human cardiac and skeletal muscles than in the liver and none was found in kidney. These data formed the basis for the hypothesis that increased serum ALT2 activity could be attributed to nonhepatic events such as skeletal muscle damage in humans.[22] This hypothesis differed from that of Yang and colleagues,[23] who suggested that ALT2 level elevation in the serum of rats was caused by hepatic induction events originating from the mitochondria rather than from nonhepatic tissue such as skeletal muscle.[23] It is unclear whether discrepancies in ALT2 isozyme localization in the rat and human liver are due to species differences or other factors such as reagent specificity or analytical methodology. In either case, the value of ALT isozyme measurements in addressing the issue of specificity is still considered to be of high value.

### Levels of ALT Isozyme Elevations With and Without Hepatic Injury

Using experimental hepatotoxicants, such as acetaminophen and carbon tetrachloride, in mice and rats, it has been shown that serum levels of ALT1 and ALT2 isozymes are elevated with hepatic injury as measured by cyclosporine-induced inhibition of enzymatic activity and Western blot analysis.[17,23] Further, in rats, the elevation in serum ALT1 isozyme activity was significantly higher than that of ALT2. In these studies, the results of activity-based assays for ALT1 and ALT2 seemed to correlate well with protein levels. In addition to classic hepatotoxicants, ALT isozyme levels have also been tested in hepatic adaptation models involving metabolic processes such as gluconeogenesis. To examine this statement, mice were treated with 25 to 75 mg/kg of dexamethasone for 1 to 3 days. Glycogen accumulation was shown to induce gluconeogenesis without associated histologic evidence of hepatic injury.[24] In treated mice, total liver and serum ALT activities were significantly elevated compared with the control group, and elevation was mostly noted for ALT2 in both the liver and blood. Similarly, using a mouse model of methionine and choline deficiency–induced nonalcoholic fatty liver disease, elevations in both ALT1 and ALT2 isozyme activities were observed.[17] Interestingly, no significant necrosis was noted by histopathologic examination in this model, rather mostly steatosis was observed, suggesting that the elevation of ALT isozyme levels may not be solely due to hepatic injury.

## NUCLEIC ACID BIOMARKERS

There has been significant interest in circulating messenger RNA (mRNA) and micro-RNA (miRNA) as clinical biomarkers for several diseases.[25–28] The advantages to using this genomic biomarker platform include (1) the high sensitivity of these assays, because they use polymerase chain reaction (PCR)-based amplification technology and eliminate the challenges associated with protein-based biomarkers, such as post-translational modifications or lack of suitable antibodies or reagents; (2) easier trans-latability than protein-based biomarkers, because the mRNA/miRNA gene signatures related to hepatotoxic events may be similar across species; and (3) the ability to establish the mechanistic basis of the hepatic injury, because changes at the molecular level could reflect pathway alterations leading to toxicity.

A recent study demonstrated the potential of circulating miRNA as biomarkers of DILI in an acetaminophen-dosed mouse model.[27] In this study, the investigators identified differential miRNA expression profiles in both liver tissue and plasma of controls and acetaminophen-overdosed mice. Levels of miRNAs that were found to decrease in the liver were increased in the plasma of treated mice. For example, levels of miR-122 and miR-192 were elevated in plasma, whereas they were decreased in the liver. In contrast, levels of miR-710 and miR-711 were increased in liver but decreased in plasma. Both miR-122 and miR-192 showed dose- and time-dependent changes in plasma that were consistent with changes in serum ALT and histologic evidence of hepatic injury, suggesting the utility of miRNAs as sensitive and specific biomarkers of liver injury.[27]

Recently, the role of liver-specific mRNA was investigated in rats treated with hepa-totoxic doses of galactosamine and acetaminophen.[28] Serum mRNA analysis performed using quantitative PCR suggested that liver-specific mRNA levels were significantly increased in serum at doses that did not cause changes in liver histopa-thology or in serum activities of hepatocellular serum leakage enzymes such as ALT and AST. The increased concentrations of liver-specific mRNA for haptoglobin, albumin, and fibrinogen polypeptides were noted much earlier and at lower doses of hepatotoxicants compared with the increase in activity of serum transaminases or the histologic evidence of liver damage. In addition, increased concentrations of mRNA in serum were both dose and time dependent. Although these mRNAs may be more sensitive and specific biomarkers than ALT, their true utility may be, as the investigators suggest, is in identifying mechanisms of liver injury based on their specific signature profiles within serum.[29] In addition, these markers may be useful tools both in preclinical studies and in clinical situations to identify whether a drug has the potential to induce DILI.

## MISCELLANEOUS HEPATIC BIOMARKERS
### Arginase 1

Arginase type 1 is a purportedly liver-specific hydrolase that catalyzes arginine catabolism to urea and ornithine and has been tested as a candidate biomarker for liver injury in a thioacetamide model of hepatotoxicity in rats.[29] In this study, significant increases in serum arginase 1 activity relative to serum ALT and AST activities correlated well with histopathologic findings. In addition, elevations in arginase I activity occurred much earlier than the histologic manifestation of hepatic damage. Similarly, evaluation of arginase 1 in studies with human liver grafts found the enzyme to be a more specific indicator of liver function than other serum markers.[30] In this liver transplant model, normalization of serum arginase 1 activity occurred much earlier than that of other enzymes.

### Glutathione-S-Transferase α

Glutathione-S-transferases (GSTs) are members of the family of phase II detoxification enzymes that catalyze the conjugation of glutathione to reactive metabolites during phase I of the metabolism. Compounds that themselves are reactive or that can generate reactive metabolites have the potential to induce GST synthesis, exemplifying a protective mechanism in response to administration of drugs and other xenobiotics. GSTα is 1 of the 4 GST isozymes (together with GST φ, μ, and θ) that are expressed in humans and other mammals. Based on GSTα expression in human hepatocytes (approximately 5% of total soluble protein), this enzyme has been tested for its utility as a hepatic biomarker in humans and rats.[31] Because GSTα is generated in response to oxidative stress in vivo, it is mainly expressed within the centrilobular zone of the hepatic parenchyma. Consequently, GSTα concentration is significantly increased when there is damage to the centrilobular area caused by toxicants such as thioacetamide and bromobenzene.[31] In rats dosed with either of these toxicants, significant elevations of GSTα concentration compared with serum ALT and AST were detected and correlated well with histologic findings. GSTα also seems to be translatable clinically based on a study of 9 patients with self-administered acetaminophen overdose, in whom significant elevations were observed in comparison to serum ALT, and there was a strong correlation with histologic findings.[32]

Other hepatic biomarkers reported in the literature include high mobility group box 1,[8] osteopontin,[33] serum F protein or hydroxyphenylpyruvate dioxygenase,[12] and cytochrome c.[34] These biomarkers are not discussed because there are limited data in the context of DILI, and as biomarkers, they seem to have limited advantages over currently available serum transaminases.

## APPROACHES AND CHALLENGES IN DISCOVERING TRANSLATABLE BIOMARKERS TO IDENTIFY IDIOSYNCRATIC HEPATOTOXICITY SIGNALS

It is clear from the list of biomarkers discussed in this article that there are no prodromal biomarkers of DILI. The presently used traditional serum aminotransferase enzymes detect injury only after it has occurred, and in the author's opinion, these enzymes cannot detect potential idiosyncratic signals. Thus, it is critical to understand whether there are biomarkers that can determine why only select patients develop DILI and whether the injury is caused by sluggish adaptive mechanisms or unknown processes that render the patients tolerant. Are there preclinical species that are more susceptible to DILI than others and if so what are the underlying mechanisms? These are important questions that will need to be addressed in the context of translatable animal models.

Clearly, the biomarkers used to date in preclinical toxicity studies have neither been able to detect clinically observable idiosyncratic hepatotoxicity nor seem to show promise. It remains to be seen whether newer approaches to translatable biomarker discovery can identify idiosyncratic toxicities that are not detected using standard toxicity-testing protocols. It is possible that idiosyncratic signatures are being missed during preclinical studies. It is also likely that rodents do in fact manifest changes in measured biomarkers but quickly adapt, resulting in lack of histopathologic and clinical pathologic abnormalities at terminal end points. The identification of biomarkers unique to human idiosyncratic signals and not anchored to histopathologic and clinicopathologic changes is critical to recognize idiosyncratic DILI preclinically. These biomarkers may include nucleic acids (miRNA/mRNA), proteins, and metabolites detectable either in blood or urine and require new experimental designs and application of hepatic injury and adaptation/regeneration end points in a temporal fashion. The selection of compound, dose, and experimental design could prove challenging because to identify the correct dosage preclinically, it is necessary to select end points for the assessment of idiosyncratic hepatotoxicity, in which by definition, clinical signs and histopathologic end points are not observed. Additional challenges include the need for extensive biomarker assay validation and altered study designs to select the appropriate samples and time points for biomarker analysis and performance, because biomarker response needs to be robust and translatable (**Fig. 2**).

Method validation for a hepatic biomarker assay is challenging and includes determining sensitivity, specificity, accuracy, and precision. Assay validation should be

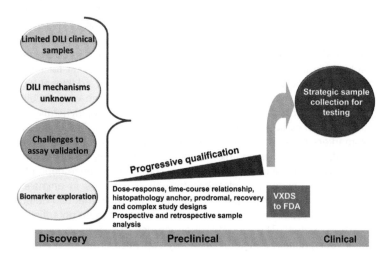

**Fig. 2.** Challenges in discovery, validation, and qualification of translatable biomarkers of DILI. The 4 main challenges are indicated on the left. Progressive qualification depends on the amount of biomarker data needed for decision making within preclinical or clinical applications. The rigor for biomarker qualification of analytes that can predict DILI is much higher and may include longer study designs, multiple time points, and recovery group assessments. FDA, Food and Drug Administration; VXDS, voluntary exploratory data submission.

differentiated from biomarker qualification, which is an evidentiary rolling process of linking a specific biomarker to a phenotypic end point such as a disease or histologic correlate. The level of assay validation depends on the stage of drug development and thus "fit for purpose." In other words, significantly less time and resources are allocated to assay validation during biomarker discovery and early preclinical drug development than during a regulatory toxicology study or clinical trial or before acceptance by regulatory authorities (see **Fig. 2**). To this end, there is guidance by regulatory agencies to effectively and proactively apply predictive and clinically translatable biomarkers during drug development.[18] Clearly, if such biomarkers are discovered, their use and interpretation in the context of drug toxicity early in drug discovery and development will enhance the "speed" to market of safer drugs and will also enable earlier attrition of compounds. A biomarker qualification process that has been initiated by the US Food and Drug Administration (FDA) encourages the voluntary submission to regulatory authorities of contextual applications of new biomarkers by academia, industry, and consortia.[18] This is successfully exemplified by the recent submission of data on novel renal biomarkers by the Critical Path Institute PSTC to the European Medicines Agency and the FDA, which resulted in the approval and acceptance of these novel biomarkers during preclinical drug development.[35] Thus, biomarkers showing promise toward addressing the current gaps in accurately predicting DILI in exploratory studies will potentially have a forward path for regulatory approval and routine testing in preclinical toxicity studies and clinical trials.

## SUMMARY

Idiosyncratic DILI is a leading cause for the withdrawal of marketed drugs in the United States and the failure of investigational drugs in clinical trials. It is not clear whether elevations of serum ALT levels detected clinically are due to impending DILI or are nonspecific signals resulting from hepatic ALT induction or adaptive mechanisms or originating from nonhepatic sources such as skeletal muscle. Although research efforts to address these concerns have shown some promise, there is at present no single biomarker that can effectively address this gap in ALT utility. Existing preclinical testing models are also poor at detecting idiosyncratic hepatotoxicants. At present, ALT is considered the reference marker of predictive DILI, and in combination with serum total bilirubin (in humans), ALT is also the reference marker for idiosyncratic DILI. Although ALT is a sensitive biomarker of intrinsic DILI, additional biomarkers are needed to add value and enhance specificity. New serum enzyme biomarkers are being qualified to improve detection of both predictive and idiosyncratic DILI. Additional strategies under evaluation that could add specificity to ALT include assessment of novel biomarkers generated mostly by hypothesis-driven discovery approaches. New experimental approaches and biomarker assay platforms are needed to identify compounds in preclinical animal models; these compounds cause hepatotoxicity in humans even when changes in classical toxicity end points in animals are not observed. It is also equally important to generate biomarkers that can detect underlying mechanisms of liver injury so that such mechanisms can be potentially avoided during drug development. This would reduce the risk of liver injury caused by new drugs under investigation in clinical trials and by approved drugs on the market.

## REFERENCES

1. Abboud G, Kaplowitz N. Drug-induced liver injury. Drug Saf 2007;30(4):277–94.
2. Zimmerman HJ. Drug-induced liver disease. In: Schiff E, editor. Schiff's diseases of the liver. Baltimore (MD): Lippincott-Raven; 1999. p. 973–1064.

3. Senior JR. Monitoring for hepatotoxicity: what is the predictive value of liver "function" tests? Clin Pharmacol Ther 2009;85:331–4.
4. Watkins PB. Biomarkers for the diagnosis and management of drug-induced liver injury. Semin Liver Dis 2009;29:393–9.
5. Shenton JM, Chen J, Uetrecht JP. Animal models of idiosyncratic drug reactions. Chem Biol Interact 2004;150(1):53–70.
6. Uetrecht J. Immunoallergic drug-induced liver injury in humans. Semin Liver Dis 2009;29:383–92.
7. Uetrecht J. Idiosyncratic drug reactions: past, present and future. Chem Res Toxicol 2008;21:84–92.
8. Adams DH, Ju C, Ramaiah SK, et al. Mechanisms of immune mediated liver injury. Toxicol Sci 2010;115:307–21.
9. Boelsterli UA, Hsiao CJ. The heterozygous Sod2(+/−) mouse: modeling the mitochondrial role in drug toxicity. Drug Discov Today 2008;13(21–22):982–8.
10. Deng X, Stachlewitz RF, Liguori MJ, et al. Modest inflammation enhances diclofenac hepatotoxicity in rats: role of neutrophils and bacterial translocation. J Pharmacol Exp Ther 2006;319(3):1191–9.
11. Uetrecht JP. New concepts in immunology relevant to idiosyncratic drug reactions: the "danger hypothesis" and innate immune system. Chem Res Toxicol 1999;12(5):387–95.
12. Ozer J, Ratner M, Shaw M, et al. The current state of serum biomarkers of hepatotoxicity. Toxicology 2008;245(3):194–205.
13. Ozer J, Chetty R, Kenna G, et al. Enhancing the utility of alanine aminotransferase as a reference standard biomarker for drug-induced liver injury. Regul Toxicol Pharmacol 2009;56:237–46.
14. Ozer J, Chetty R, Kenna G, et al. Gaps for qualifying biomarker candidates of drug induced liver injury. Biomark Med 2010;4:475–83.
15. Amacher DE. Serum transaminase elevations as indicators of hepatic injury following the administration of drugs. Regul Toxicol Pharmacol 1998;27(2):119–30.
16. Ramaiah SK. A toxicologist guide to the diagnostic interpretation of hepatic biochemical parameters. Food Chem Toxicol 2007;45(9):1551–7.
17. Ozer JS, Reagan WJ, Schomaker S, et al. Translational biomarkers of acute drug-induced liver injury: the current state, gaps and future opportunities. In: Vaidya VS, Bonventre JV, editors. Biomarkers of medicine, drug discovery and environmental health. 1st edition. John Wiley & Sons, Inc; 2010. p. 203–27.
18. Goodsaid FM, Frueh FW, Mattes W. Strategic paths for biomarker qualification. Toxicology 2008;245:219–23.
19. Amacher DE, Adler R, Herath A, et al. Use of proteomic methods to identify serum biomarkers associated with rat liver toxicity or hypertrophy. Clin Chem 2005; 51(10):1796–803.
20. Ferre N, Camps J, Prats E, et al. Serum paraoxonase activity: a new additional test for the improved evaluation of chronic liver damage. Clin Chem 2002; 48(2):261–8.
21. Kawai M, Hosaki S. Clinical usefulness of malate dehydrogenase and its mitochondrial isoenzyme in comparison with aspartate aminotransferase and its mitochondrial isoenzyme in sera of patients with liver disease. Clin Biochem 1990; 23(4):327–34.
22. Lindblom P, Rafter I, Copley C, et al. Isoforms of alanine aminotransferases in human tissues and serum—differential tissue expression using novel antibodies. Arch Biochem Biophys 2007;466(1):66–77.

23. Yang RZ, Park S, Reagan WJ, et al. Alanine aminotransferase isoenzymes: molecular cloning and quantitative analysis of tissue expression in rats and serum elevation in liver toxicity. Hepatology 2009;49(2):598–607.

24. Reagan WJ, Park S, Goldstein R, et al. Hepatic ALT1 and 2 proteins are differentially regulated by dexamethazone treatment in mice. Society of Toxicology Meeting Abstract 2008.

25. Liu L, Zhong S, Yang R, et al. Expression, purification, and initial characterization of human alanine aminotransferase (ALT) isoenzyme 1 and 2 in high-five insect cells. Protein Expr Purif 2008;60(2):225–31.

26. Bala S, Marcos M, Szabo G. Emerging role of microRNAs in liver diseases. World J Gastroenterol 2010;15:5633–40.

27. Wang K, Zhang S, Marzolf B, et al. Circulating microRNAs, potential biomarkers for drug-induced liver injury. Proc Natl Acad Sci U S A 2009;106:4402–7.

28. Wetmore BA, Brees DJ, Singh R, et al. Quantitative analyses and transcriptomic profiling of circulating messenger RNAs as biomarkers of rat liver injury. Hepatology 2010;51:2127–39.

29. Murayama H, Ikemoto M, Fukuda Y, et al. Advantage of serum type-I arginase and ornithine carbamoyltransferase in the evaluation of acute and chronic liver damage induced by thioacetamide in rats. Clin Chim Acta 2007;375:63–8.

30. Ikemoto M, Tsunekawa S, Tanaka K, et al. Liver-type arginase in serum during and after liver transplantation: a novel index in monitoring conditions of the liver graft and its clinical significance. Clin Chim Acta 1998;271:11–23.

31. Giffen PS, Pick CR, Price MA, et al. Alpha-glutathione- S-transferase in the assessment of hepatotoxicity–its diagnostic utility in comparison with other recognized markers in the Wistar Han rat. Toxicol Pathol 2002;30:365–72.

32. Beckett GJ, Foster GR, Hussey AJ, et al. Plasma glutathione- S-transferase and F protein are more sensitive than alanine aminotransferase as markers of paracetamol (acetaminophen)-induced liver damage. Clin Chem 1989;35(11):2186–9.

33. Banerjee A, Burghardt RC, Johnson GA, et al. The temporal expression of osteopontin (SPP-1) in the rodent model of alcoholic steatohepatitis: a potential biomarker. Toxicol Pathol 2006;34(4):373–84.

34. Miller TJ, Knapton A, Adeyemo O, et al. Cytochrome c: a non invasive biomarker of drug-induced liver injury. J Appl Toxicol 2008;28:815–28.

35. Dieterle F, Sistare F, Goodsaid F, et al. Renal biomarker qualification submission: a dialog between the FDA-EMEA and Predictive Safety Testing Consortium. Nat Biotechnol 2010;28:455–62.

# Protecting Animal and Human Health and the Nation's Food Supply through Veterinary Diagnostic Laboratory Testing

Claire B. Andreasen, DVM, PhD

KEYWORDS
- Animal health • Veterinary laboratory
- US foreign animal disease • Zoonotic disease
- Clinical pathology laboratory

Veterinary clinical pathologists often have an emphasis on and expertise in diagnostic laboratory testing in the areas of hematology, clinical chemistry, and cytology; but laboratory testing also may require oversight in the areas of microbiology, parasitology, toxicology, and molecular diagnostics, to name a few. Because knowledge of various disciplines is needed for the investigation and integration of information to make a diagnosis and determine disease severity and effect, the veterinary clinical pathologist is a vital part of the animal health diagnostic team. Veterinary clinical (and anatomic) pathologists, as diagnosticians and researchers, have an important role in disease detection in animals that provide our food, by detecting diseases that are emerging and exotic to the United States, zoonotic diseases, and noninfectious conditions. Veterinary clinical pathologists also need knowledge of foreign animal diseases (FADs) to differentiate FADs from similar endemic diseases.[1,2] Many of the diseases foreign to the United States are endemic in other countries, and globalization, resulting in movement of human beings, animals, and animal products, can result in a disease incursion and establishment in the United States, as occurred with West Nile Virus.

Examples of investigations by veterinary clinical pathologists and veterinary diagnostic laboratories include the verification and diagnosis of: (1) an emerging fungal disease, such as that caused by *Cryptoccocus gattii*[3]; (2) influenza, using samples for surveillance[4,5]; (3) a reportable disease, such as equine piroplasmosis; (4) dogs

Author has nothing to disclose.
Department of Veterinary Pathology, College of Veterinary Medicine, Iowa State University, 16th and University Boulevard, Ames, IA 50011, USA
*E-mail address:* candreas@iastate.edu

Clin Lab Med 31 (2011) 173–180
doi:10.1016/j.cll.2010.11.002            labmed.theclinics.com

with renal and/or liver chemistry abnormalities with a suspect diagnosis of leptospirosis and potential zoonotic disease transmission to the owners[6,7]; (5) clinical pathology test alterations associated with a bioterrorist agent, or an intentional or accidental toxicosis, such as that occurred with melamine in feed (see the article by Puschner and Reimschuessel elsewhere in this issue for further exploration of this topic)[8]; (6) bacteria that cause plague, anthrax, mycobacteriosis, or tularemia; (7) leishmaniasis in Foxhounds in the United States, a zoonotic disease undergoing immunopathologic studies and prevention strategies[9]; (8) animals as reservoirs of zoonotic diseases in the United States or diseases associated with global travel[10,11]; and (9) serum biochemical abnormalities in food animals that can indicate a feed mixing problem with resulting negative economic effects for livestock producers and consumers. The veterinary clinical pathologist is one of the many key laboratory health professionals who have an expanding role in identifying changes and patterns in disease incidence as well as assisting in the confirmation of disease outbreaks. A recent example that involved clinical pathologists, veterinary specialists, laboratory professionals, and clinical pathology and molecular diagnostics laboratories was the confirmation of H1N1 in the bronchoalveolar lavage of a cat.[12]

The following discussion shows the importance and role of state, federal and international agencies related to disease reporting in the United States to ensure accurate and timely communication and several aspects of laboratory protocols and assay proficiency among state diagnostic laboratories. With the historical occurrence of infectious agents accidentally introduced into previously disease-free countries, especially agents that affect livestock, and 75% of new emerging infectious diseases in humans being zoonotic, the consequences and scope are tremendous, and disease identification and verification by veterinary diagnostic professionals is imperative.

## LABORATORY ACCREDITATION, REGULATION, AND PROTOCOLS

Veterinary laboratories are not required to have accreditation by the federal law; however, there are several agencies and associations involved in accreditation and validation of laboratories conducting veterinary/animal laboratory testing. Human medical laboratories are required to follow federal laws passed in 1988, named as the Clinical Laboratory Improvement Amendments, which standardize assays run on human samples; however, this is not required for animal samples.[13] It is problematic for veterinary sample quality assurance regulation and surveillance if samples are analyzed by human medical laboratories or other types of laboratories that do not report to veterinary regulatory agencies. Accreditation for state veterinary diagnostic laboratories is available via inspection and certification by the American Association of Veterinary Laboratory Diagnosticians (AAVLD), but at present, this accreditation does not extend to commercial, private, or university laboratories not contained within state diagnostic laboratories.[14] The requirements are available on the AAVLD Web site and can be followed as protocols and best practices, but certification is performed by the AAVLD organization to assure compliance.[15] For clinical pathology laboratories, quality assurance and validation also may be done through the instrument supplier or private quality assurance agencies or by implementing the quality assurance guidelines of the American Society for Veterinary Clinical Pathology.[16]

Veterinary laboratories may be required to institute Good Laboratory Practices (GLPs) for drug tests, research assays, or surge capacity test procedures, if GLP is not already a part of the laboratory standard operating procedures. It should be noted that different companies and agencies may vary in their requirements for GLP testing, so before initiating the GLP protocols, it is important to request the relevant protocols from that agency or company. Basic concepts for GLP consist of documented testing protocols, equipment monitoring and records, unalterable test results with multiple validation points, and secure storage of records for specific periods to ensure consistency and reliability of results.[17] Many of these principles are outlined by the Organisation for Economic Co-operation and Development, which is an international agency that strives to define best practices that have an effect on a sustainable global economy.[18] In the future of testing validation in the United States, there may be more compliance using standards from the International Organization for Standardization (ISO).[19,20] This organization is a developer, publisher, and promoter of international standards for 163 countries and functions as a nongovernmental consortium that bridges public and private sectors to harmonize process standards. Sometimes, the standards are adopted as law through treaties or national standards and include review of processes, monitoring, records, output review, regular review of process and quality systems, and continual improvement plans. Companies or organizations can be audited and certified or registered as conforming to ISO standards. This certification does not guarantee the product but assures that an ISO process is being followed. There is also an ISO standard that is specific for accreditation of medical laboratories, and the European College of Veterinary Clinical Pathology requires many of these standards in laboratories that train veterinary clinical pathologists.[20]

Chain of custody/evidence may be required in legal cases, with the overarching goal that evidence is admissible in a court of law by documented continuity of possession and proof of integrity of collected evidence. All laboratory personnel should be versed in the requirements for chain of custody and have a standard operating procedure, but in daily operations, accurate records and secure control of specimens should be a part of laboratory protocols. These specimens are usually submitted by law enforcement agents. The key requirements in chain of custody protocols are: (1) documentation of all transfers of the submitted materials to other personnel; (2) secure storage of specimens to ensure that no tampering can occur; (3) photographic documentation; and (4) detailed written records of findings. Often, the procedures need to be witnessed and signed by 2 individuals to ensure documentation.

Also, laboratories should use universal precautions to provide barriers of protection (commonly gloves, face masks, gowns) against blood-borne and air-borne infectious diseases, especially when a zoonotic disease is suspected. These precautions are more commonly used in human medical laboratories because of the human-to-human transmission risk, but veterinary laboratories also should use applicable barrier protection via laboratory protocols and personal protective equipment when handling specimens. The World Health Organization and Centers for Disease Control and Prevention (CDC) have published guidelines and recommendations for universal precautions under various conditions.[21,22] Veterinary laboratories may be required to meet certain standards by their occupational health and safety offices.

In recent years, US law regulates the possession of select agents that are pathogens or biologic toxins as declared by the US Department of Health and Human Services (HHS) or by the US Department of Agriculture (USDA) to have the "potential to pose a severe threat to public health and safety."[23,24] The Select Agent Program was established to satisfy requirements of the USA PATRIOT Act (Uniting and Strengthening America by Providing Appropriate Tools Required to Intercept and Obstruct Terrorism Act) and the Public Health Security and Bioterrorism Preparedness and Response Act of 2002, which were enacted after the September 11, 2001 attacks and the subsequent 2001 intentional anthrax exposures. Under these laws, it is required that the United States improve its ability to prevent, prepare for, and respond to acts of bioterrorism and other public health emergencies that could threaten either public health and safety or agriculture. Individuals possessing, using, or transferring agents or toxins that are deemed as a severe threat to public, animal or plant health, or animal or plant products, must notify either the Secretary of the Department of HHS or the Secretary of the USDA and follow established protocols. USDA and CDC maintain the Select Agents lists and administer the Select Agent Program, which regulates the laboratories that possess, use, or transfer select agents within the United States.[25]

## INTERACTIONS OF VETERINARY LABORATORIES WITH STATE, FEDERAL, AND INTERNATIONAL AGENCIES

The variation in test/assay types and location of veterinary clinical pathology laboratories and other laboratories engaged in animal testing complicates the ability to provide a responsive integrated network for animal disease reporting. Laboratories may be located in state veterinary diagnostic laboratories, universities, private commercial laboratories, or in some cases, human hospital laboratories that still perform veterinary clinical pathology procedures. The use of various laboratory information management systems impairs a uniform reporting system for ease of data exchange and communication. However, there are several integrated agencies for animal disease reporting, and new efforts are being made to coordinate reporting and summary information. The reporting chain generally starts with a sample submission from a veterinarian to the laboratory and then the notification of the appropriate state, federal, or international agency. Reportable diseases vary from state to state, and policies often contain deadlines for reporting; therefore, each state's requirements should be reviewed. Briefly, if a veterinary practitioner reports a disease to the state veterinarian as a potential animal disease foreign to the United States (a critical first step), a trained FAD diagnostician is sent to investigate. Most often, veterinary practitioners are the ones to report a suspected FAD or disease exotic to the United States, but livestock producers or county extension agents may also directly contact state and federal officials.

Federal disease surveillance is overseen by USDA. The USDA Animal and Plant Health Inspection Service (APHIS) provides leadership in ensuring the health and care of animals and plants.[26] The USDA National Veterinary Services Laboratories (NVSL) located in Ames, Iowa and the Foreign Animal Diseases Diagnostic Laboratory at Plum Island, New York (also part of the NVSL) are the national veterinary diagnostic reference and confirmatory laboratories. The USDA receives disease status information of other countries from the World Organisation for Animal Health.[27] Each of these agencies maintains a list of reportable animal diseases. The Office International des Epizooties (OIE) was created to coordinate international animal disease reporting through an agreement signed in 1924. In May 2003, this became the World Organisation for Animal Health, but the historical acronym OIE was retained. OIE is the intergovernmental organization responsible for improving animal health worldwide. It is recognized as a reference organization by the World Trade Organization, and at present, there are a total of 177 member countries and territories. The OIE is headquartered in Paris, France and maintains permanent relations with 36 other international and regional organizations with regional and subregional offices in every continent. The OIE is placed under the authority and control of delegates designated by the governments of all member countries. Immediate reporting to the OIE is required for diseases listed by OIE that are not present in the United States, as well as for changes in OIE-listed pathogens, such as new strains, increases in mortality or morbidity, and alterations in disease epidemiology or other atypical emerging diseases.

State, federal, and international agencies involved in disease reporting maintain Web sites with extensive information on the role of these agencies. Many of the diseases foreign to the United States and emerging animal diseases are zoonotic and can cause serious public health problems, including loss of life. In recent years, there have been numerous examples of accidental introduction of diseases foreign to animals of United States, zoonotic diseases, and the emergence and reemergence of infectious diseases in the United States and Canada. A few examples in North America within the last 10 years are bovine spongiform encephalopathy, West Nile Virus, contagious equine metritis, monkey pox, highly pathogenic avian influenza, exotic Newcastle Disease, and New World screwworm in a dog, to name a few.[26,28] Because agriculture accounts for 13% of the US gross domestic product and 18% of domestic employment, an outbreak of FAD or zoonotic disease would significantly affect the US economy.[26] Therefore, the emphasis often has been on detecting infectious diseases, but the role of the clinical pathologist is not restricted to that area, because, as mentioned, problems in feed mixing or chemical toxicities can also often result in abnormal data seen by the clinical pathologist.

## THE NATIONAL ANIMAL HEALTH LABORATORY NETWORK

The National Animal Health Laboratory Network (NAHLN) is a cooperative effort between 2 USDA agencies, APHIS and National Institute of Food and Agriculture, and the American Association of Veterinary Laboratory Diagnosticians (AAVLD) to coordinate animal disease surveillance, testing, and reporting.[29] Initially, 12 state veterinary diagnostic laboratories were designated to participate in the program, which has now expanded to include other laboratories. NAHLN laboratories focus on different diseases using common testing methods and software platforms to process diagnostic requests and share information. The training, proficiency testing, assistance, materials, and prototypes for diagnostic tests are overseen by the NVSL. NAHLN laboratories perform routine diagnostic tests for endemic animal diseases; provide targeted surveillance and response testing for FADs; and participate in the development of new assays. The networking of these laboratories provides an infrastructure of accessible sites that can conduct validated disease surveillance for rapid early detection and high-volume testing during an outbreak, followed by assay documentation of disease eradication. Once an FAD is detected, NVSL may be assisted by NAHLN in testing suspect herds, determining the extent of the outbreak, and conducting postincident disease surveillance. US laboratories classified as OIE international reference laboratories may be requested by the OIE to assist during exotic disease outbreaks in other countries.[26]

The key elements listed by the NAHLN are:

1. Increased and more flexible capacity for laboratory support of routine and emergency animal disease diagnosis, including in case of bioterrorism events
2. Standardized rapid diagnostic techniques used at state, regional, and national levels
3. Secure communication, alert, and reporting systems
4. Modern equipment and experienced personnel
5. National training, proficiency testing, and quality assurance
6. Upgraded facilities that meet biocontainment and physical security requirements
7. Regional and national animal health emergency training exercises (scenario tests) to test and evaluate the communication and reporting protocols of the network.[29]

The NAHLN also contributes to wider societal goals, including protecting human health by decreasing the risk of zoonotic diseases; protecting animal health to decrease environmental risk and negative economic effect; lessening the risk of disease transmission between wildlife and livestock; supporting confidence in the livestock food supply of the United States; and maintaining the confidence of global trading partners.

## SUMMARY

The current detection system for animal diseases requires coordination between veterinarians; veterinary medical laboratories; and state, federal, and international agencies, as well as associated private sectors. Effective responses require that all steps in the process are followed and implemented. The effect on the food supply of the United States from animal products can be marked because animal and human health is affected, especially if a zoonotic disease is involved or when trade import or export restrictions result from a disease incident. The USDA-APHIS Veterinary Services works with partners to coordinate responses during an FAD and as the recovery after a disease outbreak is contained and resolved. The OIE sets standards to determine when a country is disease free after an outbreak. The knowledge and roles of the veterinary laboratories and all associated professionals are vital to detect, monitor, and confirm diseases and conditions that affect animal and human health, and the animal-origin food supply of the United States.

## REFERENCES

1. Spickler AR. Emerging and exotic diseases of animals—fact sheets. Section 2. In: Spickler AR, Roth JA, Galyon J, et al, editors. Emerging and exotic diseases of animals. 4th edition, 2nd printing. Ames (IA): CFSPH/IICAB, Iowa State University; 2010. p. 78–320.
2. Andreasen CB, Sorden SD. Images of emerging and exotic diseases of animals–section 3. In: Spickler AR, Roth JA, Galyon J, et al, editors. Emerging and exotic diseases of animals. 4th edition, 2nd printing. Ames (IA): CFSPH/IICAB, Iowa State University; 2010. p. 322–67.
3. Oregon Government; Department of Human Services. Acute and communicable disease prevention. *Cryptococcus gattii.* Available at: http://oregon.gov/DHS/ph/acd/diseases/cryptococcus/cgattii_index.shtml. Accessed October 19, 2010.
4. Holt DE, Mover MR, Brown DC. Serologic prevalence of antibodies against canine influenza virus (H3N8) in dogs in a metropolitan animal shelter. J Am Vet Med Assoc 2010;237:71–3.
5. Hayward JJ, Dubovi EJ, Scarlett JM, et al. Microevolution of canine influenza virus in shelters and its molecular epidemiology in the United States. J Virol 2010; 84(24):12636–45.
6. Gautam R, Wu CC, Guptill LF, et al. Detection of antibodies against Leptospira serovars via microscopic agglutination tests in dogs in the United States, 2000–2007. J Am Vet Med Assoc 2010;237:293–8.
7. Greenlee JJ, Bolin CA, Alt DP, et al. Clinical and pathologic comparison of acute canine leptospirosis caused by two strains of *Leptospira kirschneri* serovar grippotyphosa. Am J Vet Res 2004;65:1100–7.
8. Brown CA, Jeong KS, Poppenga RH, et al. Outbreaks of renal failure associated with melamine and cyanuric acid in dogs and cats in 2004 and 2007. J Vet Diagn Invest 2007;19:525–31.
9. Gibson-Corley KN, Hostetter JM, Hostetter SJ, et al. Disseminated *Leishmania infantum* infection in two sibling foxhounds due to possible vertical transmission. Can Vet J 2008;49:1005–8.

10. Jimenez-Coello M, Ortega-Pacheco A, Guzman-Marin E, et al. Stray dogs as reservoirs of the zoonotic agents *Leptospira interrogans, Trypanosoma cruzi,* and *Aspergillus spp.* in an urban area of Chiapas in southern Mexico. Vector Borne Zoonotic Dis 2010;10:135–41.
11. Spickler AR, Dvorak G. Technical fact sheets for selected zoonotic diseases of companion animals. In: Dvorak G, Spickler AR, Roth JA, editors. Handbook for zoonotic diseases of companion animals. 1st edition. Ames (IA): CFSPH, Iowa State University; 2008. p. 63–266.
12. Sponseller BA, Strait E, Jergens A, et al. Influenza A pandemic (H1N1) 2009 virus infection in domestic cat. Emerg Infect Dis 2010;16:534–7.
13. US Department of Health and Human Services. Centers for Medicare and Medicaid Services. CLIA Brochures. Available at: http://www.cms.gov/CLIA/05_CLIA_Brochures.asp. Accessed October 19, 2010.
14. The American Association of Veterinary Laboratory Diagnosticians. Available at: http://www.aavld.org/mc/page.do;jsessionid=61283FDA663B408AF53997 AE3B54ED3F.mc0?sitePageId=27915. Accessed October 19, 2010.
15. The American Association of Veterinary Laboratory Diagnosticians. Accreditation. Available at: http://www.aavld.org/mc/page.do?sitePageId=33930&orgId=aavld. Accessed October 19, 2010.
16. American Society for Veterinary Clinical Pathology. Quality assurance guidelines. Available at: https://asvcp.org/pubs/qas/index.cfm. Accessed October 19, 2010.
17. Rodrigues G. Liquid-delivery quality assurance in clinical laboratories—navigating regulations and standards for liquid-delivery verification [online]. MLO Med Lab Obs 2006. p. 48–51. Available at: http://www.mlo-online.com/articles/1206/1206special_feature_QC.pdf. Accessed October 19, 2010.
18. Organisation for Economic Co-operation and Development. Environment directorate. Good laboratory practices. Available at: http://www.oecd.org/document/4/0,3343,en_2649_34381_2346175_1_1_1_1,00.html. Accessed January 20, 2011.
19. International Organization for Standardization. Available at: http://www.iso.org/iso/home.html. Accessed October 19, 2010.
20. Freeman KP, Bauer N, Jensen AL, et al. Introduction to ISO 15189: a blueprint for quality systems in veterinary laboratories. Vet Clin Pathol 2006;35:157–71.
21. Centers for Disease Control and Prevention. Biosafety in microbiological and biomedical laboratories (BMBL). 5th edition. Government Printing Office. Available at: http://www.cdc.gov/biosafety/publications/bmbl5/index.htm. Accessed October 19, 2010.
22. World Health Organization. Available at: http://www.who.int/en/. Accessed October 19, 2010.
23. US Department of Health and Human Services. Select agent information. Available at: http://grants.nih.gov/grants/policy/select_agent/index.htm. Accessed October 19, 2010.
24. United States Department of Agriculture; Animal and Plant Health Inspection Service. Agricultural select agent program. Available at: http://www.aphis.usda.gov/programs/ag_selectagent/. Accessed October 19, 2010.
25. USDA-APHIS and CDC. National select agent registry. Available at: http://www.selectagents.gov/. Accessed October 19, 2010.
26. Spickler AR, Lofstedt J. Agencies involved in the response to outbreaks of foreign animal diseases. In: Spickler AR, Roth JA, Galyon J, et al, editors. Emerging and exotic diseases of animals. 4th edition, 2nd printing. Ames (IA): CFSPH/IICAB, Iowa State University; 2010. p. 30–40. Chapter 3.

27. World Organisation for Animal Health (OIE). Available at: http://www.oie.int/eng/en_index.htm. Accessed October 19, 2010.
28. Spickler AR, Galyon J, Roth JA. Descriptions of recent incursions of exotic animal diseases. In: Spickler AR, Roth JA, Galyon J, et al, editors. Emerging and exotic diseases of animals. 4th edition, 2nd printing. Ames (IA): CFSPH/IICAB, Iowa State University; 2010. p. 52–76. Chapter 5.
29. United States Department of Agriculture; Animal and Plant Health Inspection Service. National Animal Health Laboratory Network. A state and federal partnership to safeguard animal health. Available at: http://www.aphis.usda.gov/animal_health/nahln/. Accessed October 19, 2010.

# Toxicosis Caused by Melamine and Cyanuric Acid in Dogs and Cats: Uncovering the Mystery and Subsequent Global Implications

Birgit Puschner, DVM, PhD[a],*, Renate Reimschuessel, VMD, PhD[b]

**KEYWORDS**

- Melamine • Cyanuric acid • Acute renal failure • Crystals
- Food adulteration • Toxicosis

A large crisis of contamination of pet food began in February of 2007, when numerous cases of acute renal failure in dogs and cats were associated with the ingestion of a variety of dog and cat food products.[1] By late March 2007, 471 cases of renal failure in dogs and cats, with an estimated 104 deaths, were considered a direct result of ingestion of contaminated pet food.[2] During the recall of cat and dog food that followed, the largest ever in North America, the total number of dogs and cats sickened and killed by food contaminants was speculated to have been in the thousands. As the crisis unfolded, several major commercial pet-food companies recalled more than 1000 potentially contaminated product lines and the Food and Drug Administration (FDA) enforced an import alert on certain food ingredients from China.[3] The district offices of the FDA and the Center for Veterinary Medicine (CVM), which regulates the manufacture and distribution of animal food and drugs, received more than 18,000 phone calls.

During the investigation of this major outbreak, the contaminants were identified as melamine and melamine analogues. Additional research efforts led to a proposed mechanism of toxic action; clinical, laboratory, pathologic, histologic, and toxicologic

The authors have nothing to disclose.
[a] Department of Molecular Biosciences, School of Veterinary Medicine, University of California, 1120 Haring Hall, Davis, CA 95616, USA
[b] Center for Veterinary Medicine, Office of Research, Food and Drug Administration, 8401 Muirkirk Road, Laurel, MD 20708, USA
* Corresponding author.
E-mail address: bpuschner@ucdavis.edu

Clin Lab Med 31 (2011) 181–199
doi:10.1016/j.cll.2010.10.003
0272-2712/11/$ – see front matter

diagnostic criteria; and an identification of the source of the contamination. The contamination was not limited to pet food because by-products from pet-food manufacturing in the United States and Canada were incorporated into fish, chicken, and swine feed. This factor, in return, required the development of sensitive analytical methods for the detection of melamine and melamine analogues in tissues and a careful assessment of the risk to human health associated with eating pork, chicken, fish, and eggs from animals that had been inadvertently exposed to contaminated feed.[4] In addition, animal deaths associated with melamine and melamine analogue were also diagnosed in Europe, South Africa, and Asia. Further research revealed that deaths in cats, dogs, and pigs induced by melamine and melamine analogue occurred as early as 2003 in Spain (pigs) [5] and Korea (dogs and cats),[6] making this a global event. In late 2008, dogs died of renal failure associated with melamine and melamine analogue in Italy.[7]

On September 9, 2008, melamine was identified as the causative agent for urinary tract calculi and renal failure in infants in China.[8] At least 6 infants died, 294,000 infants were diagnosed with urinary tract stones, and 51,900 infants were hospitalized.[9] It is assumed that melamine was deliberately added to milk and milk products to boost the apparent protein level. In stark contrast to renal failure in dogs, cats, and pigs induced by melamine and melamine analogue, exposure to melamine alone resulted in clinical and subclinical urolithiasis, with rare cases of obstructive renal failure in infants. Coingestion of cyanuric acid was not necessary for the onset of disease.

The goal of this article is to provide a description and analysis of these events to emphasize the importance of veterinary diagnostic and toxicology laboratories in this type of investigation and in the broader arena of global food safety.

## TIME LINE AND EPIDEMIOLOGY

In early 2007, consumer complaints were being received regarding cats falling sick soon after consuming certain brands of cat food. The California Animal Health and Food Safety Laboratory (CAHFS) of the School of Veterinary Medicine, University of California–Davis, received what turned out to be an index case involving 2 cats presented to a southern California veterinary clinic on February 28, 2008. The indoor cats were 6 and 11 years old, from the same household, and simultaneously diagnosed with acute renal failure. The owner was suspicious of a food contaminant because both cats vomited within 1 hour of being fed recently purchased pouches of cat food. In the following 24 hours, both cats became anorexic and lethargic, developed polydipsia and polyuria, and were presented to a veterinary clinic. A diagnosis of acute renal failure was established. The more severely affected cat died despite treatment, including hemodialysis. The other cat received supportive care and slowly recovered, but continued to have reduced renal function. The diagnosis at the time was acute renal failure from an unknown cause. Typical causes, including ethylene glycol, oxalic acid, and heavy metal toxicities, were ruled out by toxicologic testing.

The acute illness of these 2 cats, and death in one of them, occurred at a time when Menu Foods Inc was receiving numerous consumer complaints about sick and dying cats that had access to various food products from Menu.[10] In addition, on March 6 and 7, 2007, acute renal failure and deaths were reported in a large number of cats from a quarterly premarket palatability study that was conducted on behalf of Menu Foods Inc.[11] In response to increased consumer complaints and concerns about a possible contamination of pet food, Menu Foods Inc issued a voluntary recall on March 16, 2007. In the following days, multiple laboratories conducted testing for a broad array of chemicals. On March 22, FDA's Forensic Chemistry Center in Cincinnati, OH as well as CAHFS identified melamine in samples of recalled pet food.

Melamine was also detected in food samples (pouches) ingested by both cats of the index case. On March 23, 2007 the New York State Agricultural Laboratory reported the finding of a rodenticide called aminopterin in recalled pet food.[12] However, this compound was not detected by either FDA or CAHFS, and was quickly dismissed as a possible cause for the numerous incidents of renal failure in dogs and cats. On March 26, 2007 FDA's Forensic Chemistry Center detected additional compounds related to melamine in recalled pet food; these included cyanuric acid, ammelide, ammeline, and ureidomelamine (the last 3 are referred to as melamine analogues).

On March 30, 2007, the FDA officially announced the finding of melamine in the recalled pet-food products. On April 3, 2007, the FDA was sent images from veterinary pathologists at Michigan State University showing crystals in the kidney of a dog that had consumed contaminated pet food. Because the crystal morphology resembled that of uric acid crystal spherulites occasionally seen in human gout, scientists at the FDA hypothesized that the crystals may have characteristics similar to urate crystals; specifically, that they may cause a syndrome similar to acute uric acid nephropathy and that they may dissolve in formalin. To test the hypothesis, pathology reports submitted to the FDA were reviewed to identify cases for which frozen tissues were available. A case from the University of Florida was identified and samples were received at the FDA on April 13, 2007. The case was from a cat in a household of 7 cats, 6 of which were affected by contaminated pet food. In slices of kidney examined by wet mount, abundant crystals were seen; those crystals, when left in formaldehyde, dissolved over time. This information was shared with the veterinary diagnostic laboratory community via a conference call with the American Veterinary Medical Association (AVMA) on April 23, 2007. As a consequence, sample collection recommendations specified freezing of samples in addition to routinely fixing in formalin.

On April 13, 2007, Proctor and Gamble contacted the FDA to report preliminary results of their study of melamine toxicosis in rats. In this study, rats were given melamine, ammeline, ammelide, and cyanuric acid at a ratio of 10:1:1:1.[13] Crystals were not observed in histopathologic sections of kidney. FDA scientists suggested a melamine/cyanuric acid ratio of 1:1 and to examine kidneys fresh rather than after routine fixation in formaldehyde. Tissues from the cat submitted by the University of Florida were examined using Raman spectroscopy by the FDA's Forensic Chemistry Center and contained melamine-cyanurate.[14]

On May 1, 2007, the finding of cyanuric acid in the recalled pet-food products was announced publicly and an interaction between melamine and cyanuric acid was suspected of being responsible for crystal formation. Initially, wheat gluten, imported from China, was believed to be the source of contamination because it was the common ingredient to all incidents. But in early April, it was shown that the contaminated feed ingredient was wheat flour, not wheat gluten. On April 9, 2007, the CAHFS laboratory confirmed another case of acute renal failure caused by a pet food that was not on the initial recall list. This confirmation resulted in expansion of the recall list. On April 16, a second commodity, rice protein concentrate, was identified as being contaminated and additional pet food was recalled. Later in the investigation, it was again confirmed that the so-called rice protein consisted primarily of wheat flour. By mid-April 2007, it became apparent that the distribution of contaminated pet food was not restricted to North America. Concurrently, it became known that several dogs and cats in Cape Town and Johannesburg, South Africa, had, in the previous 2 or 3 months, developed renal failure associated with melamine-cyanuric acid, and a recall of pet food was initiated. The South African investigation revealed several incidents between October 2006 and June 2007 that were traced back to several pet-food manufacturing plants.[15] According to a survey conducted in April 2007 by the

Veterinary Information Network (VIN), the total number of deaths of dogs and cats in the United States because of exposure to pet food contaminated with melamine and cyanuric acid at that time was probably between 2000 and 7000.

In late April 2007, pet-food waste, primarily contaminated with melamine alone, was incorporated into swine and poultry rations that were subsequently consumed by approximately 56,000 swine[16] and 2.5 to 3.0 million chickens in the United States.[17,18] Meat from animals fed contaminated pet food also was consumed by humans, but definitive data on the risk to human health were lacking. The CAHFS Toxicology Laboratory rapidly developed a method to determine the concentrations of melamine in porcine urine and muscle tissue.[19] During this time, fish feed was also contaminated and fed to fish at 160 hatcheries and 2 aquaculture farms. Scientists at the CVM-FDA began feeding studies in edible fish to provide tissues for method development for melamine and cyanuric acid.[20–22]

On May 25, 2007, data generated from the analysis of porcine samples by the CAHFS Laboratory, and surveys of melamine residues in fish commodities by the FDA provided crucial information to the FDA for conducting a human health risk assessment for consumption of melamine-contaminated meat.[4] This interim risk assessment indicated that melamine residues in edible tissues of animals exposed to melamine were unlikely to pose a human health risk.

Based on identification of melamine and cyanuric acid as the causative agents for renal failure in dogs and cats in North America in 2007, outbreaks of renal failure in Asia in 2003[6] and 2004[23] could also be solved because they shared the same causation. In addition, incidents of renal failure in pigs in Spain between 2003 and 2006[5] and in Thailand in 2007[24] could be linked to exposure to melamine and melamine analogues. Thus, although pet food contaminated with melamine and melamine analogues resulted in a major outbreak of renal failure in the United States in 2007, similar outbreaks occurred in Europe and Asia as early as 2003.

## COMMUNICATION AMONGST VETERINARIANS, VETERINARY DIAGNOSTIC LABORATORIES, AND VETERINARY ASSOCIATIONS

Officially, Menu Foods Inc issued a voluntary recall on March 16, 2007. According to the FDA, Menu Foods Inc received the first consumer complaint about a pet death on February 20, 2007. Data from a premarket palatability study,[11] in which cats died of acute renal failure, became available in early March 2007. Additional studies conducted in dogs confirmed deaths associated with renal-failure after consumption of certain pet food in early March (Birgit Puschner, unpublished data, 2007). Unlike with human illnesses and the public health role of the Centers for Disease Control and Prevention, there is no centralized system for surveillance and distribution of data of illnesses in pets. At that time, the CVM-FDA received reports of adverse drug events but did not routinely receive reports of clusters of illness in pets. The newly formed portal for reporting adverse events on the FDA Web site should help with such events in the future.[25]

However, in 2007 an increased incidence of renal failure in dogs and cats in the United States was primarily communicated through various veterinary organizations and their mailing list servers. Amongst these, the AVMA, the American College of Veterinary Internal Medicine, the American Association of Veterinary Laboratory Diagnosticians (AAVLD), VIN, and the American Board of Veterinary Toxicology played important roles in sharing as much information as possible about the ongoing diagnostic investigation of this major outbreak. Communications among these groups, the FDA, and scientists from the pet-food industry were key to providing data on cases and sharing preliminary results to guide the efforts toward understanding the mechanism of toxicity. The FDA continuously updated the list of recalled products with almost daily additions from March 16, 2007 to April 26, 2007, and the FDA Emergency Operations Center coordinated the agency efforts. Veterinarians posted clinicopathologic findings of pets known to have been exposed to recalled pet food and later, after the recall in mid-March, posted images of crystals identified in urine sediments and postmortem renal lesions. At the time, veterinary clinical pathologists were already certain that the crystals did not match any of the commonly diagnosed crystals in animals and that the lesions were clearly distinguishable from those seen in ethylene glycol or lily intoxication; however, because of the absence of a centralized surveillance or notification system for veterinarians, an accurate count of pet death and disease resulting from the 2007 contamination will never be known. As mentioned earlier, a survey conducted by VIN has estimated the total number of contamination-related deaths in dogs and cats in the United States to be between 2000 and 7000. A separate survey conducted between April 5, 2007 and June 6, 2007 by the AAVLD identified 235 cats and 112 dogs that had developed renal failure induced by melamine-cyanuric acid.[26] The survey conducted by AAVLD had stringent criteria for case inclusion, whereas the VIN survey was conducted by asking practitioners to estimate numbers of patients affected. In the AAVLD survey, the mortality was 61% in cats and 74% in dogs; however, many of the cases included in the survey were provided by veterinary diagnostic laboratories and thus postmortem cases are likely overrepresented.

## CLINICAL AND DIAGNOSTIC FINDINGS IN TOXICOSIS
### Clinical Findings

Dogs and cats exposed to toxic amounts of melamine and cyanuric acid generally develop inappetence with or without vomiting within 12 hours of exposure.[11,27] Once an animal develops renal dysfunction, polydipsia, polyuria, weakness, lethargy, and dehydration are usually noticed by the pet owner.

### Laboratory Findings

The laboratory findings in melamine-cyanuric acid toxicosis are consistent with acute renal failure.[27,28] Melamine and cyanuric acid in the diet do not seem to have dose-dependent laboratory effects.[27] Published clinical pathology data exist for cats, but there are limited data for dogs with melamine-cyanuric acid toxicosis. In cats, increased serum urea (>100 mg/dL) and creatinine (>8 mg/dL) concentrations can be detected as early as 36 hours after exposure to toxic amounts of melamine and cyanuric acid.[11,14] In addition, hyperphosphatemia (>9 mg/dL), hyperkalemia (>6 mmol/L) and a urine-specific gravity of less than 1.035 are seen in cats with impaired renal function. Laboratory abnormalities reported in dogs with melamine-cyanuric acid poisoning include azotemia, leukocytosis, neutrophilia, hyperphosphatemia, hyperkalemia, and decreased total $CO_2$ concentration.[28]

Melamine-cyanuric acid crystals are green to gold-brownish, rounded, platelike, and easily detected by microscopic examination of urine sediment.[11,27,29] The University of Guelph, Canada played an important role in the initial crystal analysis.[30] In mid-April 2007, the veterinary Laboratory Services Division, University of Guelph added melamine and cyanuric acid to cat urine (from an unexposed cat) and showed crystal formation.[30] The composition of the generated in vitro crystals matched crystals from pets affected by the recalled pet food when compared by infrared spectroscopy. Crystal formation and composition was also confirmed by micro-Raman spectroscopy.[14]

### Gross and Histopathologic Findings

On gross examination, kidneys from animals that die of melamine-cyanuric acid poisoning are often enlarged.[11,13,27] On sectioning, yellow-brown precipitates can be seen with the naked eye, particularly in the medulla.[13,14,27] By magnified inspection the precipitates can be visualized as fine dots to 0.1-cm-long threads extending from the papilla of the medulla into the obscured corticomedullary junction, and running in parallel with the medullary rays. Unstained touch impression smears of the cut surface of the kidney contain fan-shaped to amorphous crystals that are birefringent. In wet mount preparations of thin (approximately 0.5-mm) slices of kidney compressed between 2 slides, crystals can be seen within renal tubules (**Fig. 1**). This technique can be used to show even a few crystals in a large piece of tissue compared with the lower chance of finding crystals in the small sample size of cryosections (6 μm).

Histologically, melamine-cyanuric acid poisoning results in the formation of unique polarizable crystals within the lumina of collecting ducts and within proximal and distal tubules.[23,27–29,31] Crystals are translucent, pale yellow to clear, 10 to 40 μm and occasionally up to 80 μm in diameter, and fanlike, starburst prism-shaped, or globular (**Fig. 2**). They resemble urate spherulites seen in human gout.[32] Many cases from the 2003, 2004, and 2007 melamine-cyanuric acid intoxications in dogs and cats describe the characteristic crystals as pinwheels because they consist of 2 or more distinct concentric rings with linear striations that look like radiating spokes.[6,11,23,28]

The type of fixative and length of immersion play an important role when evaluating a kidney for the presence of melamine-cyanuric acid crystals.[14] Crystals do not dissolve in renal tissue that is fixed for 24 hours in either 95% alcohol or 10% buffered formalin. However, in renal tissue kept in 10% buffered formalin for 6 weeks, crystals dissolve.[23] Also, melamine-cyanuric acid crystals cannot be visualized in kidney tissues fixed for 24 hours in Bouin fixative.[27] Therefore, in suspected melamine-cyanuric acid poisoning cases, tissues should be fixed in 95% alcohol, or in 10% buffered formalin, for only short periods (1–3 hours). Special staining techniques can be used to differentiate melamine-cyanuric acid crystals from other crystals in histologic sections. Melamine-cyanuric acid crystals stain pale golden brown with hematoxylin and eosin (H&E), stain positively with Oil Red O and Gomori methylamine silver, and do not stain with Van Kossa or Alizarin Red S.[14,28]

Histologic lesions consistent with tubular necrosis are observed in poisoned animals. In addition, proliferation of tubular epithelial cells, interstitial edema, acute tubulitis, renal interstitial fibrosis, and lymphoplasmacytic interstitial nephritis can be seen, depending on the chronicity of the melamine-cyanuric intoxication.[6,11,23] Although extrarenal lesions were not identified in cats experimentally exposed to melamine and cyanuric acid, extrarenal lesions were described in naturally occurring cases. These lesions included oral ulcers and gastric mineralization, likely secondary to uremia. Melamine-cyanuric acid poisoning does not lead to characteristic lesions in other organs.[14,23]

### Toxicologic Findings

The key toxicologic finding in an animal with suspected melamine-cyanuric acid poisoning is the detection of melamine and melamine analogues in biologic specimens from the animal, and in the food. As soon as melamine and analogues were identified as the causative agents in 2007, several analytical methods were developed to accurately identify melamine, cyanuric acid, ammeline, and ammelide in the urine, serum, milk, kidney, and food. Melamine and analogues can be identified within several hours in urine or serum of a pet suspected to have been exposed to these compounds. Any concentration is significant and requires further evaluation, because these

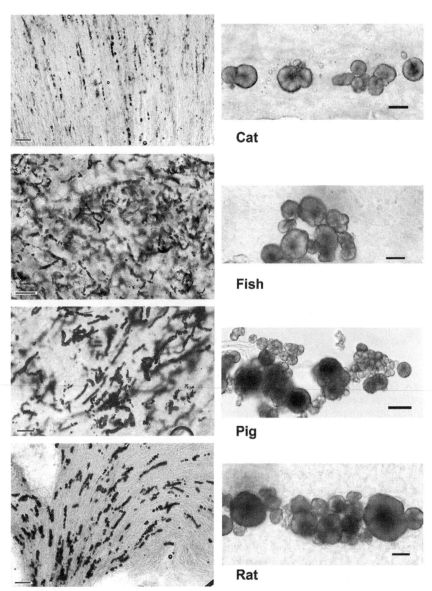

**Fig. 1.** Comparative wet-mount preparations of melamine-cyanuric acid crystals in cat, fish, pig, and rat kidneys. Small slices of kidney (either fresh or thawed) were compressed between 2 slides. Crystals in these preparations are similar to those found in urine sediment specimens. The cat was a patient that died after eating contaminated pet food. The experimental animals had been fed melamine and cyanuric acid 1:1 at 400 mg/kg bw (catfish and pig) or 200 mg/kg bw (rat). (*Left*) Crystals can be seen lined up in renal tubules, resulting in tubular obstruction (bars = 200 μm). (*Right*) Crystal morphology is similar in all species. Small, needlelike, golden-to-brown crystals are in radial arrangements that form a spherulite (bars = 20 μm). Crystals vary from 10 to 100 μm in diameter, with most in the 20- to 40-μm range. Rat kidneys *courtesy of* Dr Gamboa da Costa, National Center for Toxicologic Research/FDA.

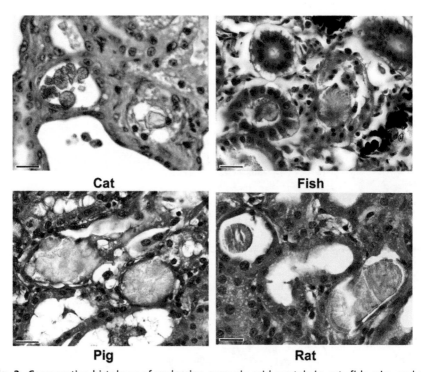

**Fig. 2.** Comparative histology of melamine-cyanuric acid crystals in cat, fish, pig, and rat kidneys. Crystal spherulites are present in the tubule lumen, sometimes abrading the tubular epithelium, as seen in the fish micrograph. Crystals typically are golden brown; some are paler and others have eosinophilic concentric laminations, as seen in the rat micrograph. Crystals vary in size and shape, forming tubular agglomerates that also may be spherical or fan-shaped. (H&E, bars = 20 μm.) (Rat kidneys *courtesy of* Dr George P. Daston, Proctor and Gamble, Cincinnati, OH.)

compounds should not be present in biologic specimens. Analytical methods are capable of detecting melamine and cyanuric acid at concentrations as low as 0.5 μg/ml in serum, urine, and milk. Pets poisoned during the 2007 outbreak often had concentrations of more than 100 μg/ml of melamine in urine or serum. Post mortem, kidney tissue can be analyzed for these compounds to confirm the presence of melamine and analogues and reach an accurate diagnosis. As is true for urine, serum and milk, analytical methods are able to detect melamine and cyanuric acid concentrations as low as 1 μg/g in kidney. This level of sensitivity is more than sufficient considering that pets that died of melamine-cyanuric acid poisoning in 2003, 2004, and 2007 had kidney melamine and cyanuric acid concentrations greater than 100 μg/g, and in many cases greater than 1000 μg/g.[6,13,27]

Many veterinary diagnostic laboratories now provide routine testing for melamine and analogues. In addition, crystal formation from melamine in combination with other melamine analogues was studied in vitro and analyzed by micro-Raman spectroscopic analyses.[14] Crystals form spontaneously when pure solutions of melamine and cyanuric acid are mixed. Spontaneous crystal formation was not detected for mixtures of melamine and ammeline, ammeline and cyanuric acid, or ammelide and cyanuric acid. Raman spectrometry was also successfully applied to confirm that crystals from a cat that had died during the 2007 outbreak were composed of melamine-cyanuric acid.[14]

## RESEARCH ON THE TOXICITY OF MELAMINE AND CYANURIC ACID
### Toxicity Studies in Cats

In mid-April 2007, shortly after melamine and cyanuric acid were identified in recalled pet food and considered possibly responsible for acute renal failure in pets, a toxicity study in cats was conducted at the University of California–Davis.[27] This study was warranted because melamine and cyanuric acid are relatively nontoxic if given individually, but toxicity data for the substances in combination was lacking. In addition, whereas there are limited data on the toxicity of melamine and cyanuric acid in dogs, rats, and mice, there were no data for cats. Illnesses and deaths associated with the pet food recalled in 2007 appeared to affect cats more than dogs and thus a study in cats was deemed necessary to provide scientific evidence that would explain the cause of the outbreak.

The oral median lethal dose ($LD_{50}$) of melamine has been reported to be 3100 mg/kg body weight (bw) in male rats and 3900 mg/kg bw in male mice.[33] In dogs, melamine administered orally at 125 mg/kg bw was reported to cause diuresis, but no other effects were found.[34] Sodium cyanurate, administered for at least 100 days in the drinking water at 700 mg/kg bw and 2200 mg/kg bw to rats and mice, respectively, caused bladder calculi and associated bladder epithelial hyperplasia, but had no other adverse effects.[35] Of 3 dogs continuously fed a diet containing 8% monosodium cyanurate, 2 died after 16 months and 21 months, respectively, whereas the third dog was killed at the end of the 2-year study.[36] Kidney fibrosis and focal dilation were noted in all 3 dogs. When the dietary concentration of monosodium cyanurate was reduced to 0.8% and fed daily for 6 months, no adverse clinical signs or renal lesions were noted.

The study in cats showed that a combination of melamine and cyanuric acid results in acute renal failure. Even after a single oral dose of the combination (32 mg/kg bw each of melamine and cyanuric acid), cats developed anorexia, vomiting, depression, and acute renal failure within 24 to 36 hours of exposure. Higher dosages of 121 mg/kg bw and 181 mg/kg bw each of melamine and cyanuric acid did not seem to result in dose-dependent clinicopathologic effects. In contrast, the extent of lesions did generally correlate with the dose and included tubular damage, interstitial edema, and crystals. The clinical, clinicopathologic, pathologic, and histopathologic findings in the study cats matched those described in cats that developed renal failure associated with the consumption of adulterated pet food.[11,23] The dosage of 32 mg/kg bw melamine and 32 mg/kg bw cyanuric acid corresponds to a dietary concentration of 0.2% melamine and 0.2% cyanuric acid. Considering the wide range of concentrations of melamine and cyanuric acid detected in recalled pet food (from 10 mg/kg to more than 3000 mg/kg), it is likely that illness and death can occur at a lower dose than 32 mg/kg bw melamine combined with 32 mg/kg bw cyanuric acid. However, there are no data on the minimum dose of melamine and cyanuric acid that causes renal failure in cats, or the ratio of melamine and cyanuric acid required to result in crystal formation in vivo. Melamine and cyanuric acid, but not ammeline or ammelide, were detected in kidney tissue of cats administered melamine and cyanuric acid.[27] In addition, only cyanuric acid was detected in the kidney of a cat administered cyanuric acid alone. These findings are in agreement with previous kinetic studies showing that melamine and cyanuric acid are not metabolized, but rather are excreted unchanged in urine.[35,37,38]

Micro-Raman spectroscopic analysis was used to determine the composition of crystals in kidney from a cat that died of renal failure after consuming recalled pet food.[14] Spectra of the crystals were compared with spectra obtained from the recrystallization of pure melamine and melamine analogue compounds and melamine-cyanurate complex crystals formed in vitro. Crystals from the cat were consistent with melamine-cyanurate complex crystals. The fact that melamine and cyanuric acid combine rapidly into a lattice structure via hydrogen bonds is considered a major driving force behind crystal formation.[39,40] This reaction is the basis for gravimetric and turbidimetric methods used to determine the levels of cyanuric acid and chlorinated isocyanurates in swimming pools.[41] The formation of insoluble melamine-cyanurate crystals seems to be pH dependent, similar to uric acid crystal formation in acute uric acid nephropathy in humans and animals.[42] Precipitation of intrarenal uric acid crystals occurs when urine pH is less than 5.5 and when increasing amounts of uric acid are present.[43,44] Thus, the acidic urine of cats and dogs provides favorable conditions for the formation of insoluble melamine-cyanurate crystals, leading to physical obstruction of renal tubules and an increase in intrarenal pressure, similar to the pathogenesis of uric acid nephropathy.[45] The pH-dependent formation of melamine-cyanurate crystals in animals also explains their predominant deposition in the distal nephron. Although intrarenal obstruction seems to play a significant role in the pathogenesis of induced renal failure induced by melamine-cyanurate, inflammation, obstruction by proteinaceous material secondary to casts, and renal vasoconstriction also may contribute.

### Toxicity Studies in Other Species

Melamine and cyanuric acid, administered together orally to rats at 50 mg/kg bw each for 3 days, resulted in increases in serum urea and creatinine concentrations and kidney weight as well as crystal deposition in the kidney.[31] When the doses of melamine and cyanuric acid were reduced to 5 mg/kg bw each, nephropathy was not observed in histologic sections stained with H&E. Melamine and cyanuric acid given individually at 50 mg/kg bw did not result in adverse effects. However, rats given 12 mg/kg bw per day for 3, 7, and 14 days developed renal crystals in increasing amounts over time.[46] When rats were administered a mixture of 400 mg/kg bw melamine and 40 mg/kg bw each of cyanuric acid, ammeline, and ammelide, or a mixture of 400 mg/kg bw melamine and 400 mg/kg bw cyanuric acid, orally for 3 days, serum urea and creatinine concentrations and kidney weight increased.[13] Rats orally given up to 100 mg/kg bw ammeline or 100 mg/kg bw ammelide alone did not develop renal effects. When rats were fed contaminated pet food from the 2004 outbreak in Asia at levels of 50% to 100% of the total diet for 12 weeks, nephrotoxicity was observed.[47] At the 100% level, the corresponding mean daily doses of cyanuric acid were 38.3 and 60.3 mg/kg bw for males and females, respectively. The mean daily melamine doses at the 100% level were 260 and 410 mg/kg bw for males and females, respectively. In this subchronic study, male rats appeared to be more sensitive to the toxic effects of the combination of melamine and cyanuric acid than females. The FDA is currently conducting an NOAEL (no observed adverse effect level) study in rats in collaboration with the National Toxicology Program. This study helps define threshold levels for developing crystals in kidneys following coingestion of melamine and cyanuric acid.

Pigs orally administered a combination of melamine and cyanuric acid of 400 mg/kg bw each developed anorexia, dehydration, lethargy, and anuria and had increased serum urea and creatinine concentrations.[14,48] Typical melamine-cyanurate crystals and renal tubular changes were seen post mortem. Clinical changes were not observed in pigs treated with 400 mg/kg bw of either melamine or cyanuric acid. In a recent FDA NOAEL study, pigs fed melamine and cyanuric as low as 10 mg/kg bw (of each compound) developed renal crystals.[49]

Fish (tilapia [Oreochromis spp], channel catfish, [Ictalurus punctatus] rainbow trout [Oncorhynchus mykiss], Atlantic salmon [Salmo salar]) given an oral mixture of melamine and cyanuric acid (400 mg/kg bw each) for 3 days developed large numbers of typical melamine-cyanurate crystals in their kidneys, but, in general, did not show clinical signs of distress. Two fish died of renal failure, but most survived, likely because gills (rather than kidneys) function as the main excretory organ for nitrogenous waste.[14] No renal crystals were seen in fish given 400 mg/kg bw of melamine or cyanuric acid separately. Trout given oral melamine at doses of 20 mg/kg bw for 3 days followed 6 days later with a single dose of 20 mg/kg bw cyanuric acid did develop melamine-cyanurate crystals.[14] Excretion of many chemicals is slower in fish than in mammals.[50]

In fish, because melamine residues persist in tissues after exposure has stopped, formation of melamine-cyanurate crystals is possible when subsequent exposure to cyanuric acid alone occurs. This finding has not been studied or confirmed in mammals, and the relevance of these data to mammals is unknown. Concentrations of melamine and cyanuric acid in muscle tissue are higher in fish that were given each compound individually than when given a mixture of melamine and cyanuric acid. Formation of melamine-cyanuric acid complex in the gut as well as in the renal tubules likely leads to decreased bioavailability for tissue deposition.

Limited data exist on the toxicity of the melamine-cyanurate complex. The acute oral $LD_{50}$s of melamine-cyanurate complex in rats and mice is 4110 mg/kg bw and 3461 mg/kg bw, respectively.[51] In that study, the oral $LD_{50}$s of melamine alone were 6000 mg/kg bw in rats and 4282 mg/kg bw body in mice, whereas the oral $LD_{50}$s of cyanuric acid were 7667 mg/kg bw in rats and 3378 mg/kg bw in mice. Therefore, the melamine-cyanurate complex is more toxic than melamine or cyanuric acid alone; but the melamine-cyanurate complex is less toxic than when the 2 chemicals are coadministered as individual compounds. Preliminary studies at CVM indicated that catfish dosed with melamine-cyanurate complex at a 400 mg/kg bw for 3 days do not develop crystals in their kidneys (Renate Reimschuessel, unpublished data, 2010).

Data on the toxicity of the combined administration of other melamine analogues, such as ammeline and ammelide, are also limited. Sheep dosed daily with a mixture of ammeline and ammelide at a total nonprotein nitrogen dose of 200 to 300 mg/kg bw developed anorexia, excessive urination, and diarrhea.[52] Clinical signs began approximately 4 weeks after the first dose and 15 of 30 sheep died between days 39 and 59 of the study. The renal tubules of these sheep contained round crystals that had radiating streaks and were birefringent with polarized light.[52] In contrast, sheep given a single oral dose of ammeline (647–1887 mg/kg bw) or ammelide (696–1823 mg/kg bw) developed no adverse clinical signs. However, conclusions about the melamine analogue data from the sheep studies should be drawn with caution, because the chemical purity in those studies was not reported and the methods to quantify all analogues present were not so refined in the 1960s as they are now. An investigation of acute renal failure of pigs in Spain between 2003 and 2006 suggested that a combination of ammeline and ammelide was responsible for these outbreaks.[5] Therefore, any combination of melamine analogues in food and feed must be carefully evaluated as a potential nephrotoxicant in animals. Because of the similar chemical structure among melamine analogues, it is possible that ammeline and ammelide can substitute for melamine and cyanuric acid in the formation of crystals.

## ANALYTICAL METHODS FOR THE ANALYSIS OF MELAMINE AND ANALOGUES IN FOOD AND BIOLOGIC MATRICES

Without the discovery of melamine and melamine analogues by analytical methodologies in suspect feed, the cause for the recall of pet food would have not been discovered. Therefore, the importance of analytical chemists in toxicologic and food safety investigations should be emphasized. Whenever outbreaks occur that may be linked to a common food source or environmental condition, systematic analytical testing is critical for excluding a compound from consideration. In addition, technologies suitable for detecting unknown compounds are essential for discovering new entities.

Melamine and melamine analogues are nitrogen-rich compounds. Illegal addition of these compounds to food occurs in part because the most commonly used methods for protein analyses in the food industry, the Kjeldahl and Dumas methods, cannot distinguish between nitrogen from protein sources and nitrogen from nonprotein sources. An incorrectly high protein measurement provides an economic incentive for adulteration with melamine and melamine analogues.

Melamine is used in the manufacture of melamine resins,[53] but has also been marketed as a fertilizer because of its high nitrogen content.[54] In the United States and Europe, melamine is not approved to be directly added to food. Melamine is a metabolite of cyromazine, which is used as an insect growth regulator for the control of fly larvae by feed-through application. Methods for the detection of residues of cyromazine and its metabolite melamine have been applied to vegetable crops.[55] Biuret is approved as a feed additive for ruminants in the United States and may contain up to 30% cyanuric acid, a by-product of its manufacture. Dichloroisocyanurate, which rapidly degrades to free chlorine and cyanuric acid, is used for water disinfection.

Before the 2007 outbreak in North America, several analytical methods had been developed for the analysis of melamine and cyanuric acid, but most of those were based on the detection of residues in crops or water.[56–58] As soon as melamine was discovered as an adulterant in recalled pet food, several FDA laboratories and veterinary diagnostic laboratories jointly developed analytical methods based on gas chromatography (GC) or liquid chromatography (LC) coupled with mass spectrometry (MS).[59] LC-MS/MS and GC-MS/MS are the methods of choice because of their high sensitivity and selectivity. The current method of choice for analysis of feed and feed ingredients for melamine and cyanuric acid is based on a novel chromatographic method that is based on hydrophilic interaction chromatography.[60]

In addition to the analysis of food and feed ingredients, analysis of muscle tissue for melamine residues became important when it was discovered that pet-food waste had been fed to swine, poultry, and fish.[19–21] The rapidly developed LC-MS/MS method provided critical information to the United States Department of Agriculture and the FDA in performing a risk assessment[4] because it allowed for accurate quantitation of melamine in pork muscle tissue at a low analytical detection limit of 1.7 ng/g. During the investigation of the pet-food recall, analysis of biologic specimens from pets suspected of having become ill or died of exposure to melamine and melamine analogues became important to the veterinary community. A suspect diagnosis could be confirmed by the detection of melamine and cyanuric acid in serum, urine, or kidney.[61] These methods are now well established and routinely offered by many veterinary diagnostic toxicology laboratories.

## GLOBAL FOOD-SAFETY IMPLICATIONS
### Global Outbreak Investigations of Pets and Pigs

Outbreaks associated with melamine and melamine analogue in pets and pigs have been confirmed from North America,[11,23] Korea,[6,62] Taiwan,[62] the Philippines,[62] Spain,[5] Thailand,[24] South Africa,[15] and Italy.[7] Melamine adulteration of foodstuffs had been reported in the 1980s, in potato meal in Germany,[63] and in both meat and fish meals in Italy.[64] However, this information was not widely known in those pre-Internet times. The fact that the incidence of melamine adulteration in imported products in Italy went from more than 70% in 1979 to 5% in 1987 shows the importance of an active surveillance program.

## Melamine-induced Nephropathy in Children

Starting in September of 2008, a sharp increase in the number of children diagnosed with kidney calculi and renal failure was noted in China. In contrast to the outbreaks of renal failure in dogs and cats induced by melamine-cyanuric acid in previous years, the urinary tract calculi of affected children consisted of uric acid and melamine at a molar ratio from 1.2:1 to 2.1:1; cyanuric acid was not detected in these calculi.[9,65–70] Infants were exposed to melamine alone, whereas animals from the adulteration episode were exposed to melamine and cyanuric acid and possibly ammeline and ammelide. Thus, there is a significant difference in the pathogenesis of renal failure induced by melamine between infants in 2008 and pets in 2007. In animals, melamine and cyanuric acid form renal crystals that result in nephropathy similar to acute uric acid nephropathy. In infants, melamine-uric acid stones form, which can cause obstructive renal failure. Infants are considered at greater risk for forming stones because they have higher urinary uric acid concentrations than adults.[71] Uric acid crystals and calculi form in the kidney when urine pH is less than 5.5, with increasing uric acid concentration, and with ongoing metabolic acidosis and dehydration.[43,72,73] The early effects of ingesting high doses of melamine alone have not been adequately characterized. Experiments have shown that weanling rats given more than 1.6% melamine in the diet develop uric acid-melamine stones within 1 month.[74] Presumably, these stones form from some type of crystal, likely melamine-urate or other types of crystals (probably melamine-cyanurate), but neither the morphology nor abundance of such crystals has been characterized. Microcrystals have been identified in kidney and urine sediment of rats dosed with melamine, but crystal composition was not determined.[74,75]

According to a report from the Chinese Ministry of Health from December 1, 2008, 22,384,000 examinations were conducted in infants with suspect melamine exposure. As of November 27, 2008, 294,000 infants had been diagnosed with urinary tract stones and sandlike calculi, 51,900 infants had been hospitalized, and 6 deaths had been confirmed.[76] It is assumed that more children developed urinary tract stones, but remained asymptomatic. The source of the illness was traced back to intentional addition of melamine to infant formula. One gram of melamine added to 1 L of milk leads to an apparent 0.4% increase in protein content.[77] Global distribution of infant formula contaminated with melamine resulted in at least 47 countries receiving such products.[78] The response taken by regulatory agencies varied greatly among countries, from doing nothing to testing all imported Chinese milk products, to banning the import of all milk and milk products from China. Although 6 infants died during the 2008 outbreak, the overall prognosis for melamine-uric acid exposure is considered good for infants who receive treatment. However, chronic studies in rats showed that melamine may induce bladder carcinoma.[74,75,79,80] Because data on long-term effects of melamine in humans do not exist, long-term follow-up of infants who recovered from obstructive nephropathy induced by uric acid-melamine is critical to gaining insight into long-term renal function and cancer incidence.

Because of the effect of milk contamination in China on food safety worldwide, many countries introduced limits for melamine in infant formula and other foods[81] and assessed a tolerable daily intake (TDI) value for melamine. A TDI does not imply that adulteration of food with melamine is acceptable. The World Health Organization established a TDI of 0.2 mg/kg bw of melamine that is applicable to humans of all ages.[76,82] In addition, an allowable concentration of 0.9 mg/L of melamine in drinking water was recently derived.[83] However, these data are applicable for exposure to melamine alone. If humans are exposed to mixtures of melamine and melamine analogues, calculi formation may occur at lower doses compared with relatively pure melamine exposure. However, there are insufficient data to allow the calculation of a health-based guidance value for coexposure to melamine analogues. Recently, the FDA reported NOAELs for crystal formation in 2 fish species. The single-dose NOAEL for catfish was 10 mg/kg bw, whereas trout had a lower NOAEL of 2.5 mg/kg bw. NOAELs for multiple daily dosing regimens of 4 days and 14 days were 2.5 and 0.5 mg/kg bw, respectively, for both species. Renal crystals did not form in catfish fed 0.1 mg/kg bw of each compound for 28 days, a dose comparable with 2.5 ppm of melamine and cyanuric acid in the feed.[84] Preliminary data from another NOAEL study indicated that crystals form in pigs fed diets containing 10 mg/kg bw melamine and 10 mg/kg bw cyanuric acid for 7 days.[85] Studies are currently in progress at the FDA to determine the NOAELs in rats after coexposure to melamine and cyanuric acid for prolonged periods.

## SUMMARY

Feedstuffs are vulnerable to chemical contamination. Because of the global nature of the food supply, increased surveillance of raw materials, animal feed, and human food is critical to rapidly detecting contaminants and assessing their risk. The intentional addition of melamine and melamine analogues to food and feed ingredients resulted in major outbreaks of poisoning associated with melamine and/or melamine analogue in animals and humans between 2003 and 2008. Although melamine or melamine analogues alone are unlikely to result in acute illness in animals, melamine alone can lead to stone formation with uric acid in children and animals. In animals, nephropathy induced by melamine-cyanurate (dogs, cats, pigs, fish) or ammeline-ammelide (pigs) crystals can lead to renal failure. Veterinary diagnostic laboratories, and in particular toxicology laboratories, play an essential role in monitoring for food- and feed-related outbreaks. Veterinary diagnostic laboratories integrate disease investigation with surveillance of animal health and thus can identify risk factors that may precede public health events.

## REFERENCES

1. Anonymous. Melamine pet food recall of 2007. Last updated April 30, 2009. Available at: http://www.fda.gov/AnimalVeterinary/SafetyHealth/RecallsWithdrawals/ucm129575.htm. Accessed May 12, 2010.
2. Anonymous. 104 deaths reported in pet food recall. New York Times; 2007. Available at: http://www.nytimes.com/2007/03/28/science/28brfs-pet.html. Accessed May 12, 2010.
3. Weise E, Schmitt J. FDA limits Chinese food additive imports. USA Today; 2007. Accessed May 12, 2010.
4. Anonymous. Interim melamine and analogues safety/risk assessment. Last updated May 22, 2009. Available at: http://www.fda.gov/ScienceResearch/SpecialTopics/PeerReviewofScientificInformationandAssessments/ucm155012.htm. Accessed May 12, 2010.
5. Gonzalez J, Puschner B, Perez V, et al. Nephrotoxicosis in Iberian piglets subsequent to exposure to melamine and derivatives in Spain between 2003 and 2006. J Vet Diagn Invest 2009;21:558–63.

6. Yhee JY, Brown CA, Yu CH, et al. Retrospective study of melamine/cyanuric acid-induced renal failure in dogs in Korea between 2003 and 2004. Vet Pathol 2009; 46:348–54.
7. Cocchi M, Vascellari M, Gallina A, et al. Canine nephrotoxicosis induced by melamine-contaminated pet food in Italy. J Vet Med Sci 2010;72:103–7.
8. ProMED-mail. Infant kidney stones – China: Gansu, milk powder suspected, request for information. 10 Sept 2008: 20080910.2828. 2008. Available at: http://www.fda.gov/ScienceResearch/SpecialTopics/PeerReviewofScientificInformationand Assessments/ucm155012.htm. Accessed May 12, 2010.
9. Sun Q, Shen Y, Sun N, et al. Diagnosis, treatment and follow-up of 25 patients with melamine-induced kidney stones complicated by acute obstructive renal failure in Beijing Children's Hospital. Eur J Pediatr 2010;169:483–9.
10. Burns K. Witnesses at congressional hearing talk about timing, imports, and surveillance. J Am Vet Med Assoc 2007;230:1601–2.
11. Cianciolo RE, Bischoff K, Ebel JG, et al. Clinicopathologic, histologic, and toxicologic findings in 70 cats inadvertently exposed to pet food contaminated with melamine and cyanuric acid. J Am Vet Med Assoc 2008;233:729–37.
12. Kerley D, Childs D. Pet food maker to take financial responsibility for pet deaths from poisoning. ABC News; 2007. Accessed May 14, 2010.
13. Dobson RL, Motlagh S, Quijano M, et al. Identification and characterization of toxicity of contaminants in pet food leading to an outbreak of renal toxicity in cats and dogs. Toxicol Sci 2008;106:251–62.
14. Reimschuessel R, Gieseker CM, Miller RA, et al. Evaluation of the renal effects of experimental feeding of melamine and cyanuric acid to fish and pigs. Am J Vet Res 2008;69:1217–28.
15. Reyers F. Melamine-contaminated pet food. The South African experience. Veterinary News; 2007.
16. Anonymous. USDA clears swine for processing. 2007. Available at: http://www.usda.gov/wps/portal/usda/usdahome?contentidonly=true&contentid=2007/05/0144.xml. Accessed May 15, 2010.
17. Anonymous. Transcripts of FDA Press conference on the pet food recall. 2007. Available at: http://www.fda.gov/downloads/NewsEvents/Newsroom/MediaTranscripts/UCM123617.pdf. Accessed August 17, 2010.
18. Anonymous. FDA: Melamine-tainted poultry, fish safe for humans. 2007. Available at: http://www.cnn.com/2007/HEALTH/05/18/pet.food.poultry.index.html. Accessed May 14, 2010.
19. Filigenzi MS, Tor ER, Poppenga RH, et al. The determination of melamine in muscle tissue by liquid chromatography/tandem mass spectrometry. Rapid Commun Mass Spectrom 2007;21:4027–32.
20. Karbiwnyk CM, Andersen WC, Turnipseed SB, et al. Determination of cyanuric acid residues in catfish, trout, tilapia, salmon and shrimp by liquid chromatography-tandem mass spectrometry. Anal Chim Acta 2009;637:101–11.
21. Andersen WC, Turnipseed SB, Karbiwnyk CM, et al. Determination and confirmation of melamine residues in catfish, trout, tilapia, salmon, and shrimp by liquid chromatography with tandem mass spectrometry. J Agric Food Chem 2008;56:4340–7.
22. Smoker M, Krynitsky AJ. Interim method for determination of melamine and cyanuric acid residues in foods using LC-MS/MS: Version 1.0. Laboratory Information Bulletin No. 4422 October 2008. Melamine and cyanuric acid residues in foods Last updated 2010. Available at: http://www.fda.gov/Food/ScienceResearch/LaboratoryMethods/DrugChemicalResiduesMethodology/ucm071673.htm. Accessed July 12, 2010.

23. Brown CA, Jeong KS, Poppenga RH, et al. Outbreaks of renal failure associated with melamine and cyanuric acid in dogs and cats in 2004 and 2007. J Vet Diagn Invest 2007;19:525–31.

24. Nilubol D, Pattanaseth T, Boonsri K, et al. Melamine- and cyanuric acid-associated renal failure in pigs in Thailand. Vet Pathol 2009;46:1156–9.

25. Anonymous. Report a problem. 2010. Available at: http://www.fda.gov/AnimalVeterinary/SafetyHealth/ReportaProblem/default.htm. Accessed July 14, 2010.

26. Rumbeiha W, Agnew D, Maxie G, et al. AAVLD survey of pet food-induced nephrotoxicity in North America, April to June 2007. In: Programs and abstracts of the 50th Annual Meeting of the American Association of Laboratory Animals Diagnosticians. Reno (NV), October 20–22, 2007.

27. Puschner B, Poppenga RH, Lowenstine LJ, et al. Assessment of melamine and cyanuric acid toxicity in cats. J Vet Diagn Invest 2007;19:616–24.

28. Thompson ME, Lewin-Smith MR, Kalasinsky VF, et al. Characterization of melamine-containing and calcium oxalate crystals in three dogs with suspected pet food-induced nephrotoxicosis. Vet Pathol 2008;45:417–26.

29. Osborne CA, Lulich JP, Ulrich LK, et al. Melamine and cyanuric acid-induced crystalluria, uroliths, and nephrotoxicity in dogs and cats. Vet Clin North Am Small Anim Pract 2009;39:1–14.

30. Anonymous. Urgent bulletin: pet food recall. 2007. Available at: http://www.labservices.uoguelph.ca/urgent.cfm. Accessed May 22, 2010.

31. Kim CW, Yun JW, Bae IH, et al. Determination of spatial distribution of melamine-cyanuric acid crystals in rat kidney tissue by histology and imaging matrix-assisted laser desorption/ionization quadruple time-of-flight mass spectrometry. Chem Res Toxicol 2010;23:220–7.

32. Fiechtner JJ, Simkin PA. Urate spherulites in gouty synovia. J Am Vet Med Assoc 1981;245:1533–6.

33. Melnick RL, Boorman GA, Haseman JK, et al. Urolithiasis and bladder carcinogenicity of melamine in rodents. Toxicol Appl Pharmacol 1984;72:292–303.

34. Lipschitz WL, Stokey E. The mode of action of three new diuretics – melamine, adenine and formoguanamine. J Pharmacol Exp Ther 1945;83:235–49.

35. Hammond BG, Barbee SJ, Inoue T, et al. A review of toxicology studies on cyanurate and its chlorinated derivatives. Environ Health Perspect 1986;69:287–92.

36. Hodge HC, Panner BJ, Downs WL, et al. Toxicity of sodium cyanurate. Toxicol Appl Pharmacol 1965;7:667–74.

37. Allen LM, Briggle TV, Pfaffenberger CD. Absorption and excretion of cyanuric acid in long-distance swimmers. Drug Metab Rev 1982;13:499–516.

38. Mast RW, Jeffcoat AR, Sadler BM, et al. Metabolism, disposition and excretion of [14C]melamine in male Fischer 344 rats. Food Chem Toxicol 1983;21:807–10.

39. Xu W, Dong MD, Gersen H, et al. Cyanuric acid and metamine on Au(111): structure and energetics of hydrogen-bonded networks. Small 2007;3:854–8.

40. Whitesides GM, Mathias JP, Seto CT. Molecular self-assembly and nanochemistry: a chemical strategy for the synthesis of nanostructures. Science 1991;254:1312–9.

41. Canelli E. Chemical, bacteriological, and toxicological properties of cyanuric acid and chlorinated isocyanurates as applied to swimming pool disinfection – review. Am J Public Health 1974;64:155–62.

42. Tolleson WH. Renal toxicity of pet foods contaminated with melamine and related compounds. In: Programs and abstracts of the 235th National Meeting of the American Chemical Society. New Orleans (LA), April 6–10, 2008.

43. Tiu RV, Mountantonakis SE, Dunbar AJ, et al. Tumor lysis syndrome. Semin Thromb Hemost 2007;33:397–407.

44. Davidson MB, Thakkar S, Hix JK, et al. Pathophysiology, clinical consequences, and treatment of tumor lysis syndrome. Am J Med 2004;116:546–54.
45. Conger JD. Acute uric acid nephropathy. Med Clin North Am 1990;74:859–71.
46. Kobayashi T, Okada A, Fujii Y, et al. The mechanism of renal stone formation and renal failure induced by administration of melamine and cyanuric acid. Urol Res 2010;38:117–25.
47. Chen KC, Liao CW, Cheng FP, et al. Evaluation of subchronic toxicity of pet food contaminated with melamine and cyanuric acid in rats. Toxicol Pathol 2009;37:959–68.
48. Ensley S, Imerman P, Copper V, et al. Determination of serum and tissue melamine and/or cyanuric acid concentrations in growing pigs. In: Programs and abstracts of the 50th Annual Meeting of the American Association of Laboratory Animal Diagnosticians. Reno (NV), October 20–22, 2007.
49. Puschner B, Reimschuessel R, Stine CB. Melamine contamination and pathology. In: Programs and abstracts of the 147th American Veterinary Medical Association Annual Convention. Atlanta (GA), July 31 to August 3, 2010.
50. Reimschuessel R, Stewart L, Squibb E, et al. Fish drug analysis – Phish-Pharm: a searchable database of pharmacokinetics data in fish. AAPS J 2005;7:E288–327.
51. Babayan AA, Aleksandryan AV. Toxicological characteristics of melamine cyanurate, melamine and cyanuric acid. Zh Eksp Klin Med 1985;25:345–9.
52. Mackenzie HI, Van Rensburg IBJ. Ammelide and ammeline as non-protein nitrogen supplements for sheep. J S Afr Vet Med Assoc 1968;39:41–5.
53. Anderson FA. Final report on the safety assessment of melamine/formaldehyde resin. J Am Coll Toxicol 1995;14:373–85.
54. Shelton DR, Karns JS, McCarty GW, et al. Metabolism of melamine by Klebsiella terragena. Appl Environ Microbiol 1997;63:2832–5.
55. Patakioutas G, Savvas D, Matakoulis C, et al. Application and fate of Cyromazine in a closed-cycle hydroponic cultivation of bean (Phaseolus vulgaris L.). J Agric Food Chem 2007;55:9928–35.
56. Briggle TV, Allen LM, Duncan RC, et al. High performance liquid chromatographic determination of cyanuric acid in human urine and pool water. J Assoc Off Anal Chem 1981;64:1222–6.
57. Fiamegos YC, Konidari CN, Stalikas CD. Cyanuric acid trace analysis by extractive methylation via phase-transfer catalysis and capillary gas chromatography coupled with flame thermoionic and mass-selective detection. Process parameter studies and kinetics. Anal Chem 2003;75:4034–42.
58. Toth JP, Bardalaye PC. Capillary gas chromatographic separation and mass spectrometric detection of cyromazine and its metabolite melamine. J Chromatogr 1987;408:335–40.
59. Anonymous. GC-MS method for screening and confirmation of melamine and related analogs. 2007. Available at: http://www.fda.gov/AboutFDA/CentersOffices/CVM/WhatWeDo/ucm134743.htm. Accessed May 26, 2010.
60. Heller DN, Nochetto CB. Simultaneous determination and confirmation of melamine and cyanuric acid in animal feed by zwitterionic hydrophilic interaction chromatography and tandem mass spectrometry. Rapid Commun Mass Spectrom 2008;22:3624–32.
61. Filigenzi MS, Puschner B, Aston LS, et al. Diagnostic determination of melamine and related compounds in kidney tissue by liquid chromatography/tandem mass spectrometry. J Agric Food Chem 2008;56:7593–9.
62. Anonymous. Pedigree brand dog food recalled in Asia after illnesses reported. 2004. Available at: http://findarticles.com/p/articles/mi_m0WDP/is_2004_March_15/ai_114410165/. Accessed May 26, 2010.

63. Bisaz R, Kummer A. Determination of 2,4,6-triamino-1,3,5-triazine (melamine) in potato proteins. Mitt Geb Lebensmittelunters Hyg 1983;74:74–9.
64. Cattaneo P, Ceriani L. Melamine contents in animals meals. Tecnica Molitoria 1988;39:29–32.
65. Lam CW, Lan L, Che X, et al. Diagnosis and spectrum of melamine-related renal disease: plausible mechanism of stone formation in humans. Clin Chim Acta 2009;402:150–5.
66. Zhu SL, Li JH, Chen L, et al. Conservative management of pediatric nephrolithiasis caused by melamine-contaminated milk powder. Pediatrics 2009;123: e1099–102.
67. Liu JM, Ren A, Yang L, et al. Urinary tract abnormalities in Chinese rural children who consumed melamine-contaminated dairy products: a population-based screening and follow-up study. CMAJ 2010;182:439–43.
68. Sun N, Shen Y, He LJ. Histopathological features of the kidney after acute renal failure from melamine. N Engl J Med 2010;362:662–4.
69. Wen JG, Li ZZ, Zhang H, et al. Melamine related bilateral renal calculi in 50 children: single center experience in clinical diagnosis and treatment. J Urol 2010; 183:1533–7.
70. Wang IJ, Chen PC, Hwang KC. Melamine and nephrolithiasis in children in Taiwan. N Engl J Med 2009;360:1157–8.
71. Fathallah-Shaykh S, Neiberger S. Uric acid stones. E-medicine. Updated July 8, 2008. Available at: http://emedicine.medscape.com/article/983759-overview. Accessed May 28, 2010.
72. Hall PM. Nephrolithiasis: treatment, causes, and prevention. Cleve Clin J Med 2009;76:583–91.
73. Kravitz SC, Diamond HD, Craver LF. Uremia complicating leukemia chemotherapy; report of a case treated with triethylene melamine. J Am Med Assoc 1951;146:1595–7.
74. Heck HD, Tyl RW. The induction of bladder stones by terephthalic acid, dimethyl terephthalate, and melamine (2,4,6-triamino-s-triazine) and its relevance to risk assessment. Regul Toxicol Pharmacol 1985;5:294–313.
75. Ogasawara H, Imaida K, Ishiwata H, et al. Urinary bladder carcinogenesis induced by melamine in F344 male rats: correlation between carcinogenicity and urolith formation. Carcinogenesis 1995;16:2773–7.
76. Organization WH. Toxicological and health aspects of melamine and cyanuric acid: report of a WHO expert meeting in collaboration with FAO, supported by Health Canada, Ottawa, Canada, 1–4 December, 2008. Geneva (Switzerland): World Health Organization; 2009.
77. Hau AK, Kwan TH, Li PK. Melamine toxicity and the kidney. J Am Soc Nephrol 2009;20:245–50.
78. Gossner CM, Schlundt J, Ben Embarek P, et al. The melamine incident: implications for international food and feed safety. Environ Health Perspect 2009;117:1803–8.
79. Okumura M, Hasegawa R, Shirai T, et al. Relationship between calculus formation and carcinogenesis in the urinary bladder of rats administered the non-genotoxic agents thymine or melamine. Carcinogenesis 1992;13:1043–5.
80. Cremonezzi DC, Diaz MP, Valentich MA, et al. Neoplastic and preneoplastic lesions induced by melamine in rat urothelium are modulated by dietary polyunsaturated fatty acids. Food Chem Toxicol 2004;42:1999–2007.
81. Akesson MT, Point CC, di Caracalla VT. Proposed draft maximum levels for melamine in food and feed. In: Joint FAO/WHO CCoCiF, editor. 2010. CX/CF 10/4/5. Available at: http://www.cclac.org. Accessed July 14, 2010.

82. Anonymous. International experts limit melamine levels in food – new guidance to help improve food safety provided by UN Food Standards Commission. 2010. Available at: http://www.who.int/mediacentre/news/releases/2010/melamine_food_20100706/en/index.html. Accessed July 12, 2010.
83. Bhat VS, Ball GL, McLellan CJ. Derivation of a melamine oral reference dose (RfD) and drinking-water total allowable concentration. J Toxicol Environ Health B Crit Rev 2010;13:16–50.
84. Reimschuessel R, Evans ER, Stine CB, et al. Renal crystal formation after combined or sequential oral administration of melamine and cyanuric acid. Food Chem Toxicol 2010;48(10):2898–906.
85. Reimschuessel R, Evans ER, Stine CB, et al. Fish – a non-mammalian model for determining a "No Observable Effect Level" (NOEL) for crystal formation in kidneys after exposure to melamine and cyanuric acid. In: Programs and abstracts of the 238th National Meeting of the American Chemical Society. Washington, DC, August 16–20, 2009.

# A Novel Educational Tool for Teaching Diagnostic Reasoning and Laboratory Data Interpretation to Veterinary (and Medical) Students

Holly S. Bender, DVM, PhD*, Jared A. Danielson, PhD

KEYWORDS

• Clinical pathology • Case based learning • Problem solving
• Diagnostic reasoning • Expert thinking • Cognitive tool
• Learning • Software design and development

Readers of *Clinics in Laboratory Medicine* no doubt share an interest in laboratory science and clinical pathology, but it is likely that few dreamed of becoming laboratorians while growing up. More often, interest in clinical pathology is piqued by particular courses or instructors or when we discover the compelling power of laboratory data to uncover and clarify hidden disease. Experienced diagnosticians, veterinarians, and physicians, with expertise developed over years of diligent study and practice, become increasingly adept at learning to trace back through a cascade of data abnormalities, using logic to connect them to underlying mechanisms of disease and ultimately identifying failing organ systems. They also learn to value data that assure of healthy organ

The contents of this article were partially developed under a grant from the Learning Anytime Anywhere Partnerships (LAAP), a program of the Fund for the Improvement of Postsecondary Education (FIPSE), US Department of Education, as well as 2 grants from the US Department of Agriculture (USDA) Higher Education Challenge program in addition to seed funding from Virginia Tech and Iowa State University. However, these contents do not necessarily represent the policy of the Department of Education or USDA, and you should not assume endorsement by the Federal Government.
The authors have nothing to disclose.
Department of Veterinary Pathology, College of Veterinary Medicine, Iowa State University, 1600 South 16th Street, Ames, IA 50011, USA
* Corresponding author.
*E-mail address:* hbender@iastate.edu

Clin Lab Med 31 (2011) 201–215
doi:10.1016/j.cll.2010.10.007
0272-2712/11/$ – see front matter © 2011 Elsevier Inc. All rights reserved.

labmed.theclinics.com

function. It can provide immense satisfaction to use diagnostic reasoning skills to uncover answers hidden in laboratory data and by doing so, provide a rational foundation for effective treatment, often sparing patients pain, suffering, and invasive additional diagnostic procedures.

It takes many years of deliberate practice to become an expert in complex disciplines.[1] Articles spanning 4 decades have explored how expert diagnosticians develop their expertise, how they think, and how best to teach diagnostic reasoning.[2–11] In a recent extensive review of this research, Norman[12] shows how this inquiry has generally shifted from an exploration of general problem-solving strategies to how and what diagnosticians remember and mental representations of knowledge. The outcome has been inconclusive, leading Norman to declare that "there is no such thing as clinical reasoning; there is no one best way through a problem."[p426] Considering the complexity of laboratory medicine and understanding expertise in this area, it is easy to appreciate the amount of time and effort needed for mastery. The author (H.S.B.) started to truly appreciate the difficulty of developing expertise in laboratory medicine when first attempting to teach novices (ie, students) the art and science of clinical pathology in the early 1980s. My experience in teaching a course to second-year veterinary students was the genesis of the Diagnostic Pathfinder, a software tool designed by our research group to help students learn to interpret laboratory data. Today, the Diagnostic Pathfinder is used by clinical pathology faculty at 11 veterinary schools in the United States and Canada, a veterinary diagnostic laboratory, as well as one Australian and two European veterinary schools. It also has been adapted to teach clinical pharmacology, toxicology, and parasitology at our institution. The Diagnostic Pathfinder also has strong applicability for teaching medical students laboratory data interpretation.

This article first outlines the barriers to learning laboratory data interpretation. Second, it outlines the Diagnostic Pathfinder and how it addresses each of these barriers. Third, it presents the theoretical underpinnings of the Diagnostic Pathfinder, providing evidence that supports its value in the cognitive process of diagnostic reasoning. We invite readers to contact us for more information about the Diagnostic Pathfinder.

## TEACHING AND LEARNING THE PROCESS OF LABORATORY DIAGNOSIS

Laboratory diagnosis is taught in many different courses and settings in both veterinary and medical curricula. Some curricula start with an introductory course in clinical pathology, and in other programs, laboratory diagnosis is integrated into various organ systems or medicine courses. Regardless of the approach, the ultimate goal of introductory clinical pathology courses is to facilitate proficiency in the interpretation of clinical pathology data. This article focuses on early courses in clinical pathology in which students encounter large amounts of laboratory data for the first time and need to develop proficiency in diagnostic reasoning.

### Clinical Pathology in the Veterinary Curriculum

Before the introduction of Diagnostic Pathfinder, we had a successful introductory clinical pathology course with many useful teaching strategies. Taking the lead from our mentors, my coinstructor and I designed the course around a set of approximately 100 cases of increasing complexity. With these cases (then on paper), students applied their new knowledge and practiced their diagnostic skills in realistic scenarios before practicing on real patients during their clinical years. Concepts of clinical pathology were first introduced in a lecture format and grounded in basic physiology and pathophysiology. We used a systems approach to introduce the key concepts of clinical pathology, incrementally starting with the erythron, where after establishing a foundation in red cell physiology and health, we moved on to lectures on alterations of erythrocytes and their associated laboratory data in disease. Carefully timed homework assignments of simple cases worked on paper illustrated hemorrhage, hemolysis, anemia of renal failure,and so on, giving students the opportunity to apply the knowledge of erythrocyte kinetics, for example, and to build their new skills. Interactive in-class discussions of homework cases enabled students to refine their diagnostic proficiency and deepen understanding. Lectures concerning leukocytes followed the erythrocyte section, and the accompanying homework cases grew in complexity. Cases targeting leukocyte concepts also included erythrocyte data as "fair game" when our paper patients afflicted by inflammatory diseases developed anemia of chronic disorders. The remaining systems were stepped-in using a similar format. We chose cases carefully to introduce new concepts incrementally, while repeating previous concepts, each time in a different case scenario; cases became progressively more complex.

### Challenges in Learning Diagnostic Reasoning

For years, these students (novices) had watched their clinical mentors (experts) glance at laboratory reports and arrive at a diagnosis seemingly instantaneously, and they were eager to acquire similar lightning-fast analytical skills. The tie between the assigned cases and their goal of becoming diagnosticians was immediately clear, requiring little prodding or explanation from their teachers. We saw students become intensely engaged both intellectually and emotionally as they learned to formulate and communicate their diagnostic rationale.

To some students, it was a joy from the beginning as they learned to crack the code inherent in becoming a diagnostician. To many, however, once the cases became challenging, it became a difficult and frustrating transition from a training system in which rote memorization was the predominant learning strategy to one where complex thinking and problem solving was required. Although there was general agreement among students concerning the value of case studies, the prospect of changing learning strategies after 20 or more years of academic success was excruciating for many. Students struggling with the change in learning strategies grappled with the difficult combination of high emotional engagement with the cases and little initial success in solving them. Some were certain that their first awkward attempts at solving cases were a litmus test indicating their dismal future as veterinary diagnosticians.

Despite assurances that their skills would surely improve with practice and the abundance of cases to work on, those who struggled with the transition to this new learning strategy saw enormous disparity between themselves and the stars of the class who seemed to "get it" with ease. Frustration turned to anger. Some confided a resistance to even begin their homework, or at best made feeble efforts. Some students admitted a growing resentment at the panic that ensued after reading the initial history, because when they did so, the diagnosis did not pop into their minds immediately as it seemed to for their mentors. To cope with this situation, struggling students would read the history, jump to a diagnosis and then look at the data. Laboratory data that supported their presumptive diagnosis were included in the rationale; however, data refuting this diagnosis were often ignored. Of course, this led to more frustration when the struggling students' diagnoses were completely and repeatedly unrelated to their instructor's. When my coinstructor and I tried to dissuade students from this approach, they often complained about the difficulty in learning clinical pathology and wished it could be more like anatomy, where one either knows a structure or does not. Cases with laboratory data require a different strategy; much more is involved, requiring a different approach whereby rote memorization is not sufficient.

### The Challenge of Assessment

An important complication inherent in using case-based problem solving is that it is difficult to reward students directly with credit for keeping up with their homework. Grading detailed case solutions for 100 or more students is an insurmountable task for instructors with many competing faculty duties. However, without accountability for completing homework assignments, students tend to resort to their usual methods of learning by memorizing and cramming before examinations, then often performing poorly.

In class, we reviewed the diagnostic rationale of each case the day it was due, but by then, the stars were surging ahead and those who struggled were losing interest, resulting in more anger, more resentment, and no eye contact with their instructors in the halls. However, eventually, persistence paid off with seemingly countless discussions, demonstrations, and alternate explanations of the diagnostic process. Predictably, each year, after about half to two-thirds of the semester had passed, clarity ultimately came. At that time, all was well and most students had gained a respectable level of proficiency. Then, without fail, several students would approach me to explain their new understanding with enthusiasm and to ask why I had not ever explained how to approach the diagnostic process!

## MEETING EDUCATIONAL CHALLENGES WITH THE DIAGNOSTIC PATHFINDER

There had to be a better and less stressful way to learn for all concerned. So began a multidisciplinary partnership of extraordinary people who brought their talents and skills to build a remarkable computer program. The Diagnostic Pathfinder software emerged from the instructional process described earlier and built on its strengths. The primary goal was to approach the instructional problems described with a well-designed solution using computer technology. The specific goals were to (1) gate the process of completing the homework cases, thereby preventing students from jumping to conclusions before evaluating all the data, (2) require students to name all the abnormalities in the data with the proper medical terminology, (3) require students to form hypotheses of the underlying pathophysiologic mechanisms in an outline format using drag-and-drop technology to place supporting data beneath each mechanism, (4) require completion of this outline before making a diagnosis, and (5) give students credit for submitting a solution online before case discussions (**Table 1**). Because we were unable to identify existing software that addressed these goals, we developed the Diagnostic Pathfinder.

### Design, Development, and Implementation of the Software Tool

In 1997, we formed a multidisciplinary Biomedical Informatics Research Group to create the instructional and interface design of the software and to evaluate its effectiveness on student and faculty users. The design process began with faculty and student interviews to refine and extend the vision as well as to define how to make it work as a software program. Filmed observations documented students as they created solutions for their paper cases, skipping over data and jumping to the diagnosis, thereby confirming the need to gate this process and require completeness. This front-end analysis led to the creation of paper prototypes for multiple iterations of interface design and usability testing. The software was first piloted as a homework

**Table 1**
**Main instructional challenges in interpreting laboratory data and how these challenges are addressed by the Diagnostic Pathfinder**

| Instructional Challenge | Pathfinder Element to Address the Challenge |
| --- | --- |
| Students jump to conclusions before evaluating all the data | Gate the process of completing cases; students must identify and name data abnormalities and then complete their rationale before making a diagnosis |
| Students must learn new vocabulary, especially in an introductory class | Require students to name all data abnormalities using proper medical terminology |
| Students struggle to make connections between seemingly disparate clinical findings, data abnormalities, and pathophysiologic mechanisms of disease | Require students to form hypotheses of the underlying pathophysiologic mechanisms in an outline format using drag-and-drop technology to place supporting data beneath each mechanism |
| Students need incentive (credit) to engage in meaningful practice | Give students credit for submitting a solution online before case discussions in the classroom |

tool by a group of 10 veterinary students at Virginia Polytechnic Institute and State University; it was used to demonstrate the diagnostic process to the class and to lead case discussions. The second part of the project involved dissemination of the software to clinical pathologists teaching comparable courses at veterinary schools at the University of Wisconsin, University of California-Davis, and University of Guelph. In addition, we piloted a continuing education program for veterinary practitioners at the Veterinary Information Network, an online education source.

### A Brief Demonstration of the Software

Participating instructors can enroll students in the Diagnostic Pathfinder via the Internet from anywhere in the world. We prefer the institutional e-mail address as a login ID so that students are readily identified by affiliation. Students download the software to their computers via a link to the Iowa State University College of Veterinary Medicine (ISU-CVM) server. The Pathfinder is a Java (Sun Microsystems, Inc, Santa Clara, CA, USA)-based application, which once installed, can run online or offline, needing to connect only for initial installation and case submission. Once logged in, the student opens a case from a list in their course. We typically assign 72 cases for homework in the clinical pathology course at the ISU-CVM.

The first window typically contains a picture of the patient and a short text description of history, signalment, and physical examination findings (**Fig. 1**). Using the mouse, the student selects relevant data and clicks the *Record Observation* button, which causes the selected data to appear under *Observations and Data Abnormalities*. Additional observations can be recorded in a notes field or as free text. Once all the relevant physical findings are noted, the student clicks on the next tab, *Lab Data* (**Fig. 2**). The format of the lab data window is designed to resemble a routine clinical laboratory data report on which the default assessment for all laboratory data is *Normal*. The student starts with the basic task of identifying laboratory data values that are outside the reference interval. Then, the student must correctly name each data abnormality using the proper medical term, which takes basic cognitive skills that are typically not difficult for veterinary students but which help them learn medical terminology. Some students

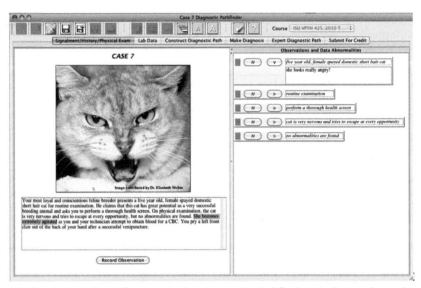

**Fig. 1.** The first window of a case in the Diagnostic Pathfinder. Students select relevant history, signalment, and physical examination findings, which then appear in the right-hand column under Observations and Data Abnormalities, where they are identified with an H for history.

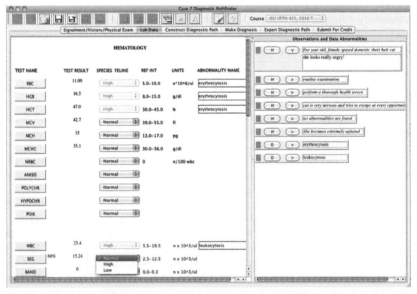

**Fig. 2.** The Lab Data window. Test names are abbreviated on buttons, which can be clicked to reveal the full name of the test. Pull-down menus are used to assess data as normal, high, or low. Correct assessment causes the cursor to jump into an Abnormality Name box where the appropriate medical term must be typed in and spelled accurately. Correctly named data abnormalities are automatically added to the list in the right-hand window where they are identified with a D for data.

report this as a good way to relieve tension associated with not yet knowing the diagnosis, as it eases them into the process of forming a diagnostic rationale. If the abnormality is named correctly, it is appended to the growing list of observations and data abnormalities. If the data abnormality is named incorrectly or misspelled, the system returns feedback requiring that the student try again and correct it. Faculty authors can allow as many synonyms as desired for the names of laboratory data abnormalities; the system requires the student to type in one of them. If the student tries 3 times without success, they can ask the system to show them the correct term and then type it to proceed. We elected this option so that students would not become stuck at this point if they could not correctly name a data abnormality. All abnormal data must be identified and named; the system does not allow a student to jump ahead to the diagnosis before doing so.

Once all the data abnormalities are assessed and named properly, the student is allowed to move on to the *Diagnostic Path Constructor* window (**Figs. 3** and **4**), which is where they formulate the diagnostic rationale (the *diagnostic path*) that connects data abnormalities to the underlying pathophysiologic mechanisms of disease. This is the central and most important part of the Diagnostic Pathfinder. Here, the student enters a hypothesis as a *New Mechanism* to explain the underlying pathophysiologic mechanism of one or more associated data abnormalities. Mechanisms are free text

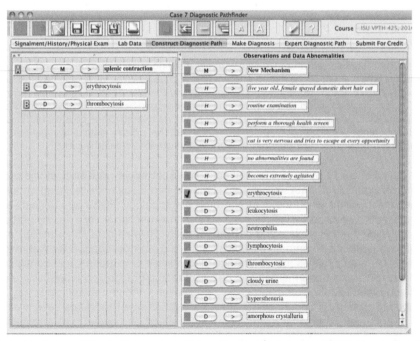

**Fig. 3.** The Diagnostic Path Constructor window. Students enter a hypothesis as a mechanism to explain the observations and data abnormalities. A New Mechanism can be dragged into place from the right side or can be created by right clicking in the appropriate area on the left or by using a button on the toolbar. The diagnostic path in the left window is created by the drag and drop of elements from the right window by holding down the mouse button on the blue square. In this case, "splenic contraction" is the mechanism (M) hypothesized to explain 2 data (D) abnormalities, erythrocytosis and thrombocytosis. As each data abnormality is dragged into place, it is checked off on the list to the right.

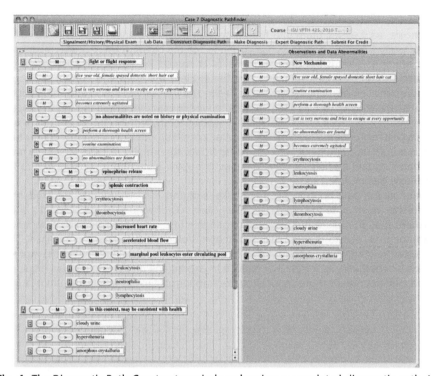

**Fig. 4.** The Diagnostic Path Constructor window showing a completed diagnostic path. In this example, a fight or flight response (epinephrine release) accounts for the physical findings of agitation and nervousness and is supported by the lack of other clinical abnormalities. The splenic contraction data grouping has been dragged beneath the physical findings; the splenic contraction and leukocyte data groupings are related to the physical findings by the intervening mechanism of epinephrine release. The urinary data abnormalities are grouped separately because they can be observed in otherwise healthy cats.

and are not checked by the system for accuracy, spelling, or plausibility at this point. Each observation and data abnormality is moved into place under existing or newly named mechanisms using the drag-and-drop methodology. Placement beneath and to the right of a mechanism indicates support for that mechanism or a causal relationship between the mechanism and data abnormality. Related data abnormalities may be grouped under a common mechanism, providing stronger support for that mechanism. Data abnormalities may be dragged individually or in groups, and contiguous and noncontiguous abnormalities can be selected and dragged together using shift-click, control-click, or command-click combinations. Abnormalities also may be dragged in repeatedly under several alternate mechanisms if there are several alternate hypotheses. Additional mechanisms are created as needed and arranged in a hierarchical path to explain all observations and data abnormalities.

Students tie the observations and data abnormalities together into a coherent explanation based on the hypothesized pathophysiologic mechanisms (see **Fig. 4**). Each parent-child data grouping can be collapsed and dragged as a unit or selected as a group and dragged into place. The rationale now begins to tell a story. In the example illustrated, the apparently healthy cat is agitated, resulting in a fight or flight response that causes a release of epinephrine and results in contraction of the spleen, increased heart rate, and accelerated blood flow, mechanisms that explain the hematologic abnormalities.

A novice learner trying to interpret leukocytosis without this context might have assumed that an inflammatory response was present, or concentrated urine may have been misinterpreted as a sign of dehydration. Within this context, however, the leukocyte changes make more sense as simply demargination from tachycardia and accelerated blood flow rather than as inflammation. Furthermore, without physical findings supporting dehydration, hypersthenuria is likely an incidental finding (cats are very efficient at concentrating their urine). It is important for students to learn that some laboratory findings such as amorphous urinary crystals, although noted on laboratory reports, are often not clinically significant. This example illustrates how the *Diagnostic Path Constructor* window supports the goal of finding connections between related data, explaining the data groupings with the underlying pathophysiology, and tying together the rationale in a coherent story or diagnostic path. Unlike with paper and pencil, students can drag the data groupings around repeatedly until the rationale makes sense, expressing the story in their own personal way.

Progression to making a diagnosis is contingent on every observation and data abnormality being dragged under and thus explained by at least 1 mechanism. Once students are satisfied with their case solution, they can enter a diagnosis by clicking on the *Make Diagnosis* tab. The *Diagnosis* box that appears is a free text field and is not checked for spelling or accuracy by the system. After entering their diagnosis, students click on the *Make Diagnosis* button, which freezes their solution and causes the system to reveal the instructor's *Expert Diagnostic Path* for a side-by-side comparison while the case is fresh in the student's mind (**Fig. 5**). The expert solution may be color-coded by the faculty author to emphasize certain mechanisms. Students are then asked to self-assess how well their solution matches the instructor's solution. This self-assessment is meant only to communicate an assurance of a student's perceived competence or concern. The student also receives confirmation of on-time submission and course credit. The system awards a point for each case solution submitted on time, regardless of its quality. In-class quizzes (explained later) are used to measure mastery of the diagnostic process.

As the course progresses, cases become increasingly lengthy and complex, repeating common themes like stress leukograms and dehydration and building incrementally as

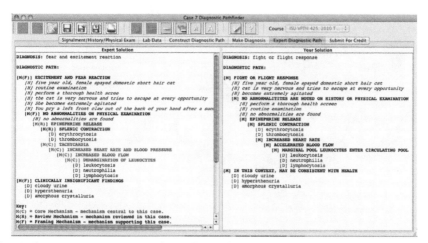

**Fig. 5.** The Expert Diagnostic Path window. After students submit their diagnosis, they receive immediate expert feedback. Their diagnostic path/case solution (on the *right*) is shown side-by-side with the instructor's (expert) solution (on the *left*).

new systems are studied. Hyperlinks to photomicrographs illustrate microscopic or gross findings (**Fig. 6**). Cases and the expert path can also be linked to e-books, medical databases such as PubMed, Web sites, virtual slides, videos, and other reference material.

Three other tools support the Diagnostic Pathfinder: the Course Manager to create courses, transfer cases, and enroll students; the Case Editor to facilitate and automate the tasks involved in case authoring or editing; and the Report Generator to quickly view student solutions and manage course credit.

## RESEARCH RESULTS AND THEORETICAL FOUNDATIONS—WHY IT WORKS

Although software tools that look nice and work as designed might be considered a useful end in and of themselves, we were committed to determining the extent to which this software actually helped alleviate the problems it was designed to address. We designed and conducted several studies to evaluate the software and the experience of students and faculty using the software.[13–15]

### Effects on Student Learning

First, we wanted to find out if students learned clinical pathology better using the Diagnostic Pathfinder and if their experience was more pleasant. We found that students who used the Pathfinder performed significantly better on case-based final examination questions than those who participated in curricular processes that used paper-based cases, but they were otherwise identical (**Table 2**).[13,15] Similarly,

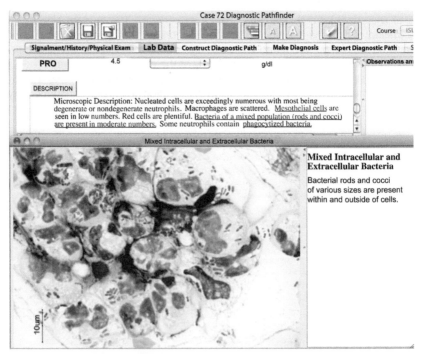

**Fig. 6.** Photomicrographs and other resources can be linked to the cases. In this example, an image of neutrophils with intracellular bacteria is linked to the microscopic description of an exudate in an animal with an effusion.

**Table 2**
Differences in percentage final examination scores obtained by students using the Diagnostic
Pathfinder compared with control students at 3 different institutions

| Study Design | Pathfinder Mean | Control Mean | P Value[a] | Effect Size[b] | References |
|---|---|---|---|---|---|
| Pathfinder vs paper-based control (Institution 1) | 87.3 ± 10.1 (n = 173) | 81.6 ± 9.8 (n = 334) | <.0005 | 0.58 | 5 |
| Pathfinder vs paper-based control (Institution 2) | 90.1 ± 6.5 (n = 126) | 85.0 ± 8.1 (n = 120) | <.0005 | 0.70 | 7 |
| Pathfinder as a supplement (Institution 3) | 87.0 ± 5.7 (n = 113) | 84.7 ± 7.1 (n = 199) | .002 | 0.36 | 7 |

[a] Independent samples $t$-test.
[b] Cohen's d.

students using the Pathfinder as a supplemental instructional strategy also outscored their counterparts participating in otherwise identical instruction.[15] Students also indicated that using the Pathfinder made their homework more enjoyable and made learning clinical pathology easier.[13,15] These results have been consistent across thousands of students at 7 veterinary colleges where evaluations have been performed one or more times (depending on the college) between 2002 and 2010.

## Mitigating the Cognitive Load

Second, we wanted to explore the effectiveness of the Diagnostic Pathfinder in mitigating the cognitive load imposed by the diagnostic reasoning process. Cognitive scientists have known for decades that there are predictable limits to the mind's capacity to process information. One of the best-known early efforts to quantify the ability to manage cognitive load came from George Miller's[16] landmark article. In attempting to unify several studies regarding what is now commonly referred to as the mind's working memory, Miller suggested that the mind can recall about 7 new stimuli, without recoding (in Miller's words, chunking) the information in some way. Sweller[17] proposed cognitive load theory as a useful framework for evaluating learning tasks in light of the limitations of the mind's working memory and in terms of the kinds of load that those learning tasks impose on cognitive processes. Given the best available current estimates of working memory limitations, cognitive load theorists work under the assumption that working memory can hold no more than 5 to 9 information elements and can actively process no more than 2 to 4 elements simultaneously.[18]

Theoretically, there are 3 kinds of loads that might be involved in a learning task. Intrinsic load is the inherently irreducible requirement of a specific cognitive task. Intrinsic load cannot be reduced without changing the task itself. For example, for an experienced clinician, diagnosing and developing a treatment protocol for a patient with hyperadrenocorticism might be easily accomplished with very little effort and therefore have very little intrinsic load. A veterinary or medical student might find the same task insurmountable unless it is simplified (changed) in some way. Such a change might entail reducing the task to manageable pieces (first considering history, then carefully examining laboratory data with reference to notes, then reviewing the pathophysiology of suspected diseases, and so forth). As the student becomes more capable, the intrinsic load of diagnostic problem solving for familiar cases/conditions is reduced for that student. Extraneous cognitive load comes from tasks that are irrelevant to or unnecessary in accomplishing the learning task. For example, poor, incomplete, or inaccurate explanations or distractions impose extraneous cognitive load. Germane cognitive load channels cognitive resources in helpful directions for learning. Clear explanations and relevant practice tasks are examples of teaching interventions that might provide germane cognitive load.

We posited that the Diagnostic Pathfinder helps students learn the difficult task of integrating clinical laboratory data by reducing extraneous cognitive load and introducing germane cognitive load. There can be little doubt that integrating clinical laboratory data to explain even a simple clinical case imposes considerable cognitive load on veterinary and medical students. They must simultaneously consider multiple disruptions in different organ systems, many potential disease processes, and, in the case of veterinary students, comparative information for multiple species. The specific ways in which we think this is accomplished has emerged through analysis of survey data from hundreds of students and interviews with faculty.[14]

First, the Pathfinder provides detailed, relevant feedback at the moment of highest interest to students—just as they have finished working through the problem, when their own solution is fresh in their mind. Although the benefit of feedback is well documented,[19,20] seeing a solution to the problem in the same format as their own solution and at the moment of highest engagement imposes germane cognitive load that is particularly powerful.

Second, the Pathfinder gates the learning task. Students first identify abnormal data and name the abnormality correctly—then they explain it. All data must be identified before it is explained, and all data must be explained before it is compared with the expert solution. This strategy reduces the intrinsic cognitive load of the overall learning task, allowing students to master these skills and combine knowledge and skills into integrated conceptual units (chunks) for later use.[21] Our studies[13,15] showed that the learning benefits achieved while using the Pathfinder were demonstrated under circumstances in which the gating requirement was no longer present (ie, taking a final examination on paper), suggesting that the individual tasks were indeed chunked during learning and the Pathfinder was not simply functioning as a "crutch" or aid.

Third, data manipulation is easy via the drag-and-drop interface. Students can easily try out multiple explanations, playing with the data until the system says what they want it to say. This feature is likely to reduce the extraneous cognitive load imposed by manipulating data in less-flexible formats (such as paper).

Fourth, the Pathfinder environment is safe for students to engage with the problems without the fear of making an embarrassing and/or high-stakes mistake. To the extent fear of mistakes or failure imposes extraneous cognitive load, it can divert students from the goal of learning.

Finally, although not an objective of our study, we found that sequencing cases from simple to more complex was instrumental in managing the intrinsic cognitive load when learning how to interpret laboratory data.[18]

## CLASSROOM IMPLEMENTATION STRATEGIES

Our university partners have implemented the Pathfinder in many different ways. The number of cases used in a single course has varied from 5 to 108. The Pathfinder has been implemented in both core courses and supplemental electives. Cases have been integrated into lecture and laboratory settings and have been used for instruction with introductory students, fourth year students, residents, and practicing veterinarians.

Pathfinder cases have been used for homework, in-class practice activities, and testing. Most instructors have used existing cases and solutions, but some have entered their own solutions, and still others have authored extensive sets of their own cases and solutions. Although Pathfinder implementations have varied, all instructors have chosen to sequence cases beginning with simple cases and gradually increasing case complexity, with later cases that usually repeat and build on themes introduced in earlier cases.

One recent major adaptation of Pathfinder use in our course at Iowa State University involved the addition of team-based learning (TBL) strategies. TBL is intended to engage students who are using the Pathfinder in helping each other gain skills in diagnostic reasoning. The TBL strategy uses teams of 6 students each, some of which engage from a satellite location in Nebraska via 2-way video technology. Approximately 6 Pathfinder cases are assigned per week as homework, following pertinent lecture material; 2 cases are due at the beginning of each case discussion session, and a third new case is assigned as an in-class quiz. The third case has learning objectives similar to one of the homework assignments but is set in a different scenario or involves a different species. For example, the homework assignment following lectures on hemolytic anemia includes a case of a cat with extravascular hemolysis caused by *Mycoplasma hemofelis* infection and a case of a horse with an intravascular hemolysis from red maple poisoning. The quiz on the following day is a case of a dog with extravascular immune-mediated hemolytic anemia. As part of the quiz, students answer 5 multiple-choice questions designed to probe deeply into their understanding of the various pathophysiologic mechanisms underlying hemolysis. The students first take the quiz individually and then again with their team. Both the individual and the team scores contribute to their grade. Team quizzes are animated and lively, as team members must arrive at a consensus solution; when doing so, they teach each other complicated concepts while communicating and convincing one another of the intricacies and correctness of their solutions.

## OUR FUTURE IN THINKSPACE

The Diagnostic Pathfinder has strong potential to facilitate learning in multiple disciplines, as well as in advanced clinical pathology courses, residency training programs, and as continuing education for veterinary practitioners. We are currently partnering with faculty in fields as diverse as toxicology, parasitology, pharmacology, internal medicine, anatomic pathology, materials science engineering, physics, horticulture, and geology, both to reengineer the Pathfinder and to combine it with other software into a more flexible and extensible learning tool. ThinkSpace is open source software based on Google Web Toolkit technology (Google, Inc, Mountain View, CA, USA). The ThinkSpace interface will allow authors to add differential diagnoses, give students the ability to select tests, and add the option to choose treatments. These expanded functionalities will enhance the applicability of the Pathfinder to other courses in which diagnostic reasoning is taught.

## SUMMARY

Several studies have shown that the use of the Diagnostic Pathfinder is associated with improved performance and student satisfaction. The Pathfinder helps learners compensate for the difficulty inherent in diagnostic problem solving by assisting them in managing cognitive load: gating the process, providing for easy manipulation of many conceptual elements in the diagnostic path, and providing timely and relevant feedback. The Pathfinder has been used successfully in a variety of settings and contexts. Although those implementations have varied, all share a common sequencing of cases from simple to complex, with later cases building on information contained in earlier cases.

## ACKNOWLEDGMENTS

Thousands of students and many faculty, staff, and administrators have contributed to the success of the Diagnostic Pathfinder. The authors wish to acknowledge and thank everyone who has helped to develop this tool or been instrumental in its support. Eric M. Mills and Pamela J. Vermeer were fundamental to the Pathfinder's development, and it would not have been completed without their involvement. Other major contributors include Laura Baseler, G. Daniel Boon (deceased), Angela Brokman, Mary Christopher, Roberta Di Terlizzi, Jeanne George, Cody Hankins, Debby Hix, Andrea Warner Honigmann, Julie Jarvinen, Karen Levitan, Richard Martin, Peggy Meszaros, Matthew Miller, Jelena Ostojic, Gary Osweiler, Paul Pion, Steven Stockham, Kristina Taylor, Seth Vredenburg, Tracy Wilkins, Darren Wood, Sonja Wiersma, and Karen Young.

## REFERENCES

1. Ericsson KA. Deliberate practice and the acquisition and maintenance of expert performance in medicine and related domains. Acad Med 2004;79(10 Suppl): S70–81.
2. Bordage G, Lemieux M. Semantic structures and diagnostic thinking of experts and novices. Acad Med 1991;66(9 Suppl):S70–2.
3. Cholowski KM, Chan LKS. Diagnostic reasoning among second-year nursing students. J Adv Nurs 1992;17(10):1171–81.
4. Hardin LE. Cognitive processes of second-year veterinary students in clinical case resolution. J Vet Med Educ 2003;30(3):236–46.
5. Stevens RH. Search path mapping: a versatile approach for visualizing problem-solving behavior. Acad Med 1991;66(9 Suppl):S73–5.
6. Schwartz W. Documentation of students' clinical reasoning using a computer simulation. Am J Dis Child 1989;143:575–9.
7. Coderre S, Mandin H, Harasym PH, et al. Diagnostic reasoning strategies and diagnostic success. Med Educ 2003;37(8):695–703.
8. Chang RW, Bordage G, Connell KJ. The importance of early problem representation during case presentations. Acad Med 1998;73(10 Suppl):S109–11.
9. Rikers RM, Loyens SM, Schmidt HG. The role of encapsulated knowledge in clinical case representations of medical students and family doctors. Med Educ 2004;38(10):1035–43.
10. Groves M, O'Rourke P, Alexander H. The clinical reasoning characteristics of diagnostic experts. Med Teach 2003;25(3):308–13.
11. Ferrario CG. Experienced and less-experienced nurses' diagnostic reasoning: implications for fostering students' critical thinking. Int J Nurs Terminol Classif 2003;14(2):41–52.
12. Norman G. Research in clinical reasoning: past history and current trends. Med Educ 2005;39(4):418–27.
13. Danielson JA, Bender HS, Mills EM, et al. A tool for helping veterinary students learn diagnostic problem solving. Educational Technology Research and Development 2003;51(3):63–81.
14. Danielson JA, Mills EM, Vermeer PJ, et al. The Diagnostic Pathfinder: ten years of using technology to teach diagnostic problem solving. In: Scott TB, Livingston JI,

editors. Leading edge educational technology. New York: Nova Science Publishers, Inc; 2008. p. 77–103.

15. Danielson JA, Mills EM, Vermeer PJ, et al. Characteristics of a cognitive tool that helps students learn diagnostic problem solving. Educational Technology Research and Development 2007;55:499–520.
16. Miller GA. The magical number seven, plus or minus two: some limits on our capacity for processing information. Psychol Rev 1956;63(2):81–97.
17. Sweller J. Cognitive load during problem solving: effects on learning. Cogn Sci 1988;12(2):257–85.
18. van Merrienboer JJ, Sweller J. Cognitive load theory in health professional education: design principles and strategies. Med Educ 2010;44(1):85–93.
19. Hattie J, Timperley H. The power of feedback. Rev Educ Res 2007;77:81–112.
20. Shute VJ. Focus on formative feedback. Rev Educ Res 2008;78(1):153–89.
21. van Gog T, Ericsson KA, Rikers RM, et al. Instructional design for advanced learners: establishing connections between the theoretical frameworks of cognitive load and deliberate practice. Educational Technology Research and Development 2005;53(3):73–81.

# Index

*Note:* Page numbers of article titles are in **boldface** type.

Clin Lab Med 31 (2011) 217–227
doi:10.1016/S0272-2712(11)00011-4
0272-2712/11/$ – see front matter © 2011 Elsevier Inc. All rights reserved.

labmed.theclinics.com

# Moving?

## Make sure your subscription moves with you!

To notify us of your new address, find your **Clinics Account Number** (located on your mailing label above your name), and contact customer service at:

**Email: journalscustomerservice-usa@elsevier.com**

**800-654-2452** (subscribers in the U.S. & Canada)
**314-447-8871** (subscribers outside of the U.S. & Canada)

**Fax number: 314-447-8029**

**Elsevier Health Sciences Division**
**Subscription Customer Service**
**3251 Riverport Lane**
**Maryland Heights, MO 63043**

*To ensure uninterrupted delivery of your subscription, please notify us at least 4 weeks in advance of move.

Printed and bound by CPI Group (UK) Ltd, Croydon, CR0 4YY

03/10/2024

01040454-0004